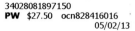

LIVING
THE GOOD
LONG LIFE

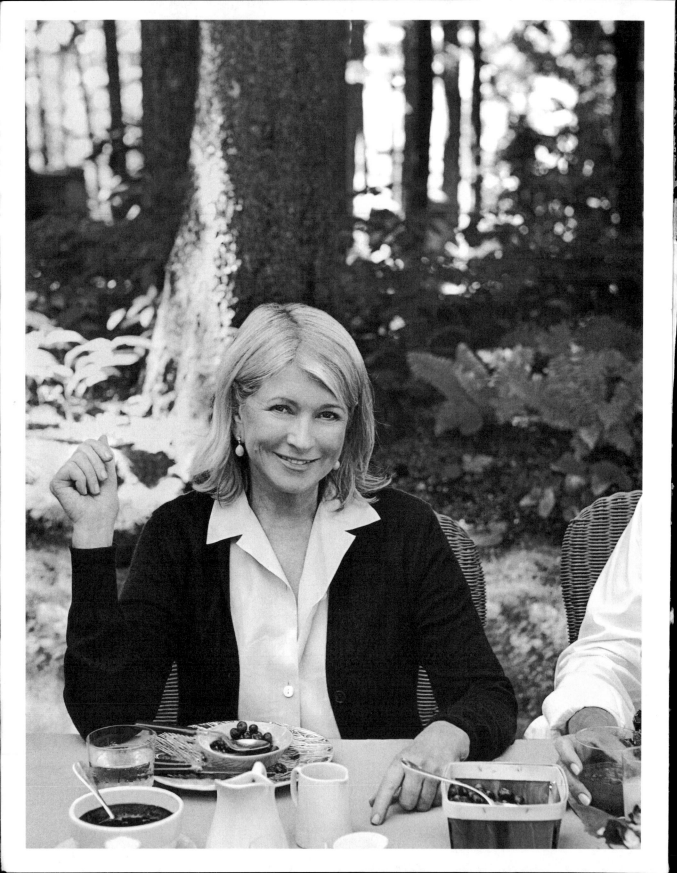

LIVING THE GOOD LONG LIFE

MARTHA STEWART

A PRACTICAL GUIDE TO
Caring for Yourself and Others

Clarkson Potter/Publishers
New York

This book is dedicated to all former, present, and future "caregivers," including my mother, Martha Kostyra. And it is also dedicated to all of us who wish to live good, long, and productive lives.

Copyright © 2013 by Martha Stewart Living Omnimedia, Inc.

All rights reserved.
Published in the United States by Clarkson Potter/Publishers,
an imprint of the Crown Publishing Group,
a division of Random House, Inc., New York.
www.crownpublishing.com
www.clarksonpotter.com

CLARKSON POTTER is a trademark and POTTER with colophon is
a registered trademark of Random House, Inc.

Library of Congress Cataloging-in-Publication Data
Stewart, Martha.
Living the good long life / Martha Stewart.
1. Older people—Health and hygiene.   2. Older people—Psychology.
3. Well-being—Age factors.   I. Title.
RA777.6.S74 2013
613'.0438—dc23   2012011827

ISBN 978-0-307-46288-6
eISBN 978-0-307-95321-6

Printed in the United States of America

Book and jacket design by Special Projects Group,
Martha Stewart Living Omnimedia
Photograph and illustration credits appear on page 390
Jacket photographs by John Dolan (front), Anna Williams (back),
and Jayne Hinds Bidaut (back flap)

10 9 8 7 6 5 4 3 2 1

First Edition

I have long been interested in the very important subjects of health and health care, with the goal of living well now and into the future. I've always sought out the best medical treatments, read as many books and articles as I could on these subjects, and asked lots and lots of questions of my doctors as well as of my friends and acquaintances in the "business" of health. I believe that being informed about all aspects of health is the best way you can prepare yourself to enjoy a good, long life.

In putting together this book, I relied on the expertise of many, including the excellent doctors and care providers at the Martha Stewart Center for Living (MSCL). I am grateful to Dr. Audrey Chun, director of MSCL, for all that she did to help define what this book could and should be, and for setting the tone in her wonderful foreword. Dr. Albert Siu, professor and chair of the department of geriatrics and palliative medicine at the Icahn School of Medicine at Mount Sinai, also greatly contributed to my understanding of the subjects covered herein. Other doctors at Mount Sinai for whose expertise I am grateful include Dr. Christine Chang, assistant professor of geriatrics and palliative medicine; Dr. Sita Chokhavatia, associate professor of medicine in the division of gastroenterology; Joan Griffiths Vega, facilitator of an Alzheimer's caregiver group and group teacher for a mindfulness-based caregiver stress-management group; Ella Jolly, geriatric psychiatric social worker; Dr. Jana Klauer, physician with an expertise in nutrition and metabolism; and Dr. Michael A. Palese, associate professor of urology and director of minimally invasive surgery. I am so thankful to Dr. Brent Ridge, former VP of Healthy Living at Martha Stewart Living Omnimedia, for his work in putting together the original proposal for this book. In researching the voluminous text, we relied on the work of Dr. Gerald Imber, author of *The Youth Corridor*; Linda Packer, MSW, LSCW, geriatric care manager and founder of Prime Life Network; and Dr. Dennis Popeo, attending psychiatrist at NYU Langone Medical Center.

I am fortunate to have a great team of doctors with whom I consult regularly, among them Dr. Albert Knapp, clinical associate professor of medicine at NYU School of Medicine; ophthalmologist Dr. Stuart Aaron; gynecologist and obstetrician Dr. Jane Galasso; dermatologist Dr. Catherine Orentreich; and Dr. Steven A. Stuchin, associate professor at NYU School of Medicine and chief of orthopedic services at NYU Hospital for Joint Diseases.

I am indebted to my personal trainer, Mary Tedesco, for all that she does to keep me in shape, as well as to James Murphy, director of the Iyengar Institute, for his yoga lessons, and to Dr. Wanda Lopez for her unique chiropractic care. In researching how to prevent falls (one of the biggest health risks for seniors), the work of Fall Stop . . . Move Strong proved invaluable, and for that I thank the group's cofounders, Celeste Carlucci and Julie Kardachi.

I have learned much over the years about financial matters, including estate planning, from my banker, Jane Heller, senior vice president of private wealth management at US Trust, Bank of America. I am also thankful to Carlyn S. McCaffrey, lawyer and partner at McDermott, Will & Emery LLP.

For a list of all who contributed to the production of this book, please turn to page 388.

CONTENTS

FOREWORD BY AUDREY CHUN, M.D. 8

INTRODUCTION 10

PART 1 HEALTHY LIVING TODAY 24

CHAPTER 1 Healthy Eating 26

CHAPTER 2 Healthy Fitness 74

CHAPTER 3 Healthy Brain 122

CHAPTER 4 Healthy Outlook 144

CHAPTER 5 Healthy Living Every Day 180

CHAPTER 6 Healthy Looks 226

CHAPTER 7 Healthy Home 258

PART 2 HEALTHY LIVING
INTO
TOMORROW 300

CHAPTER 8   Healthy Living
into the Future 302

CHAPTER 9   Healthy Caring 336

RESOURCES 374   ACKNOWLEDGMENTS 388

NOTES 381   CREDITS 390

SUGGESTED READING 387   INDEX 391

FOREWORD

BY Audrey Chun, M.D., DIRECTOR OF THE MARTHA STEWART
CENTER FOR LIVING AT MOUNT SINAI HOSPITAL

When Martha first mentioned that she wanted to write a book on aging gracefully, I was thrilled. Who better to debunk the stereotypes and to serve as a model for successful aging than the woman who has spent decades helping us see what true living can be?

I have worked with Martha as the director for the Center for Living since 2008, and sometimes people express surprise at my wanting to work in geriatrics, particularly in our youth-obsessed culture. Some even ask bluntly, "Isn't it depressing to work with old people?" In fact, it is quite the opposite. I have the privilege of taking care of patients as they transition through their last stages of life, and I am continuously awed by their lives and their narratives. They have marched for civil rights, survived the Holocaust, been true innovators of industry, produced incredible art, raised families, and adapted through some of the most profound changes of the last century. They are our parents, aunts, uncles, sisters, brothers, and friends, and it seems implausible to me that we would not be interested in the experiences they have to offer. At a time when news headlines often make me question our humanity, they renew my hope in what we can achieve as a people. Their lives and attitudes inspire me to live a purpose-filled and richer life.

The Martha Stewart Center for Living embodies the central vision of our geriatrics medical practice: whole-person care, including physical and social well-being, as well as measures to prevent disease—and then, when disease occurs, the best medical care. We strive to provide care that is comprehensive and personalized to reflect the individual patient's needs and values. The Center for Living also encourages maintaining good health through lifestyle changes by providing programs like tai chi to prevent falls and group visits to educate people on diet and exercise. If serious illness occurs, we reevaluate treatments based on the patient's goals of care and strive for the best quality of life for whatever time a person may have. We recognize this journey is not in isolation, but occurs within the context of caregivers—families and friends who need support and education as much as the patient does.

Those who have lived most successfully into this oldest age seem to have a few things in common:

- A rich social network of friends and family, both young and old.

- A meaningful and purposeful life: it's the reason to get up in the morning; meaning and purpose can be anything as long as it's important to the person—family, work, painting, volunteering, even online backgammon tournaments!

- A resilient personality—ability to recover from adversity and move on with life rather than dwell on challenges.

We are extremely fortunate to have Martha advocating for these older adults—advocating for better care and caregiver support, and breaking the stereotypes of aging with her own active and healthy lifestyle. While nobody can expect to live forever, the goal is to live the time we have with the best health and physical/mental capacity possible. This is a remarkable book because it gives practical advice on daily activities we can incorporate into our lives for healthier and better living.

From those of us who work tirelessly to promote health and respect for older adults, thank you, Martha Stewart. Only you could bring together such a comprehensive book on living!

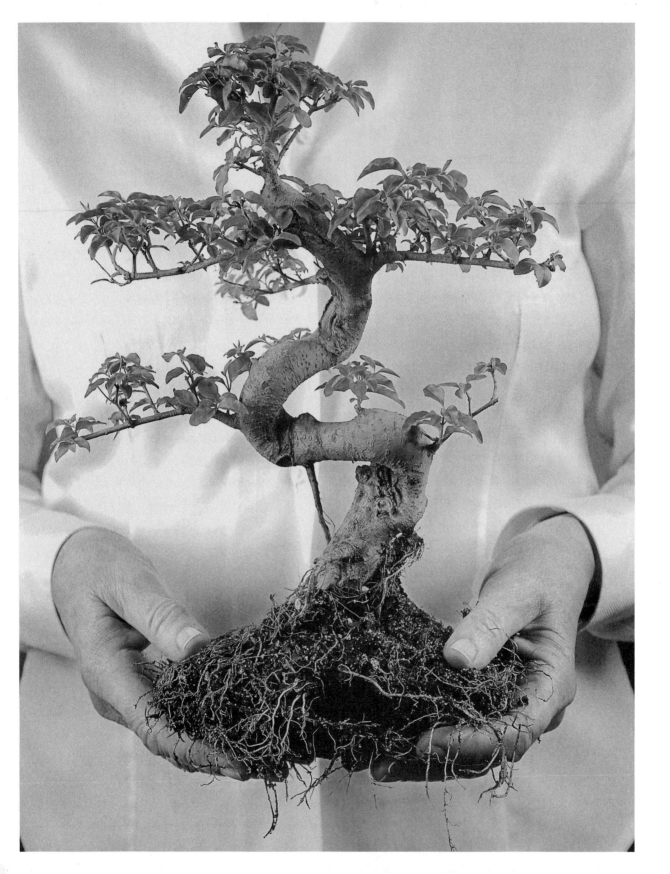

INTRODUCTION

I wrote my first book, *Entertaining,* in 1982. I was 41 years old and had never written a book before. My doctor, in the sit-down session after the physical exam exclaimed, "You are a late bloomer." I took his remarks as a vast compliment and have never forgotten that it is, indeed, never too late to start a project, never too late to embark on a new career, never too late to realize a dream. In 1982, I was actually just getting started: more than a decade later, when I was in my fifties, I launched my own company, Martha Stewart Living Omnimedia. As I complete this book, in 2013, I find myself just as active as ever, and just about to begin a new initiative that I have been dreaming about for a while. Along the way, I have been active in philanthropic endeavors, built the Center for Living at Mount Sinai Hospital, been very involved in company business, and most recently, become a doting grandmother of two.

In truth, I don't think about age much at all because there is so much to do, so many things to accomplish, and so much to look forward to. I know I am not getting younger, and there is no magic antiaging elixir or pill I can ingest, but there are definite steps to take, definite things one can do to stem the onslaught of aging and make oneself approach the coming years with grace, dignity, and good health.

When the Martha Stewart Center for Living, which facilitates access to health-care resources for older adults, opened in 2008, I chose the bonsai as my image for the process of graceful aging. Unlike a painting or sculpture, it is a work of art that is never finished.

A bonsai continues to grow and evolve over time. Indeed, the tiny potted plant, with graceful gnarled trunk and leaning boughs, embodies our feelings about aging, and when properly tended, bonsai can thrive and flourish, growing even more appealing and interesting with age. It's definitely worth noting that the older the bonsai, the more valuable and desirable. The Center is dedicated to my mother, Martha Kostyra, or "Big Martha," as my family called her. Mom passed away in 2007 at the age of 93. She had lived a full and productive life and was in good health almost until she died.

I learned so much from my mother. She taught me about the importance of home and history, family and tradition. She also taught me that growing older need not mean narrowing the scope of your activities and interests or a diminution of the great pleasures to be had in the everyday. In fact, the very opposite was true for her! These valuable lessons are very much in keeping with the Center's mission, which is not about aging. It's about living—living gracefully and healthfully with energy and enthusiasm even as we grow older.

Admittedly, it's hard to fight the tide. Our culture is obsessed with youth, and we are bombarded by antiaging messages everywhere— about our food, our exercise, our medicine, our face creams, even our dental hygiene. The ubiquitous emphasis on youth and beauty and fitness seems to leave no room for getting old.

And yet, our generation is finding the room. We've redefined aging, and most of us are entering our later years in much better shape and much more prepared than any generation before us. But I want all of us to be prepared for later life. And that means making our health and well-being a greater priority.

How do we accomplish that? It is up to each one of us. Everything we do affects how we age—from the food we eat to the frequency with which we exercise and the way we handle stress. Finding a doctor you like and trust is paramount, as is being vigilant about screenings and regular tests to be sure you have all the information you need to make smart decisions about your health.

I embrace that approach and have always been very careful to eat good wholesome food, to exercise regularly, to find wonderful doctors, and to make time for family and friends, though of course I still make some mistakes. (Eating too much is an occupational hazard!) I don't always believe what I see when I look in the mirror, or feel an ache or a pain. I'm not a fearful person, but it is in these moments that I'm reminded: healthy living never stops. You have to keep at it on a regular basis and make it a part of your lifestyle. Your health has to be a huge priority if you are going to succeed at aging gracefully.

And it's never too early or too late to start, which is very important. Some might say, "I always ate poorly." Or, "I never exercised, what's the point?" The point is that scientists have discovered all sorts of promising evidence that starting and maintaining a health regimen in middle age and beyond can extend your years, and your quality of life.

With this book, I wanted to create a guide that is a practical, no-nonsense, straightforward, important list of things to do so you can prepare to live a long life that's as good and healthy and carefree as possible. That includes how to incorporate fitness, supplements, cognitive exercises, and all the latest medical preventions and procedures—no matter your starting point. Whether you are 40, 50, 60, or beyond, these lifestyle changes are still an investment—money in the bank for staying mobile and healthy through our "platinum" years.

Caring for an aging parent or loved one can be a rewarding experience, an opportunity to help in ways great and small. But it can also exact a physical, emotional, and financial toll. In fact, it can be another full-time job. We need to find new ways to support caregivers at the same time that we help older people remain robust and vital as they age. We owe it to those who cared for us when we were young. We owe it to future generations who will help care for us when we are old. And we owe it to ourselves, so that we can continue to thrive for many, many years.

Each of us has to take charge of our own outcomes. In her autobiography, *A Backward Glance,* the great American novelist Edith Wharton wrote, "One can remain alive long past the usual date of disintegration if one is unafraid of change, insatiable in intellectual curiosity, interested in big things, and happy in small ways." I heartily agree with Mrs. Wharton's prescription for longevity. My own motto is, "When you're through changing, you're through."

Everyone can find a way to keep changing for the better—to keep growing and flourishing, like a bonsai tree. I sincerely hope you enjoy and find enrichment from this book.

Martha Stewart

HOW TO USE THIS BOOK

In the chapters ahead, you will find valuable information, ideas, and strategies you can apply as you continue to care for yourself and others. In Part 1: "Healthy Living Today," you'll find chapters on how to eat, exercise, and live for better health today, as well as chapters on protecting and improving your cognitive function, mental well-being, and appearance as you age. Part 2: "Healthy Living into Tomorrow," focuses on how to take preventive health measures in all areas of your life, and explores what it means for your health to be a caretaker—a role so many of us take on in midlife.

You may want to sit and read this handbook straight through, marking the pages that most interest you so you can develop your own, customized healthy-living game plan. Or, you may want to dive straight in to "Healthy Fitness" (Chapter 2) or "Healthy Outlook" (Chapter 4), because those are the aspects of healthy living that you're concerned with right now.

Either way, rest assured that this book is meant to become dog-eared, referenced, and referred to often. You don't need to commit all of the advice to memory, nor do you need to try to implement it all right away. Healthy living is an ongoing, ever-evolving project, much like my beloved bonsai trees or your own treasured and ever-changing home. If you try to overhaul too many aspects of your life at once, you'll find yourself overwhelmed and unable to keep up with it all. Instead, pick one small healthy habit to start practicing today, whether that's drinking more water, walking at lunchtime, or attending a weekly yoga class. Once the first habit feels like second nature (usually after two to four weeks of dedicated effort), make another change, and so on.

When you make small changes, you'll find that they are easier to incorporate and will quickly become indispensable. You'll probably also begin to notice concrete changes in how you look and feel. You should begin to sleep better, have more energy, and feel fewer aches and pains. Your weight might creep down or stabilize where it needs to be. And your eyes, skin, and hair will take on a new glow. Enjoy these changes for what they are—proof that you've made taking good care of yourself a true priority for a long, healthy life.

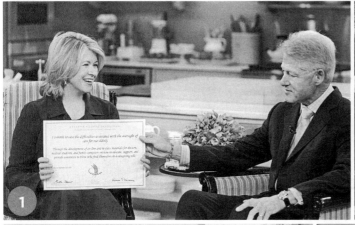

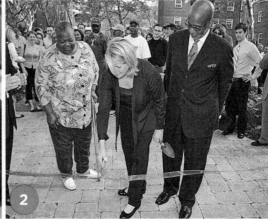

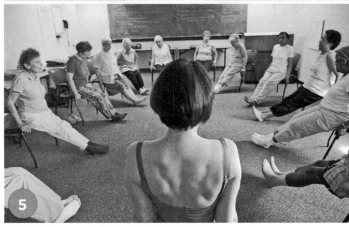

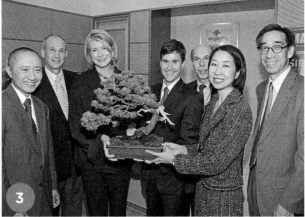

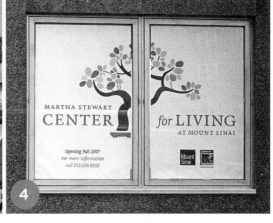

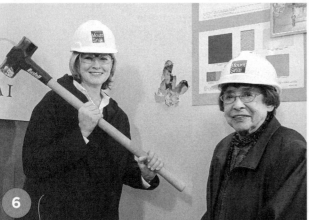

CLOCKWISE FROM TOP LEFT: (1) Announcing to former President Bill Clinton, on my show in 2007, my pledge to the Clinton Global Health Initiative to support caregivers of the elderly. (2) Cutting the ribbon at the garden at the Martha Stewart Center for Living at Mount Sinai Hospital in New York City on October 9, 2007. (3) Here I am with some of the doctors involved with opening the Center. (4) The logo for the Center is a bonsai tree, to symbolize graceful aging. (5) One of the many wellness classes offered at the Center. (6) Breaking new ground with Mom, to whom I dedicated the Center.

ESTABLISHING THE CENTER

It was in 2006 when my daughter, Alexis, asked me to meet with a geriatrician at Mount Sinai Hospital, Brent Ridge, to discuss a special project. I agreed, and the three of us—Alexis, Brent, and I—had a very interesting conversation about establishing a geriatric outpatient ward at the hospital where this very young doctor practiced. His enthusiasm for his work, his passion involving the care of older patients, and his devotion to the study of geriatric medicine and its vast possibilities for extending the lives of the aging American population in a positive, healthy, successful fashion intrigued me greatly.

Dr. Ridge and I had lots in common in our idealistic approach toward longevity and our belief that approaching old age should involve a positive, not negative, state of mind. My mother, who was in her early nineties at the time, was our unofficial but very visible "standard of perfection": a woman who had a friendly and very good outlook, with her community, with her large family (she had six children), with her church, and with her friends. She was strong, of sound mind, and had never, really, been sick. Her most interesting and, I think, strongest characteristic was her "curiosity": she read books, newspapers, and magazines, listened to news programs, watched documentaries, and went to the movies. She loved her grandchildren and spent valuable time with them. She ate well and did not smoke or drink excessively (an occasional glass of wine made her happy). She had an excellent and small group of medical experts who cared for her well. We decided to build the Center for Living in her honor.

ADDRESSING THE SENATE

U.S. SENATE SPECIAL COMMITTEE ON AGING,
APRIL 16, 2008

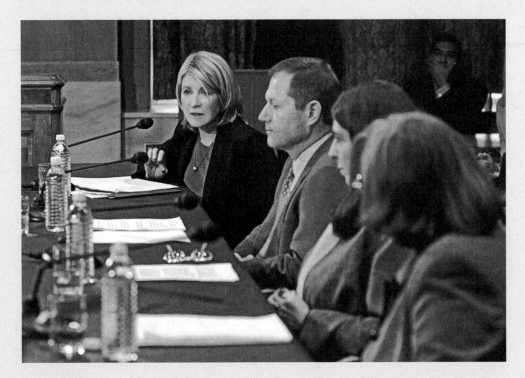

I had the unique opportunity to testify before the U.S. Senate about a pressing issue that is close to my heart: how to improve the quality of life for America's aging population and its caregivers. I continue to work to raise awareness about this topic. The more people that discuss this issue—whether with their doctors, their local politicians, or their own families—the more change is likely to occur. Acknowledging the challenges that face us all and having open discourse about them are the first steps toward finding solutions.

**Chairman Kohl, Ranking Member Smith, and members of the Committee:
I appreciate the invitation to testify before you today and am honored to be here.**

You have chosen a subject that is increasingly critical to our quality of life—not only for older Americans but for family members who care for them. I look forward to learning from the work of the Committee as it continues to examine this issue. The experience of the distinguished professionals on your panel today will be important as well.

I respond to your invitation today as a member of a family whose eyes were opened by personal experience—and to share what we have been learning at the Martha Stewart Center for Living at Mount Sinai Medical Center in New York City.

My professional life has been centered on the home, the well-being of the family, and everything that these subjects encompass. When I began working in this area more than twenty-five years ago, the subject of homemaking as it relates to families was largely overlooked, though the interest was clearly broad and the desire for information, strong. My colleagues and I soon discovered we were satisfying a deeply felt unmet need.

Today I see a similarly unmet need. Our aging relatives and the families who care for them yearn for basic information and resources. We all know this is a significant sector of our society: more than 75 percent of Americans receiving long-term care rely solely on family and friends to provide assistance. The majority of these caregivers are women, many of whom are also raising children. Often, these women are working outside the home as well.

I understand the challenges family caregivers face. My mother, Martha Kostyra, passed away last year at the age of 93. My siblings and I were fortunate that she was in good health almost until she died. Still, we came to know firsthand the number of issues that needed to be managed.

First, it's difficult, especially in smaller cities and rural locations, to find doctors experienced in the specific needs that arise with age. Think of all that this includes: the effect of medications on elderly patients; how various medicines interact with each other; warning signs for depression and onsets of other conditions increasingly common in the elderly. How do we ensure that they take their medications? How do we help structure our parents' lives so they can live independently for as long as possible? And how do we support the generation of caregivers who devote so much of themselves to their parents' aging process?

This only touches on the myriad of issues, of course. Worry is the backdrop for everything these families do: What if the parent falls? What if she leaves the burners on? What if he takes his medications twice—or forgets to take them at all?

Now I am learning even more about the physical, emotional, and financial toll that the experience can exact. Caring for an aging parent or loved one can be another full-time job. In fact, 43 percent of baby boomers have taken time off from work and 17 percent have reduced hours to help care for an aging parent. They do this at a time when their expenses are rising. One recent study found that half of those caring for a family member or friend 50 years or older are spending, on average, more than 10 percent of their annual income on caregiving expenses. Many dip into savings and cut back on their own health-care spending to cover the bill. Is it any wonder that family caregivers are at increased risk of developing depression, anxiety, insomnia, and chronic illnesses?

In the Kostyra family, we were grateful to be there for my mother, who had given so much to us and was a well-loved presence in our lives and in the lives of her thirteen grandchildren. Our experience in her final years and my resulting awareness of the issues Americans face is one of the reasons for the creation of the Center for Living. The goal of the Center, which is dedicated to my mother, is to help people to live longer, healthier, productive lives even as they age.

We have set a goal at the Center to use research and the practice of geriatric medicine to try to elevate the level of eldercare and its importance in our society. Did you know that there is currently one geriatrician to every 8,500 baby boomers? That's clearly not adequate. We are also working to develop new tools and resources for caregivers. We are collaborating with a large number of organizations and motivated, experienced individuals, many of whom have been studying these issues for years. There are numerous devoted and knowledgeable people in this arena, and we hope we can all learn from one another.

This is a field that eventually impacts most families in emotional and encompassing ways. Yet sometimes it's the simple solution that holds an answer. Not so long ago at the Center, a woman brought in her father, who had suffered a stroke two years earlier. After the stroke, he had been told he could never eat again and was placed on a feeding tube. He was devastated and depressed. He had spent his life as someone with a passion for good food, and his future looked bleak to him. At the Center, a doctor experienced in geriatric care asked the man to drink a glass of water. He did, without a problem. "If he can do this," the doctor said, "he can eat." This simple exchange improved the man's quality of life immeasurably. And I'm sure it improved the quality of his daughter's life, too, knowing that her father was happier.

I want to share with you three things I've learned from our work at the Center and that others may find useful:

- We must make an effort to coordinate care. Most older Americans have several doctors. It's important for these doctors to cooperate with one another and work closely with caregivers.

- It is important that we, as a society, recognize the stresses and challenges that caregivers face and support them as best we can. We want to ensure that their health isn't undermined by the demands of eldercare.

- We must encourage families to open up a dialogue now. Even if your older relatives are in good health, it's important to plan for a day when they might not be.

I have always been a firm believer in the role of preparation and organization in progressing toward a goal. My concern today is whether our country and our overstretched medical system can possibly meet the demands of 76 million baby boomers who will start turning 65 in the next two years. We are on the cusp of a health and caregiving crisis that must be addressed now. I know you recognize this, and that is why we are here today. I thank you for your dedication to this important matter and for the opportunity to express my thoughts.

THE TEN GOLDEN RULES FOR SUCCESSFUL AGING

It's been called the silver tsunami, and it's headed this way: by 2047, there will be more Americans over 60 than under 15. The numbers of the oldest-old, those over 85, proportionately will grow the most of any demographic. Our increasingly aged population will affect the allocation of physical, emotional, medical, and mental care in our society. And that means we, as the pioneers of this generational landscape, must do our part to redefine the implications of aging and what it means to be, act, and feel old.

Indeed, this redefinition of aging has already begun. In less than a century, we've added fifty years to human life expectancy, says Laura Carstensen, the founding director of the Stanford University Center on Longevity. It's as if, quite literally, we've earned a second lease on life—an extra half-century! Yet this new longevity poses significant emotional and psychological dilemmas that as a culture we're only beginning to address. What does this time frame mean in terms of retirement? What are the new expectations for family, childrearing, and relationships? How does this new chronology affect the definitions of old and young? Until a century ago, there was no such thing as adolescence—a life stage that is now universally accepted. What will this newly evolving second stage be called?

Perhaps we haven't established these norms because we like to avoid them. We certainly don't feel old, at least not old as we'd once conceived it, or as old as our parents seemed at our age. But denial can be risky, resulting in missed warning signs for health complications or lack of preparation for certain contingencies—a seriously debilitating illness, a death of a spouse.

Finding new meaning in aging and embracing the many gifts it brings are possible. For starters, the quality of the rest of your life is more within your control than you think. How long your parents lived is neither a death sentence nor a health insurance policy. It turns out that genes account for only about 25 percent of your health and longevity: the rest is influenced by where and how you live. These are two factors that you can control, starting now, whether you're in your forties, fifties, sixties, or beyond.

The following "Golden Rules" for successful aging have been confirmed by science and will help you achieve optimal health.

1. EAT WELL

2. MAINTAIN A HEALTHY WEIGHT

3. STAY PHYSICALLY ACTIVE

4. GET QUALITY SLEEP

5. WEAR SUNSCREEN

6. COLLABORATE WITH A GOOD PRIMARY-CARE DOCTOR REGULARLY

7. FIND YOUR PASSION

8. CONNECT WITH OTHERS

9. STOP COMPLAINING— CHANGE WHAT YOU CAN, AND ACCEPT WHAT YOU CANNOT

10. STAY CURIOUS

PART 1

HEALTHY LIVING
TODAY

CHAPTER 1   Healthy Eating 26

CHAPTER 2   Healthy Fitness 74

CHAPTER 3   Healthy Brain 122

CHAPTER 4   Healthy Outlook 144

CHAPTER 5   Healthy Living Every Day 180

CHAPTER 6   Healthy Looks 226

CHAPTER 7   Healthy Home 258

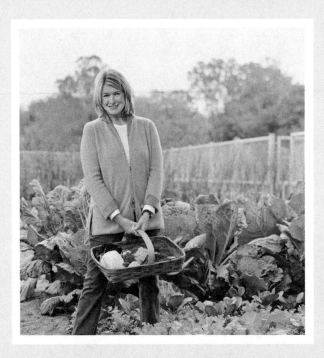

CHAPTER 1

Healthy Eating

PLAN *a better plate* 28

FOCUS *on the great eight* 31

PUT *a healthy plan in place* 43

COOK *for better health* 48

CONSIDER *your changing needs* 70

I believe in eating real food. And by *real*, I don't mean something that passes for food, that's been processed and preserved until it no longer resembles the beautiful, organic bounty that nature gives us. I grow much of what I eat because I love to have a garden. But even when I'm food shopping or eating out, the same principle applies: quality and purity matter.

Most convenience foods are just not in my vocabulary because they are full of artificial colors and flavors, and are especially high in sodium and fats. My body functions better on real food—a good diet gives me energy, keeps my weight under control, and prevents disease. No pill can do all of that. Fresh, unprocessed food is the best antiaging tool around.

When I've had a period of overindulging in rich foods, I don't diet; I never have. I don't believe in cutting out any food entirely, like butter, sugar, or cream. I just eat less of these favorite foods if I'm watching my weight. During these times, I find drinking exotic, flavorful teas, such as white peony tea from China, feels very cleansing and restorative. And every morning, I'll drink a glass of hot water with a squeeze of fresh lemon; it's a refreshing tonic that helps keep me hydrated and holds me over until I eat breakfast.

PLAN *a better plate*

Food is the most powerful—and fundamental—tool we have for leading a full, healthy, and happy life. It's also the root of our most treasured memories. Think about how satisfied you feel after sharing a leisurely and delicious Sunday lunch with family. Simple meals centered around home-cooked, unprocessed foods offer nourishment for the body and soul. Even after fixing a solo weeknight supper, you know you'll feel more content, and more cared for, if you prepare something from fresh ingredients, instead of just popping dinner out of a package.

This is because the right food can embody our culture, express our creativity, and most of all, nourish our bodies. For generations, humans subsisted on a diet that was reaped from the earth using no chemical fertilizers or pesticides, and they ate what they hunted or raised. But the increased production of processed foods over several decades has mirrored an increase in the incidence of obesity—more than 65 percent of U.S. adults are now considered overweight or obese.[1] Though the average U.S. life expectancy has climbed to nearly 80 years since World War II, we are also experiencing unprecedented rates of dietary-related diabetes, heart disease, and cancer. In short, a longer life doesn't necessarily mean a greater quality of life.

Fortunately, eating plenty of fruits, vegetables, whole grains, and legumes (while minimizing saturated fat, refined sugar, and excess calories) is the best recipe we have for health and longevity. Researchers have declared diet to be as effective as medication, ever since adults with high blood pressure were able to reduce several heart disease risk factors just by changing how and what they ate during a study by the National Institutes of Health.

The medical world is finally reaching consensus on what healthy eating looks like, and it has nothing to do with foolish fads that cut out entire food groups or that focus on eating one food (such as grapefruit) for a week. Instead, we're looking to cultures that haven't shifted wholesale to our modern grab-and-go mentality. These cultures offer compelling evidence that eating right is a powerful tool for aging well.

ADOPT A "BLUE ZONE" DIET

You may have heard of the so-called Blue Zones—longevity hot spots around the globe where residents routinely live to be 100 years and older. They also enjoy proud traditions of delectable cuisines where fresh, whole foods are revered and savored.

Two of these hot spots—the Italian island of Sardinia and the Greek island of Icaria—share similar dietary patterns, which have collectively been referred to as the "Mediterranean diet." Studied since the 1980s, the diet's basic components include lots of leafy green vegetables, whole grains, legumes, fruits, fish, and olive oil. Dairy products, typically yogurt and cheese, offer natural sources of probiotics, or friendly bacteria that keep digestion running smoothly while lowering the risk of gut-borne infection. Red meat, which is high in saturated fat, and processed foods are rarely eaten. "The Mediterranean diet protects against heart disease and other inflammatory conditions, diabetes, and many cancers," affirms Dr. Jana Klauer, a New York–based physician with expertise in nutrition and metabolism who sits on the board of Mount Sinai Hospital's Center for Living. The diet is so potent that one ten-year assessment found that people who eat a Mediterranean diet in their seventies, eighties, and nineties are half as likely to die of complications from heart disease, hypertension, or diabetes, as compared with those who eat a more modern menu full of unhealthy fats, salts, and added sugars.

In another Blue Zone, Okinawa, Japan, the cuisine is centered on fresh seafood, seaweed, soybeans, and tofu, while sweet potatoes and bitter melon—rich sources of vitamins and minerals known to reduce risk of heart disease—serve both as side dishes and as desserts. Antioxidant-rich turmeric tea also plays a starring role. And residents tend to consume fewer calories. All of these measures result in lower obesity rates for Okinawans, as well as a reduced incidence of cancer and vascular disease, than are found among their fellow Japanese.

FOLLOW THE NEW U.S. GUIDELINES

In 2011, the U.S. government finally traded its old, defunct food pyramid for a new nutritional model called MyPlate—and dietitians rejoiced. For too long, Americans have considered meat, particularly red meat, to be the star of the dinner plate, around which a meal is planned. Thanks to MyPlate, we now understand that meat is merely a side dish or source of flavoring, while vegetables, beans, and whole grains are the primary focus. When you plan a meal, imagine the produce taking up half the plate, the whole grains one quarter, and the protein—be it animal- or plant-based—only the last quarter.

As you begin to plan more meals that look like MyPlate, you'll ensure that you're eating plenty of whole grains, vegetables, fruits, beans, nuts, and healthy fats (like olive oil) every day. Vary your protein choices so that fish and seafood make an appearance at least twice a week, and more often than red meat.

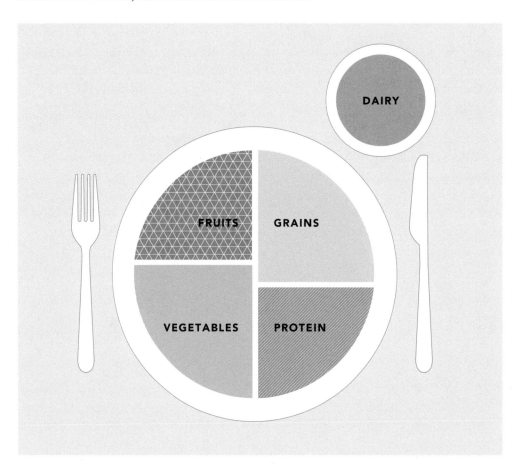

FOCUS *on the great eight*

Front-loading your diet with plant-based foods, good fats, calcium-rich ingredients, and lean animal proteins is one of the best ways to improve and maintain health. Memorize the following eight food groups to maximize nutrition.

1 FRUITS AND VEGETABLES

THE LONGEVITY-ENHANCING BENEFITS

Trace the word *vegetable* to its roots and you get "vigorous," "active," and "strong." It's no surprise, then, that a plant-based diet is high in antioxidant compounds such as vitamins C and E and beta-carotene, and flavonoids and carotenoids, which fight cancer-causing free radicals, reduce your risk of diabetes, and promote better memory and eyesight.

HOW TO GET ENOUGH

Drink fresh-squeezed juice, serve sliced vegetables for snacks with hummus or yogurt-herb dip, toss fruit into cereal or yogurt, lightly sauté seasonal vegetables in olive oil, or roast them at 400°F until just soft. Add tender, dark leafy greens such as spinach and arugula to salads; simmer heartier greens such as kale, collards, Swiss chard, and mustard greens or thinly slice them into ribbons and add to hot soup; use leafy greens in place of lettuce in sandwiches. Add grapes, chopped apples, pears, or oranges to salads and sandwich fillings such as chicken or tuna salad.

ON YOUR PLATE

Eat unlimited quantities of vegetables, with an emphasis on leafy greens. Shoot for at least five servings per day and you'll cut your risk of developing heart disease by up to 20 percent. Try to eat 1 to 2 portions of fruit per day, such as 1 small apple or orange, 1 small banana, 1/3 melon, 2 fresh figs, 1 kiwi, 1/2 cup berries, 1/2 pomegranate, 1 small nectarine, or 1 clementine.

TRY FROZEN FRUITS AND VEGETABLES

Consuming frozen produce can be an easy way to boost fruit and vegetable intake. Frozen is also healthy: the commercial flash-freezing process preserves all the vitamins and minerals in fruits and vegetables. And frozen can be even more nutritious than fresh, since often the most valuable nutrients of the latter diminish during transport and storage.[2]

Moreover, frozen fruit and vegetables are typically precut and are easy to handle. Be sure, however, that you're buying pure frozen produce that incorporates no added sugar, sauces, or unpronounceable chemicals. Or, freeze your own fruits and vegetables when they are at their peak.

2 WHOLE GRAINS

THE LONGEVITY-ENHANCING BENEFITS

As the individual seeds of grasses, grains are compact storehouses of nutrients. Switching from refined "white" grains (such as those found in most widely available bread, pasta, flour, and rice) to whole grains is an easy way to get more filling fiber, B vitamins, and vitamin E, which aids red blood cell and muscle formation. Quinoa—not technically a grain but a high-protein seed of the broad-leaf plant, cultivated by the ancient Incas and Mayans—and true grains such as barley and millet contain lots of magnesium, which helps ward off high blood pressure and osteoporosis.

HOW TO GET ENOUGH

Heart-healthy old-fashioned rolled or steel-cut oats can be cooked on the stovetop or in a microwave. Instead of white rice, try quinoa, millet, barley, or whole-grain brown rice as a filling, high-fiber side dish. (These cooked grains also make a delicious breakfast when served with low-fat milk and a dash of honey or agave nectar syrup.) Prepare large batches of grains to have on hand for the week. Experiment with soba—noodles made of buckwheat—or other whole-grain noodle varieties in your favorite pasta dishes.

ON YOUR PLATE

Aim for 3 ounces per day; a 1-ounce serving of grain is equal to 1 slice of whole-grain bread, or ½ cup of cooked pasta, quinoa, brown rice, millet, or oatmeal.

ALTERNATIVE PASTAS

Grocery store shelves are brimming with a growing assortment of alternative pastas, many made from whole grains that can help reduce your risk of stroke, heart disease, and diabetes. Here are four delicious options:

WHOLE WHEAT: The bran and germ in whole-wheat pasta contain antioxidants that combat heart disease and cancer. Several brands include flax, which contributes heart-healthy omega-3 fats and can boost the overall fiber quotient.

SOBA: Japanese for *buckwheat*, this grain offers good-quality protein, as well as the antioxidants rutin and quercetin, which are beneficial to people with high blood pressure. It also contains bone-building phosphorus.

SPELT: A good source of thiamin and niacin, pasta made from this ancient cereal grain has significantly more protein than wheat pasta.

KAMUT: Pronounced kuh-MOOT, this ancient grain leads the whole-grain pack for protein content, at 10 grams per 2 ounce serving. It also contains healthy amounts of the antioxidants vitamin E, selenium, and zinc.

3 BEANS AND LEGUMES

THE LONGEVITY-ENHANCING BENEFITS

Legumes (split peas, lentils) are pods filled with individual seeds (called pulses when dried) that are an exceptionally high source of fiber and virtually fat-free protein; when combined with grains, legumes are as nutritionally complete as animal proteins. They also contain lignans, plant-based hormones that may reduce the risk of estrogen-related cancers such as breast cancer (although their benefits may not be gender specific; they may reduce pancreatic, prostate, and colon cancers as well). Beans (pinto, kidney, garbanzo, black, and such) are also a good source of nondairy calcium, so it's especially important to eat these if you're lactose-intolerant or vegan.

HOW TO GET ENOUGH

With an ample supply of beans and grains in your pantry, a nutritious dinner is always within reach. Spread chickpea or lentil hummus on sandwiches in place of mayo or other high-fat dressings, or use as a dip for carrots, celery, or peppers. Make bean soup or toss several varieties together into a salad. Scatter beans on top of green salads or stir into broth-based soups. Mash beans with a fork, sprinkle with chopped fresh herbs, and drizzle with olive oil; serve with toasted bread or pita.

ON YOUR PLATE

Try to eat two portions per day, such as 1 cup cooked beans, or 1 cup cooked peas/legumes.

BEANS FROM SCRATCH

Although canned beans are convenient, they tend to contain higher amounts of sodium than those cooked from scratch. Consider cooking a large batch of beans and then freezing individual portions, which you can defrost as needed. When purchasing dried beans, buy from a source with a good turnover.

Don't mix newly purchased dried beans with older ones; the older they are, the longer they take to cook. If kept in a tightly sealed container in a cool place, dried beans will stay fresh for a year. Rinse dried beans before cooking and pick over to remove any small stones or twigs.

To prepare, soak beans overnight (or up to 24 hours) in the refrigerator before cooking, or "quick soak" beans by placing them in a saucepan of cold water, covered, and bring to a boil. Turn off the heat and soak beans, covered, for 1 hour. To cook, bring beans and soaking liquid to a boil in a large pot; reduce heat and simmer until beans are tender, anywhere from 30 minutes to 3 hours, depending on the type and age of beans.

4 NUTS AND SEEDS

THE LONGEVITY-ENHANCING BENEFITS

Almonds, walnuts, hazelnuts, and pumpkin seeds are nutritional powerhouses chock-full of fiber and vitamin E (good for the skin and cardiovascular system), as well as phytosterols, a type of plant-based fat that may lower cholesterol. Most nuts and seeds are between 10 to 25 percent protein, too, making them a quick-energy snack with staying power. However, because they're high in fat—albeit heart-healthy unsaturated fats—nuts and seeds should be consumed in moderation.

HOW TO GET ENOUGH

Sprinkle almonds, sunflower seeds, or walnuts on cereal, yogurt parfaits, oatmeal, salads, cooked vegetables, and brown rice or whole-wheat couscous. Make a trail mix of your favorite nuts with dried cranberries and blueberries. Buy natural varieties of peanut and almond butters—you'll get all the benefits of nuts without unnecessary added sugar. When baking, substitute up to one-fourth of the regular flour with a nut "flour" or meal, such as almond or pecan. (You can find nut flours in the baking section of larger grocery stores, or you can pulse nuts yourself in a food processor just until they reach a fine consistency.)

ON YOUR PLATE

Enjoy one 1-ounce serving of nuts and seeds per day. Examples of one portion include 20 cashews, 22 almonds, 14 walnut halves, or 32 peanuts.

CHOOSE WISELY

Some nuts do a better job at helping your heart while others may help protect your memory. The following happen to be nutritional all-stars. Choose unsalted nuts whenever possible.

WALNUTS: The only nut with a significant amount of omega-3 fatty acids, walnuts may help fight illnesses including coronary heart disease.

PISTACHIOS: These are a good source of phytosterols, which help lower cholesterol levels. They are also high in protein and beta-carotene, which is linked to vision health.

BRAZIL NUTS: One ounce exceeds the DRI (dietary reference intake) for selenium, a mineral shown to help protect against breast and protate cancers.

PEANUTS: The B vitamins niacin and folate found in peanuts help maintain a healthy heart and may decrease your risk for certain cancers; folate may also protect against cognitive decline.

ALMONDS: These are high in vitamin E, which may help protect against some cancers. Their fats are largely monounsaturated, which helps lower "bad" cholesterol and reduces the risk of heart disease.

PECANS: A native of North America, pecans contain more disease-fighting antioxidants than any other nut commonly found in the United States.

5 SEAFOOD

THE LONGEVITY-ENHANCING BENEFITS

No other protein source comes close to delivering the essential fatty acids called omega-3s as cold-water fish, including salmon, sardines, mackerel, sablefish, herring, and trout. Omega-3s have been associated with a reduced risk of stroke and heart disease, and decreased odds of depression and cognitive decline in older people. Shellfish, such as oysters, mussels, clams, and shrimp, are excellent low-fat sources of protein and of minerals such as calcium, iron, and zinc. As with small cold-water fish, they are a good choice for sustainable seafood and tend to be low in mercury.

HOW TO GET ENOUGH

Use anchovies in salads and as a sandwich filling (though anchovies can be high in sodium; consume in moderation if you have hypertension). Canned sardines and canned wild salmon (drizzled with lemon and olive oil on toasted bread) make tasty snacks. Change up a satay (broil thin strips of cod—in place of beef or lamb—on skewers) or tacos (use a flaky whitefish like halibut instead of beef or pork). If you don't like to cook fish at home, remember to order seafood when you dine out.

ON YOUR PLATE

Eat a 3- to 4-ounce portion, three times a week (a portion of fish fillet is about the size of your palm or a deck of playing cards).

THE SKINNY ON OMEGA-3 FATTY ACIDS

The omega-3s found in cold-water fish like salmon and sardines, and in flaxseed and walnuts, may have bodywide health benefits. Studies suggest that these healthy fats may lower high blood pressure and triglycerides, reduce the risk of heart attacks and depression, and help prevent age-related macular degeneration (see page 334).[3] They reduce joint inflammation, stave off dementia, and may lower the risk of colorectal cancer. There are three types: ALA (alpha-linolenic acid), EPA (eicosapentaenoic acid), and DHA (docosahexaenoic acid). Although you can take supplements to obtain all of these fatty acids, experts believe it's best to consume them through diet.

ALA: Found in flaxseed and other vegetable sources, such as canola oil, ALA reduces the incidence of coronary heart disease, according to studies.

EPA: Plentiful in cold-water fish, EPA, combined with DHA, may be particularly helpful in preventing heart disease.

DHA: Found in oily cold-water fish, DHA is particularly beneficial to eye health. Sufficient DHA in the diet may lower the risk of Alzheimer's disease. Algal oil, made from ocean algae, is a plant-based source of pre-formed DHA and can be found as a dietary supplement.

6 LEAN ANIMAL PROTEIN

THE LONGEVITY-ENHANCING BENEFITS

Protein is the body's cellular building block, containing the essential amino acids needed for good health and for helping rebuild muscle mass, which dwindles as we age. Chicken, turkey, and eggs are lower in heart-unhealthy saturated fat than red meat, and are great sources of B vitamins, which help guide the body's major metabolic processes and aid in energy production. One member of this vitamin family, B_{12}, helps maintain a healthy nervous system and a steady supply of oxygen-carrying red blood cells. Once maligned as a source of dietary cholesterol, eggs are better for you than was once thought. The yolk, in particular, contains vitamin A, folate, and choline (it's nature's best source of this nutrient), which contribute to eye health and brain function. Although the yolk contains most of the egg's cholesterol, new research has shown that only a little actually makes it into the bloodstream.[4] If your cholesterol levels are normal, eating a few eggs per week shouldn't be dangerous.

HOW TO GET ENOUGH

Substitute ground turkey in any recipe that calls for ground beef. Use leftover chicken or turkey in a sandwich or salad for lunch. Keep turkey or chicken cutlets, stored in zip-seal bags, in the freezer and use as a basis for stir-fries or sandwiches. Add chunks of cooked chicken or turkey to bean-based chilis and other stews. A hard-boiled egg makes a portable, perfect pre-workout or between-meal snack.

ON YOUR PLATE

Try to consume a 3- to 4-ounce portion of poultry three or four times a week (a portion is about the size of your palm or a deck of playing cards). Eat up to 3 eggs per week.

WATCH OUT FOR SODIUM

When choosing lean protein, avoid salt- and nitrate-filled cold cuts, and opt for cooked, unprocessed meats instead. Research shows that even small changes in salt intake can make a difference in stroke risk.[5]

In one study, those who ate 4,000 mg or more of sodium a day were at increased risk of stroke compared with those who took in 1,500 mg or less daily. For every 500-mg increase in sodium intake per day, the risk of ischemic stroke increased 17 percent. A 2-ounce portion of turkey or chicken deli meat can contain upwards of 500 mg of sodium, while a similar portion of hard salami can contain more than 1,000 mg. Read nutritional information on packages, and limit your daily sodium intake to fewer than 2,300 mg and preferably 1,500 mg a day. Watch for sodium in other processed foods, such as tomato sauce, and various canned foods, condiments, and prepared mixes.

7 CALCIUM-RICH FOODS

THE LONGEVITY-ENHANCING BENEFITS

In addition to strengthening bones, calcium is required to keep muscles (including the heart) functioning. When the body lacks calcium, it will draw it from the bones to support these vital functions. Deficiency may, therefore, result in fractures and diseases such as osteoporosis; some evidence also links calcium from food or supplements to controlling blood pressure, decreasing the risk of prediabetes, and curbing memory loss. Although calcium is nearly synonymous with dairy products, there are multiple other dietary sources of this mineral (see below).

HOW TO GET ENOUGH

Blend yogurt with fresh fruit for smoothies; combine it with homemade muesli (raw oats, dried fruits, nuts). If you eat fortified cereal, drink the milk in the bottom of the bowl; it contains many of the vitamins from the cereal. Grate or crumble a flavorful cheese (feta, bleu, Parmesan) over salads or vegetables; you won't have to add much to get a punch. Make a creamy dip for crudités by mixing plain low-fat yogurt, Dijon mustard, and curry powder.

ON YOUR PLATE

You can drink two servings of milk and fortified soymilk per day. Eat no more than 1 cup of plain yogurt daily. Limit cheese to 1 ounce a day. Choose low-fat varieties of milk, cheese, and yogurt.

GET YOUR CALCIUM—WITHOUT THE COW

Most people will develop some degree of lactose intolerance as they get older, even if in their youth they drank milk without a problem, say researchers at the National Institutes of Health. Over the years, your body stops producing large quantities of lactase, the enzyme responsible for breaking down lactose. Production generally doesn't stop entirely, but some lactose passes intact through the intestine to the colon, where it's fermented by the resident bacteria. As bacteria break down the lactose, gas is produced, which can cause bloating, cramps, and diarrhea. Avoiding dairy foods only worsens symptoms when you do indulge in, say, ice cream, because those bacteria become less efficient at breaking down lactose if they're not continuously asked to do so. What's more, our intestines become less efficient at absorbing calcium and vitamin D as we age, even though these are necessary to maintain mental alertness, memory, and good circulation. So don't skimp on calcium. If you're lactose intolerant or vegan (or just want to reduce dairy), you can meet the recommended adequate intake (or AI) of calcium for adults by consuming 1,000 mg/day of these foods recommended by the USDA:

- Fortified cereals, 1 oz = 236–1,043 mg
- Soy beverage, calcium fortified, 1 cup = 364 mg
- Sardines, 3 oz = 325 mg
- Salmon, 3 oz = about 181 mg
- Collards, cooked, ½ cup = 178 mg
- Molasses, blackstrap, 1 tablespoon = 172 mg
- Soybeans, green, ½ cup = 130 mg
- Spinach, cooked, ½ cup = 146 mg
- White beans, canned, ½ cup = 96 mg

8 GOOD FATS

THE LONGEVITY-ENHANCING BENEFITS

The days of nonfat-diet fads are gone, and it's generally recognized that fats—at least the right kinds—are good for you. Along with carbohydrates and protein, fats are one of the body's most basic nutrients. Generally, you should stick to unsaturated fats. Monounsaturated fatty acids, such as those found in olive oil and avocados, can help keep blood vessels flexible and lower total cholesterol levels, including LDL ("bad") cholesterol. Polyunsaturated fats, such as the omega-3s found in walnuts and cold-water fish, tend to reduce the body's production of cholesterol—both HDL ("good") and LDL. Not all saturated fats are necessarily bad. For instance, coconut oil contains lauric acid, a saturated fat that has antiviral, antimicrobial, and antifungal properties, and raises good HDL cholesterol (as well as bad LDL). For these reasons, cold-pressed, virgin coconut oil has been embraced by the health food community in recent years, and piqued the interest of nutritionists. However, there's still not enough evidence to prove coconut oil is actively beneficial in the way that other unsaturated vegetables oils have proven, and the American Heart Association still recommends a diet low in any saturated fats.

HOW TO GET ENOUGH

Drizzle a high-quality (unrefined) extra-virgin olive oil over salads, steamed or roasted vegetables, or baked potatoes in place of butter or bottled dressings. Substitute walnut oil for your usual olive oil in salad dressings or dip whole-wheat bread into it. Snack on whole olives or chop them and add them to salads, rice, or pasta. Chopped olives give richness to an ordinary marinara sauce, and mashed avocado makes a satisfying sandwich spread or toast topper.

ON YOUR PLATE

Use olive oil often, but not more than 1 teaspoon per meal. Limit yourself to a single portion of avocado, about a third of a whole avocado.

THE SKINNY ON FATS

Instead of trying to eliminate fat from your diet, focus on eating the right kinds. Sort through your cupboards to make sure you're not keeping unhealthy fats on hand.

UNSATURATED FATS ARE BEST There are two types of unsaturated fats: monounsaturated and polyunsaturated. Don't get too hung up on which is which. Both are called "good" fats because they improve blood cholesterol levels and fight inflammation, lowering your risk of heart disease. They are found primarily in plant foods. Omega-3 fatty acids, however, are most prevalent in fish. Called essential fats, omega-3s are an important type of polyunsaturated fat that your body can't make, so they must come from food. Daily allowance: 28–62 grams.

USE SATURATED FATS WITH CAUTION These kinds of fats come mainly from red meat, poultry with skin, and whole-milk dairy products (cheese, whole-fat milk, and ice cream) and raise levels of harmful LDL cholesterol, increasing the risk of heart disease and stroke. You don't have to eliminate them from your diet entirely (meat and dairy can be good sources of protein), but it's a good idea to keep your intake as low as possible. Daily allowance: 16–22 grams or 10 percent of daily calories.

AVOID TRANS FATS These primarily man-made fats are created through partial hydrogenation of unsaturated fats. You'll find them in packaged foods such as cookies, crackers, and snack foods. They're also used for deep-frying foods because they can be reheated repeatedly. Steer clear of trans fats, which, research shows, raise your risk of heart disease. Daily allowance: none to less than 2 grams.

STORE WISELY Remember to store salad and cooking oils in a cool, dark place. (Do not store them above the stovetop or on top of the refrigerator, or the heat will spoil them.) They'll keep longest in your fridge, though most will solidify. Just leave them at room temperature for a short period to reliquefy them before use. If you prefer to keep oils in the pantry, buy smaller quantities so you'll replace them more frequently.

MEET YOUR VITAMIN AND MINERAL NEEDS

Use this chart to ensure you're getting enough key nutrients in your diet. If not, increase your intake of the food group listed under "Good Sources" and, if necessary, consult your doctor about supplementation.[6]

NUTRIENT	WHAT YOU NEED	GOOD SOURCES
CALCIUM Helps maintain bone health and fight osteoporosis; may help protect against cancer, diabetes, and high blood pressure	**Men** 51–70 years: 800 mg/day Over 71: 1,000 mg/day **Women** 51–70 years: 1,000 mg/day Over 71: 1,000 mg/day	Low-fat dairy products, fortified orange juice, salmon with bones, leafy greens (collards, mustard, broccoli, kale), tofu
CHROMIUM Mineral that helps the body utilize insulin, the hormone that keeps blood sugar balanced; may help reduce LDL cholesterol levels	**Men** 51–70 years: 30 mcg/day Over 71: 30 mcg/day **Women** 51–70 years: 20 mcg/day Over 71: 20 mcg/day	Whole-grain breads and cereals, lean meats, eggs, wheat germ, broccoli, garlic, red wine
FOLATE Helper enzyme in the synthesis of amino acids, DNA, and RNA; prevents megaloblastic anemia	**Men** 51–70 years: 320 mcg/day Over 70: 320 mcg/day **Women** 51–70 years: 320 mcg/day Over 71: 320 mcg/day	Dark green leafy vegetables, eggs, beans, enriched and whole-grain breads and bread products, fortified ready-to-eat cereals
VITAMIN A Required for normal vision, gene expression, reproduction, embryonic development, and immune function	**Men** 51–70 years: 625 mcg/day Over 71: 625 mcg/day **Women** 51–70 years: 500 mcg/day Over 71: 500 mcg/day	Liver, dairy products, fish, darkly colored fruits, leafy vegetables
VITAMIN B$_6$ Helps body to make antibodies and hemoglobin	**Men** 51–70 years: 1.4 mg/day Over 71: 1.4 mg/day **Women** 51–70 years: 1.3 mg/day Over 71: 1.3 mg/day	Canned chickpeas, fortified cereals, organ meats, fortified soy-based meat substitutes, bananas, avocados

NUTRIENT	WHAT YOU NEED	GOOD SOURCES
VITAMIN B$_{12}$ Coenzyme in nucleic acid metabolism; prevents megaloblastic anemia	**Men** 51–70 years: 2.4 mcg/day Over 71: 2.4 mcg/day **Women** 51–70 years: 2.4 mcg/day Over 71: 2.4 mcg/day	Salmon, tuna, ground beef, beans, low-fat cottage cheese, fortified cereals, meat, fish, poultry
VITAMIN C Protects against free radicals	**Men** 51–70 years: 75 mg/day Over 71: 75 mg/day **Women** 51–70 years: 60 mg/day Over 71: 60 mg/day	Citrus fruits, tomatoes, red and green peppers, potatoes, Brussels sprouts, cauliflower, broccoli, strawberries, cabbage, spinach
VITAMIN D Helps regulate blood levels of calcium and phosphorus; helps maintain a healthy immune system	**Men** 51–70 years: 600 IU/day Over 71: 800 IU/day **Women** 51–70 years: 600 IU/day Over 71: 800 IU/day	Fish liver oils, flesh of fatty fish, eggs from hens that have been fed vitamin D, fortified milk products, fortified cereals
VITAMIN E A general antioxidant, it improves immunity in older adults	**Men** 51–70 years: 12 mg/day Over 71: 12 mg/day **Women** 51–70 years: 12 mg/day Over 71: 12 mg/day	Vegetable oils, unprocessed cereal grains, nuts, wheat germ oil, sunflower seeds
VITAMIN K Helps stimulate osteocalcin, a protein important in bone strength; involved in blood clotting	**Men** 51–70 years: 120 mcg/day Over 71: 120 mcg/day **Women** 51–70 years: 90 mcg/day Over 71: 90 mcg/day	Dark green leafy vegetables (collards, spinach, kale), Brussels sprouts, Swiss chard, parsley
ZINC Helps maintain sense of smell and taste; bolsters body's immune system	**Men** 51–70 years: 9.4 mg/day Over 71: 9.4 mg/day **Women** 51–70 years: 6.8 mg/day Over 71: 6.8 mg/day	Oysters, lobster, crab, beans, nuts

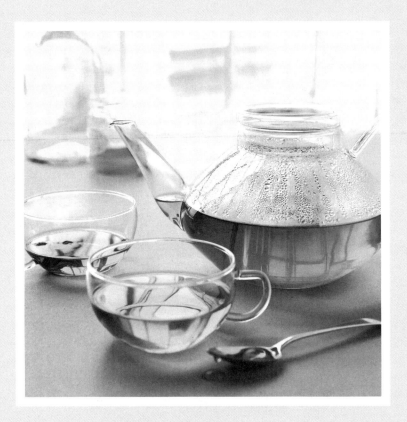

HAVE A CUP OF TEA

Practice the English custom of afternoon tea. Drink one or two cups of green or black tea accompanied by 1 or 2 ounces of low-fat cheese and a whole-grain biscuit. The tea contains polyphenols and antioxidants to help repair cell damage. The cheese contains protein, calcium, and probiotics to aid digestion. And the whole-grain biscuit is a source of fiber. The entire snack is just about 200 calories—and if you can take 15 minutes to sip in peace, you'll find it fully satisfying and restorative.

PUT *a healthy plan in place*

When it comes to nutrition, if we don't take a proactive approach, our goals are easily sabotaged. We are bound to make fewer healthful choices when we wait too long to eat, grab something on the run, or surround ourselves with the wrong foods. Here's how to avoid such traps.

GET AN OBJECTIVE OPINION ABOUT YOUR WEIGHT

First, make an appointment with your doctor to see if you're currently at a healthy weight. Two measurements that can help assess your proper weight are the body mass index (BMI) and the waist/hip ratio (WHR). Once you know the right weight range for your body type, talk to a nutritionist about healthful, nutritious ways to make that scale reading move up or down to your optimal weight. Check out the link on the Academy of Nutrition and Dietetic's homepage (www.eatright.org) to find a registered dietitian in your area, or ask your doctor for a recommendation.

As you work toward your optimal weight range, weigh yourself weekly. Tracking your weight is one screening test you can actually do at home, notes Dr. Jana Klauer. "You will stay on top of the small, one- to two-pound gains that signal that you need to change your calorie intake or your activity level. You can also keep tabs if you suddenly start to lose weight unintentionally."

Record your weight so you have an accurate history to show your doctor. Any rapid increase or decrease in weight could be the first manifestation of a more serious problem, such as congestive heart failure, edema, or depression. Every few months, use a tape measure to record the circumference of your waist. (To find the ideal spot, locate the bottom of your rib cage and the top of your hip bone; place the tape measure equidistant from these points.) Fat that accumulates around your middle is associated with an increased risk of type 2 diabetes and cardiovascular disease. A waist size of over 40 inches for men and 35 inches for women is associated with a significantly increased risk. Share your statistics with your doctor so the two of you can work together to prevent chronic conditions such as diabetes and heart disease.

STOCK A HEALTHY PANTRY

Fill your kitchen with healthful ingredients, and you'll be much more prepared to put together a nutritious meal anytime. The following tips will help you determine what to keep on hand, and what to look for on food labels.

❶ NUT BUTTERS
LOOK FOR natural versions, which have no added sugar and no hydrogenated oil, the source of unhealthy trans fats.

❷ CEREAL
LOOK FOR at least 3 grams of fiber and no more than 10 grams of sugar per serving (less is even better). And pay attention to recommended serving size—it's likely smaller than what you usually pour into your bowl.

❸ CRACKERS
LOOK FOR keywords such as "whole grain" or "whole wheat" at the top of the ingredients list and at least 3 grams of fiber per serving.

❹ PASTA AND RICE
LOOK FOR the words "100 percent whole grain" on the label for whole-wheat pasta, and 3 grams of fiber per serving. For rice, choose whole-grain varieties (such as brown, wild, red, or brown basmati); these are higher in fiber and nutrients than their more processed white cousins.

❺ OIL
LOOK FOR extra-virgin, cold-pressed olive oil, which is high in heart-healthy monounsaturated fats and contains disease-fighting antioxidants.

❻ NUTS AND DRIED FRUIT
LOOK FOR roasted, unsalted nuts for snacking. Almonds are the highest in vitamin E, and walnuts boast omega-3s. All dried fruit is a good source of fiber and potassium, but cranberries and blueberries are antioxidant superstars. Look for those with no added sugar.

❼ SALT AND SPICES
LOOK FOR opportunities to use sea salt, which is more flavorful than table salt, so you'll need less of it and still get great flavor. Limit your intake to 1,500 milligrams of sodium per day. Use spices to add flavor without adding calories. Spices also increase satiety, so you'll be less likely to overeat.

❽ CANNED TOMATOES
LOOK FOR the shortest list of ingredients on the label and the least amount of added sugar and sodium. All kinds of canned tomatoes—diced, or in a sauce or paste—will be good sources of the potent antioxidant lycopene, but tomato paste will have the highest levels because it's the most concentrated.

❾ CANNED TUNA AND SALMON
LOOK FOR light tuna, which has the lowest amount of potentially harmful mercury. For lower-calorie versions, opt for those packed in water (although tuna in olive oil has a wonderfully rich flavor). Choose canned wild salmon for one of the best sources of omega-3s.

❿ CANNED BEANS
LOOK FOR low-sodium varieties, since canned beans can be high in salt. As a general rule, more color means more nutrients, so red kidney, pinto, and black beans are extra-rich in a variety of antioxidants. But all beans are wonderful (and inexpensive) sources of protein and fiber.

⓫ CHICKEN BROTH
LOOK FOR unsalted or low-sodium broths. Opt for organic whenever possible.

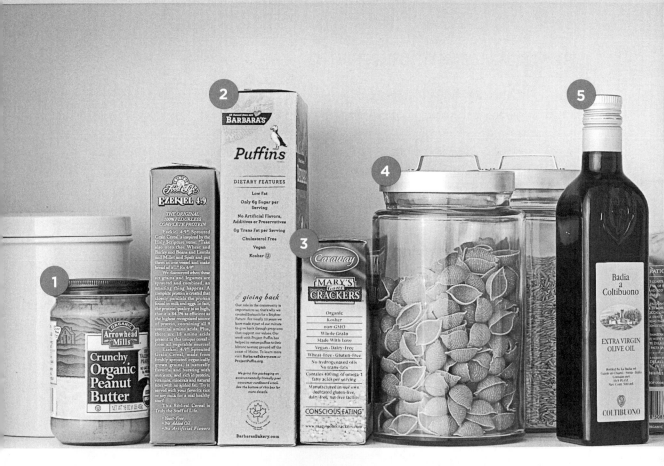

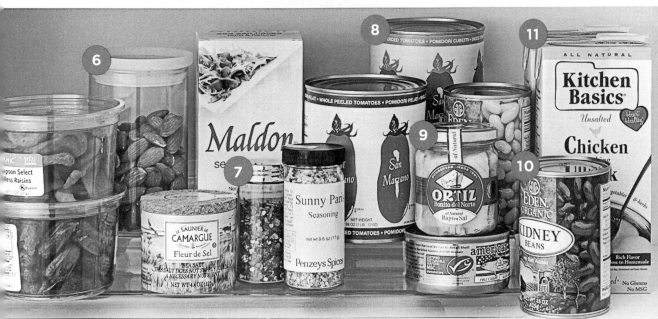

PRACTICE MINDFUL EATING

As you rebalance your plate to feature less processed, unhealthful fare and more fresh, whole foods, it's also important to slow down and savor each dining experience, taking the time to taste your food. When you eat more slowly and truly enjoy each meal, something magical happens: you feel more satisfied with less. This is important because research shows that a lean body weight is important for longevity: obesity is a primary risk factor in the development of cardiovascular disease, stroke, type 2 diabetes, high blood pressure, and many types of cancer.

The good news is that watching your weight through this kind of mindful eating is not the unpleasant experience you may remember from past dieting attempts. Yes, you probably will need to shave some excess calories from your daily diet—as we age, our metabolism slows by 5 to 7 percent per decade, and the body requires fewer calories just to maintain a healthy weight. But if you're already in your optimal weight range, you'll need to lose only 100 calories or fewer per day, per decade. If you're choosing the kinds of sustaining foods recommended in this chapter, you won't even miss the calories.

ELIMINATE EMPTY CALORIES

Eating fewer calories doesn't necessarily mean eating less food. Simply find sources of empty calories in your diet and eliminate them. Some of the most common culprits are fruit drinks, carbonated beverages, presweetened snacks and cereals, and whole-fat dairy products. If you aren't sure, try to eat food that is as close to its natural state as possible.[7]

| These easy adjustments have health benefits beyond the calories saved: | • Trade your daily 8-ounce soda for seltzer with lemon juice.
• Remove the saturated fat–soaked skin from servings of poultry (trim after cooking, so meat stays moist).
• Top pasta with lycopene-rich tomato sauces instead of cream sauces; sprinkle the dish with dried chile pepper flakes rather than grated cheese.
• Choose water-packed tuna over oil-packed. |

RETHINK YOUR MEALTIMES

If you grew up in a certain era, you were likely raised with three solid meals a day and taught to always clean your plate. However, experts now believe that smaller meals, eaten more frequently, are far better for promoting overall health and maintaining a target weight. In fact, cultures that eat smaller meals tend to be healthier overall.

Okinawans, for example, who have one of the highest percentage of centenarians on the planet, practice a natural form of portion control called "hara hachi bu," which roughly translates to "80 percent full." They pay such close attention to how food makes them feel that they're able to stop eating just before they are completely sated. This makes sense, considering it takes 20 minutes for the stomach to signal your brain that you've had enough.

In order to sustain that feeling of "80 percent full" from one meal to another, try apportioning your calories into five or six smaller meals and snacks, eaten roughly three hours apart. Doing so will keep your blood sugar steady and curb hunger, which may help you eat fewer calories overall. Consume most of your calories in the first half of the day, to fuel yourself when you're most active and burning calories most efficiently. Include a healthy protein, such as eggs, fish, yogurt, lean meats, or nuts, in most of your meals to help regulate your blood sugar.

To make food preparation easy, stock your freezer and pantry with healthy ingredients (see page 44 for ideas) that can be prepared quickly. Keeping these items on hand will serve you well if your mobility is limited, you rely on others to pick up groceries, or your day is overscheduled.

COOK *for better health*

Nothing tastes as delicious as a meal you've planned, prepared, and taken the time to enjoy. Cooking ensures that we eat well, put together meals that appeal to our personal tastes, and celebrate the bounty of the season.

It can be daunting to cook if you're suddenly single or getting in the habit after years of takeout and restaurant meals. But cooking for yourself is actually easier than cooking for others: it's quicker, less stressful, and less costly. (Over time, you'll find that stocking a healthy pantry and cooking from scratch save a significant amount of money, as well.) If it's tomato or asparagus season, you can eat asparagus or tomatoes every day. And caviar or smoked salmon for one is far less expensive than salmon or caviar for a crowd, so you can indulge yourself and benefit from the omega-3s and other good fats while you are at it.

It's worth noting that cooking is one of the few areas in life where you can have total control: you cook what you want, whenever you want. And just as important, you know exactly what you're putting into your body. So many prepared and packaged foods are high in added fats and sugars, the very things you should be minimizing. Less than one-third of the calories in home-cooked foods come from fat, while restaurant and store-bought meals derive nearly 38 percent of their calories from fat, according to the Department of Agriculture.

A solid understanding of certain basic techniques will equip you to eat for greater health and longevity. Master the easy formulas for a salad with vinaigrette, a quick soup, and three healthy cooking techniques—roasting, stir-frying, and parchment cooking—and you'll be able to produce more healthful, less-expensive, and better-tasting meals in the comfort of your own kitchen.

ESSENTIAL KITCHEN EQUIPMENT

The proper equipment always makes the job easier. You don't have to rush out and buy all the newest pots and pans available, but the following staples should prove quite useful:

- A 2-quart stove-top and ovenproof casserole with a lid
- An 8- to 12-inch skillet
- A 9½-inch oval baking dish
- A 6- to 8-quart stockpot
- A food processor or blender
- A 2-quart mixing bowl
- An 8-inch square pan
- A baking sheet

A GUIDE TO HEALTHIER EATING

Armed with a well-stocked pantry and a few simple cooking techniques, you can prepare a variety of flavorful and healthful meals that will keep you energized throughout the day. Replacing larger meals with smaller, more frequent ones needn't be a big challenge.

On the following pages you'll find 40 recipes for small meals and snacks that can be enjoyed from breakfast through dinner, plus a few healthful desserts. These recipes rely heavily on pantry staples—such as rice, oatmeal, and canned beans—along with fresh vegetables, fruits, and meats that can be purchased as you need them. When shopping for fresh ingredients, buy only what you need, particularly if you're cooking for one, to minimize waste.

Even if you're just cooking for yourself, however, you should make an effort to sit down to at least one meal each day. When you set aside time to eat in peace, you'll be more likely to find your meal satisfying and restorative—and to choose the right balance of foods.

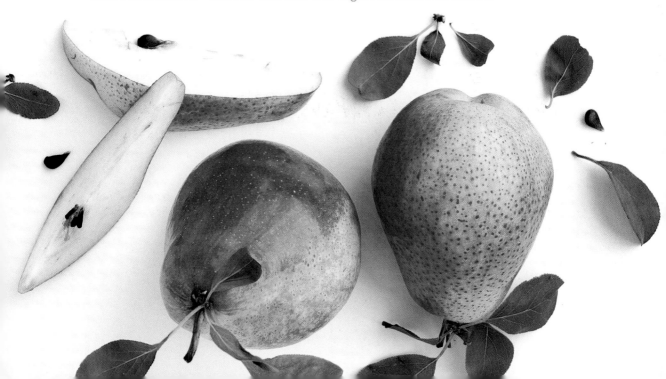

EAT THE RAINBOW

The easiest way to assure you have a varied diet is to incorporate vegetables and fruits in a broad range of colors. Aim for two to three different hues with each meal, which will also help to increase your overall intake of produce.

RED

BENEFITS: lycopene, an antioxidant that appears to reduce risk of cancer and cardiovascular disease; and anthocyanins, which protect cells from damage

SOURCES: red apples, beets, red bell peppers, cherries, red grapes, radishes, rhubarb, strawberries, raspberries, pomegranate, tomatoes, watermelon

YELLOW-ORANGE

BENEFITS: carotenoids, such as beta-carotene, which the body converts to vitamin A and are vital to healthy cell growth, bone and skin health, and immune function

SOURCES: apricots, cantaloupe, carrots, yams, sweet potatoes, yellow peppers, mango, peaches, pineapple, pumpkin, sweet corn, yellow summer or winter squash (such as butternut and acorn)

ORANGE-YELLOW

BENEFITS: flavonoids, powerful antioxidants that protect the body's cells from free radicals and help metabolize fats; and vitamin C

SOURCES: citrus fruits (oranges, lemons, grapefruits), papaya

GREEN

BENEFITS: folate (B_9), which plays an important role in cell division and helps to make red blood cells; lutein, important for eye health; and indoles, powerful cancer fighters

SOURCES: asparagus, avocado, cucumbers, spinach, kale, collard, chard, and other leafy greens, plus broccoli, artichokes, brussels sprouts, fresh herbs

BROWN

BENEFITS: terpenoids, high in antiviral and anti-inflammatory properties; and niacin (B_3)

SOURCES: mushrooms such as maitake, shiitake, and reishi

WHITE

BENEFITS: diallyl disulfide, a phytochemical that may reduce the risk of stomach and colon cancer; and allicin, which may help lower cholesterol

SOURCES: bananas, garlic, onion, chives, cauliflower, parsnips, potatoes, turnips

BLUE

BENEFITS: anthocyanins, a group of flavonoid pigments that show promise as anti-cancer and anti-inflammatory agents

SOURCES: blueberries, purple grapes, eggplant, plums, raisins

PURPLE

BENEFITS: resveratrol, a type of antioxidant that may help prevent damage to blood vessels in the heart and reduce "bad" (LDL) cholesterol

SOURCES: red and purple grapes, berries (blueberries, cranberries, blackberries), plums

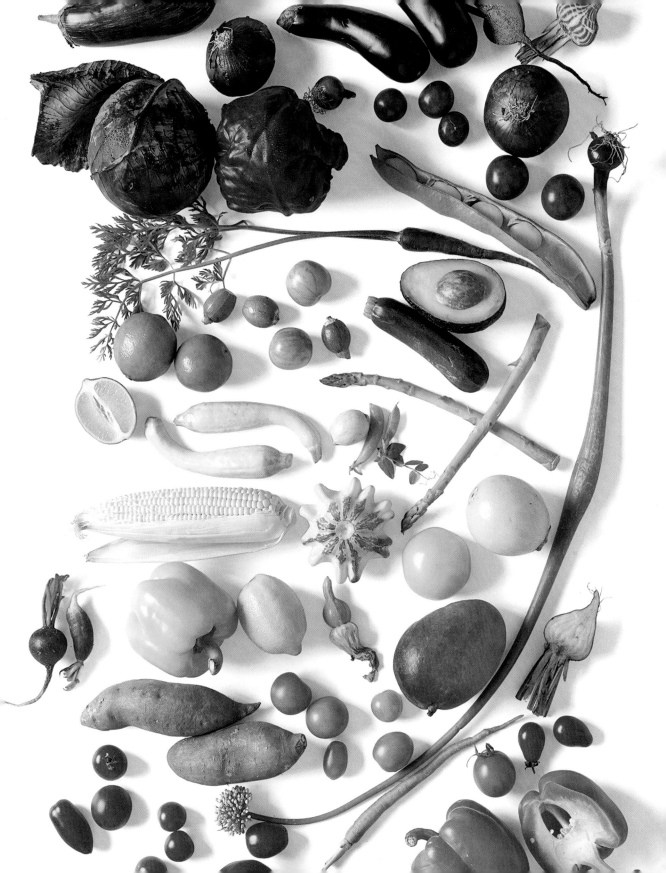

START THE DAY WITH GREEN JUICE

Every morning before I get into my car, I drink about eight
ounces of green juice. Using my trusty Breville juicer, I make
a blend of whatever fresh produce is on hand, much of which I
grow at the farm. One of my favorite combinations is spinach,
cucumber, parsley, chervil, fresh ginger, and orange peel. I
actually feel a jolt of energy when I imbibe these drinks, and I
love to share them with my friends.

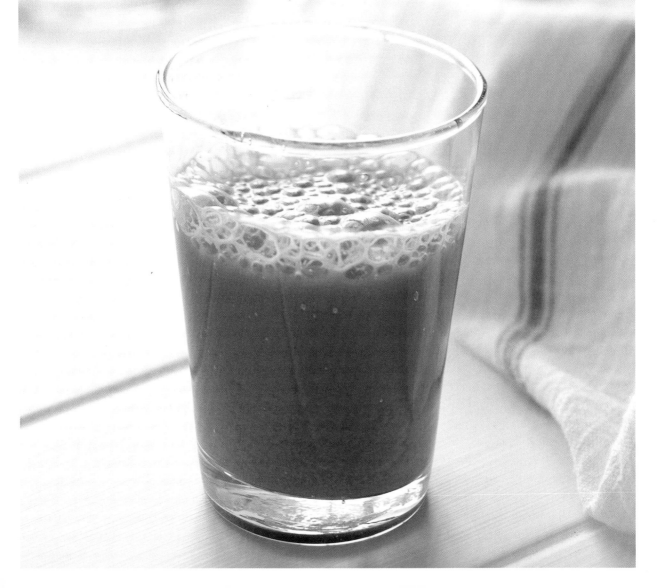

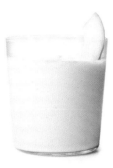

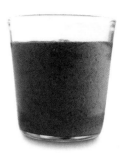

AVOCADO-PEAR SMOOTHIE

In a blender, puree ½ ripe **avocado** (pitted and peeled), ¼ cup **silken tofu** (drained), ½ cup **pear juice,** 1 tablespoon **honey,** and ¼ teaspoon **vanilla extract** until smooth. Add 1 cup **ice;** blend until smooth.

BLUEBERRY–GREEN TEA SMOOTHIE

In a blender, puree ½ cup each frozen **blueberries** and **strawberries,** ½ cup chilled unsweetened **green tea,** ¾ cup plain low-fat **yogurt,** and 2 tablespoons ground **flaxseed** until smooth.

PEACH-RASPBERRY SMOOTHIE

In a blender, puree 1 cup fresh or frozen sliced **peaches,** 1 cut-up ripe **banana,** 1 cup fresh **raspberries,** 1 cup **ice,** and ¼ cup unsweetened **almond milk** until smooth.

CARROT-GINGER SMOOTHIE

In a blender, puree 1 cut-up ripe **banana,** ½ cup **carrot juice,** ½ cup plain low-fat **yogurt,** 1 tablespoon chopped peeled **fresh ginger,** and 1 cup **ice** until smooth.

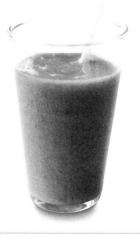

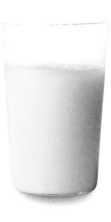

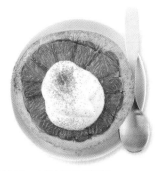

BROILED GRAPEFRUIT

Halve a red or pink **grapefruit,** and loosen segments from membranes and pith with a paring knife. Sprinkle each grapefruit half with 1 tablespoon **light brown sugar** and ¼ teaspoon ground **cinnamon.** Broil on a baking sheet until top is slightly browned, 4 to 5 minutes. Top with ½ cup plain low-fat **yogurt** and sprinkle with more cinnamon.

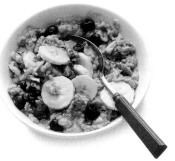

OATMEAL WITH BLUEBERRIES, WALNUTS, AND BANANAS

Bring 1 cup water to a boil; add ½ cup old-fashioned **rolled oats** and a pinch of ground **cinnamon** and **salt**; simmer until tender, 5 minutes. Stir in ¼ cup fresh or frozen **blueberries.** Top with sliced **banana** and chopped toasted **walnuts** and serve with maple syrup and skim milk, as desired.

SCRAMBLED EGGS WITH SPINACH AND TOMATOES

Whisk 2 large **eggs** in a bowl, and season with **salt** and **pepper.** Heat 2 teaspoons **olive oil** in a skillet over medium-low. Add eggs and cook, stirring frequently, until just set, 1 to 2 minutes. Stir in ¼ cup chopped **spinach** and ¼ cup halved **cherry tomatoes.** Spoon mixture into a toasted halved **pita bread.**

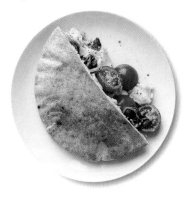

YOGURT PARFAIT

Layer 1 cup nonfat plain **yogurt,** ¾ cup **mixed fresh fruit** (such as blackberries, sliced strawberries, chopped kiwi, and orange segments), and 2 tablespoons chopped toasted **walnuts** in a glass. Drizzle with **honey.**

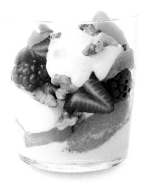

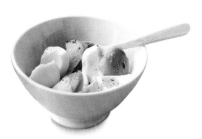

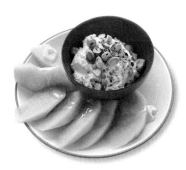

HARD-COOKED EGG WHITES WITH AVOCADO

Tear the whites of 2 **hard-cooked eggs** into bite-size pieces and put in a serving bowl. (Reserve yolks for another use.) Use a spoon to scrape pieces from ⅓ **avocado** into bowl. Season with **salt** and **pepper** and drizzle with **extra-virgin olive oil.**

CANTALOUPE WITH RICOTTA AND PISTACHIOS

In a small bowl, sprinkle ¼ cup part-skim **ricotta** with 2 tablespoons chopped shelled **pistachios.** Slice ¼ **cantaloupe** (peeled and seeded) into wedges, arrange on a plate, and drizzle with **honey,** if desired. Serve with ricotta mixture.

HOT RICE CEREAL WITH ALMONDS AND RAISINS

Bring ¾ cup cooked long-grain **brown rice,** ½ cup **milk,** and 1½ teaspoons **maple syrup** to a boil in a medium saucepan. Cook, stirring occasionally, until thickened slightly, about 3 minutes. Serve topped with chopped toasted **almonds** and **golden raisins,** and sprinkle with ground **nutmeg** or **cinnamon.**

WHOLE-GRAIN TOAST WITH GOAT CHEESE AND RASPBERRIES

Toast a slice of **whole-grain bread.** Let cool slightly and spread with 2 tablespoons fresh **goat cheese.** Top with ¾ cup **raspberries,** mash with a fork, and drizzle with a little **honey.**

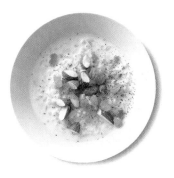

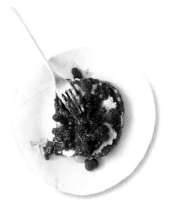

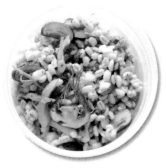

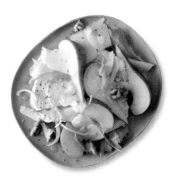

BARLEY, MUSHROOM, AND DILL SALAD

Heat 1 teaspoon **olive oil** in a skillet over medium. Sauté ½ cup sliced **white mushrooms** (stems removed) until tender, about 5 minutes. Toss together mushrooms, 1 cup cooked **pearl barley**, ½ grated peeled **carrot**, ½ thinly sliced **celery** stalk, ½ thinly sliced **scallion**, and 2 teaspoons **fresh dill** in a bowl. Drizzle a little **vinaigrette** (page 65) over top; season with **salt** and **pepper**, and toss to combine. Garnish with dill.

POACHED CHICKEN, ESCAROLE, AND PEAR SALAD

Whisk together 2 teaspoons **red-wine vinegar** and 1 tablespoon **extra-virgin olive oil;** season with **salt** and **pepper.** Arrange 1 or 2 torn **escarole** leaves, ¼ sliced **pear,** and ¼ thinly sliced **shallot** on a plate; top with 1 sliced poached **chicken breast half.** Drizzle with a little **vinaigrette** (page 65), and garnish with shaved **Pecorino cheese** and chopped toasted **walnuts.**

WHITE BEAN SALAD WITH SPICY ROASTED TOMATOES AND BROCCOLI

Preheat oven to 375°F. On a rimmed baking sheet, toss 1 cup total **broccoli** florets and chopped stems, 1 cup halved **cherry tomatoes,** 1 thinly sliced **garlic** clove, and a pinch of **red-pepper flakes;** drizzle with **extra-virgin olive oil** and season with **salt.** Roast until broccoli is tender and tomatoes are soft, 20 minutes. Let cool. Toss ½ cup cooked **white beans** (drained and rinsed) with broccoli, tomatoes, ½ cup **baby spinach,** and 2 tablespoons **vinaigrette** (page 65).

BAKED SWEET POTATOES WITH TOASTED NUTS AND ORANGES

Preheat oven to 400°F. Prick 2 small **sweet potatoes** with a fork and wrap in foil. Bake until tender, about 1 hour. Unwrap and split open with a knife. Top each with ¼ cup chopped toasted **almonds** or **pecans,** a pinch each of ground **cinnamon** and **nutmeg,** and flaky **sea salt.** Serve with **orange** wedges for squeezing on top.

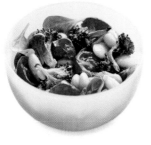

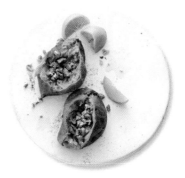

LUNCH THAT PACKS A PUNCH

One of my favorite weekday lunches is a large salad—fresh greens and fresh herbs dressed with a vinaigrette, along with a simply cooked piece of salmon drizzled with fresh lemon juice. This provides me with a tasty meal and enough protein and staying power to get through a busy afternoon—and it's heart-healthy as well.

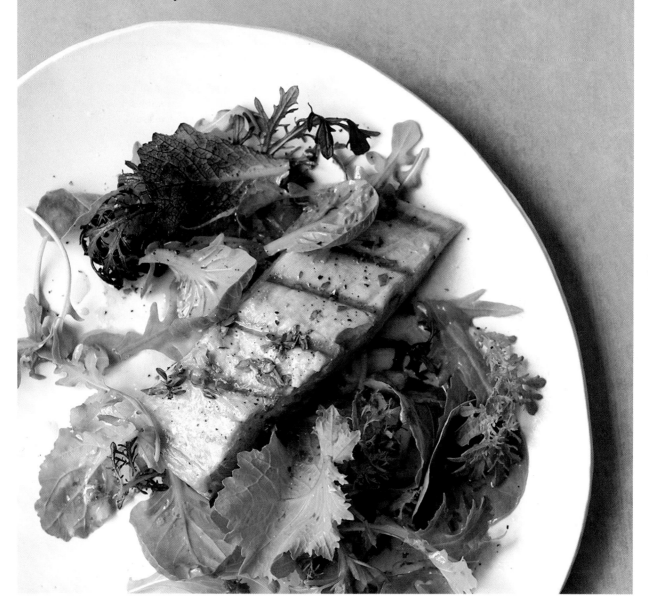

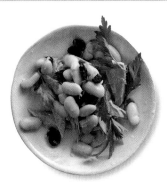

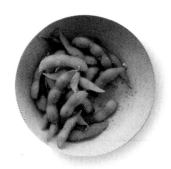

TUNA AND WHITE BEANS

Mix together ½ can **tuna** (drained), ⅓ cup cooked **cannellini** or other white beans (drained and rinsed), 1 tablespoon **raisins,** finely grated zest of ½ **lemon,** and ½ tablespoon **lemon juice.** Season with **salt** and **pepper** and toss to combine. Garnish with fresh **parsley.**

EDAMAME WITH CHILE SALT

Pulse ¼ teaspoon **red-pepper flakes** in a spice grinder until finely ground, then mix with ½ tablespoon **salt** and ¼ teaspoon **sugar** in a small bowl. Toss 8 ounces cooked frozen **edamame** with chile-salt mixture and serve warm with **lemon** wedges.

KALE DIP WITH BLANCHED PEAS

Heat 1 tablespoon **olive oil** in a skillet over medium. Add 1 thinly sliced **garlic** clove and 3 cups thinly sliced **kale** leaves. Cover; cook, stirring occasionally, until kale is tender, 3 minutes. Let cool. Puree mixture with 1 cup low-fat **cottage cheese** in a food processor. Add a pinch of **red-pepper flakes** and 1 tablespoon **lemon juice.** Refrigerate, covered, up to 3 days. Serve with blanched **sugar snap** or **snow peas.**

CHILI-LIME POPCORN

Heat 1 tablespoon **canola oil** with 3 **popcorn kernels** in a saucepan over medium. When kernels pop, add ¼ cup more kernels. Cover; cook, shaking pan, until popping slows, 3 to 4 minutes. Remove from heat; let stand, covered, 1 minute. Stir together ½ teaspoon each **chili powder** and **ground cumin,** ¼ teaspoon **salt,** and 1½ teaspoons grated **lime** zest. Sprinkle on hot popcorn; squeeze a lime wedge over, and toss to coat.

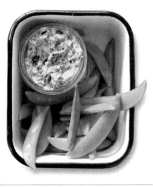

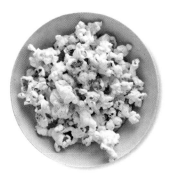

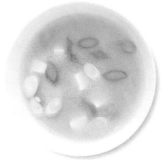

MISO SOUP

Bring 1 cup **vegetable** or **chicken stock** to a simmer in a saucepan. Add 2 ounces **silken tofu,** drained and cut into cubes, and simmer 2 minutes, just to heat through. Place 1 tablespoon **white miso** (available at Asian food stores and many supermarkets) in a small bowl and stir in ¼ cup cooking liquid until smooth. Add mixture to saucepan and cook just until soup is hot (do not let boil). Garnish with thinly sliced scallions, if desired.

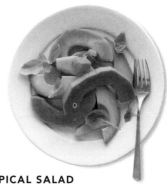

TROPICAL SALAD

Arrange 3 slices each chilled **papaya, cantaloupe,** and ripe but firm **avocado** (all peeled and seeded). Drizzle with 2 teaspoons fresh **lemon** juice and garnish with fresh **basil.**

DARK CHOCOLATE AND MIXED NUTS

Break a small bar of **dark chocolate** into bite-sized pieces. Combine with 2 tablespoons dried blueberries or raisins and ½ cup toasted **mixed nuts,** such as almonds and walnuts; pecans and cashews are other good options.

WHOLE-GRAIN CRACKER WITH HUMMUS AND CHEDDAR

Spread 2 tablespoons **hummus** over 1 large **whole-grain cracker.** Top with 1 slice **sharp cheddar** and 1 tablespoon **radish or alfalfa sprouts;** season with **pepper.**

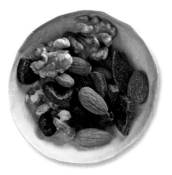

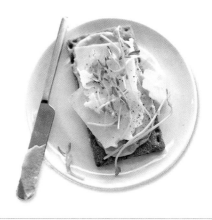

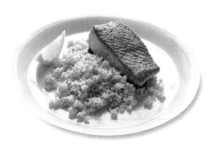

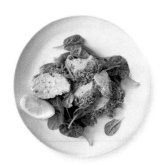

SEARED SALMON WITH BULGUR

Pat a **salmon** fillet (3 to 4 ounces) dry and season on both sides with **salt** and **pepper.** Heat 2 teaspoons **olive oil** over medium in a skillet. Add salmon and cook until opaque throughout, about 3 minutes per side. Serve with cooked **bulgur** tossed with sliced **scallions** and **lemon** wedges.

ALMOND-CRUSTED CHICKEN BREAST WITH SPINACH

Preheat oven to 425°F. Pulse ½ cup **roasted almonds,** 1 **garlic** clove, ½ teaspoon **salt,** and 3 tablespoons **extra-virgin olive oil** in a food processor to make a coarse paste. Rub mixture onto 2 boneless, skinless **chicken breast halves.** Roast until cooked through, 15 to 18 minutes. Slice and serve atop **baby spinach,** with **lemon** wedges.

PASTA WITH GREEN BEANS AND TUNA

Cook 3 ounces **fusilli** according to package instructions, adding 2 ounces trimmed **green beans** 1 minute before end. Drain. Combine 1 can (3 ounces) chunk light **tuna** (drained), 1 tablespoon **extra-virgin olive oil,** 1 tablespoon **almonds,** toasted and chopped, 2 teaspoons chopped fresh **parsley,** ½ teaspoon grated **lemon** zest, 1 teaspoon lemon juice, and 1 minced **garlic** clove; season with **salt** and **pepper.** Toss with pasta and beans.

HERB-FILLED OMELET

Whisk 3 large **eggs** in a bowl; season with **salt** and **pepper.** Heat an 8-inch skillet over medium-high. Add 1 tablespoon unsalted **butter;** heat until hot but not smoking. Add eggs and cook, tilting skillet occasionally and pulling cooked egg away from sides with a flexible spatula, until omelet is just set. Sprinkle with 1 tablespoon chopped **mixed fresh herbs,** such as tarragon, basil, chives, and parsley. Use spatula to gently fold over both sides so they overlap; slide onto plate.

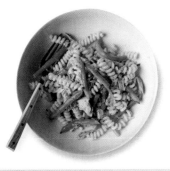

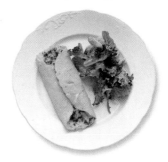

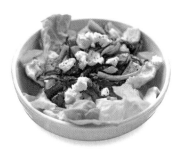

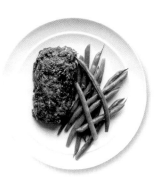

ROASTED VEGETABLE SALAD WITH GOAT CHEESE

Preheat oven to 450°F. On a rimmed baking sheet, toss 2 julienned peeled **carrots,** 1 diced **zucchini,** and 1 **red onion,** cut into wedges, with 1 tablespoon **olive oil;** season with **salt** and **pepper.** Roast until vegetables are tender, 20 minutes, tossing once. In a bowl, whisk 1 tablespoon **sherry vinegar** and 1 tablespoon oil; season with salt and pepper. Add 1 small head **Boston lettuce;** toss. Top with vegetables and crumbled **goat cheese.**

MEATLOAF WITH GREEN BEANS

Preheat oven to 375°F. In a bowl, combine 1 tablespoon plain **breadcrumbs,** 2 teaspoons **milk,** 1 tablespoon **ketchup,** 2 tablespoons grated **cheddar,** 1 thinly sliced **scallion,** and 2 tablespoons finely grated peeled **carrot;** season with **salt** and **pepper.** Add 4 ounces **ground beef** and mix. Form into a 2½-by-4-inch loaf on a rimmed baking sheet. Bake until cooked through, 30 minutes. Serve with sautéed or blanched **green beans.**

MUSHROOM AND FONTINA QUESADILLA

Heat 1 teaspoon **olive oil** in a skillet over medium-high. Cook ½ pound thinly sliced **mushrooms,** stirring occasionally, until browned, 8 minutes. Season with **salt** and **pepper.** Place mushrooms and ½ cup grated **fontina** on half of a **flour tortilla;** fold tortilla over filling. Cook quesadilla in skillet over medium until golden and cheese is melted, 3 minutes per side. Cut into wedges.

BROWN RICE WITH BLACK BEANS AND AVOCADO

Cook ½ cup long-grain **brown rice** according to package instructions; fluff with a fork and place in a bowl. Top with ½ cup cooked **black beans** (drained and rinsed) and ⅓ **avocado,** sliced into wedges. Serve with assorted garnishes such as cilantro, sour cream, shredded cheddar cheese, and chopped red onion and tomato, as desired.

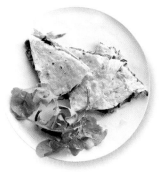

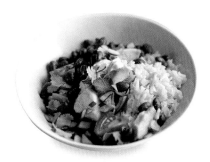

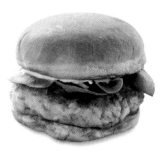

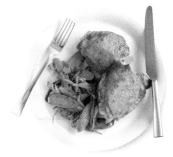

SALMON BURGER WITH SPINACH

Combine ¼ cup plain **breadcrumbs** with 1 can (7.5 ounces) **salmon** (drained and flaked), 2 tablespoons chopped **celery**, 1 tablespoon chopped **shallot,** and 1 tablespoon **mayonnaise.** Season with **salt** and **pepper;** mix well. Form into a patty; chill 10 minutes. Heat 2 teaspoons **olive oil** in a skillet over medium. Cook patty, flipping once, until browned, 8 minutes. Serve on a toasted bun with mayonnaise and **baby spinach.**

SEARED CHICKEN WITH CARROTS

Season 2 bone-in, skin-on **chicken thighs** with **salt** and **pepper;** sprinkle both sides with **flour.** Heat a skillet over medium-low. Cook chicken, skin side down, until browned, 8 to 10 minutes. Flip chicken; push to one side of skillet. Add 1 thinly sliced **shallot** and 2 thinly sliced peeled **carrots;** cook, tossing occasionally, until tender and chicken is cooked through, 10 to 12 minutes. Transfer to a plate; sprinkle vegetables with fresh parsley, if desired.

TROUT WITH ESCAROLE AND OLIVES

Heat 2 teaspoons **olive oil** in a skillet over medium-high. Season 1 skin-on **trout fillet** with **salt** and **pepper;** cook skin side up until golden, 5 minutes. Gently flip; cook until opaque throughout, 2 minutes. Transfer to a plate. Cook 3 cups trimmed **escarole** leaves, ¼ teaspoon grated **orange** zest, and 4 **green olives,** pitted and chopped, stirring, 2 minutes. Add 2 tablespoons **orange juice** and toss to coat. Serve alongside trout.

BROILED TOFU AND SNOW PEAS

Stir ½ teaspoon grated peeled fresh **ginger,** 2 teaspoons **soy sauce,** 1½ teaspoons **honey,** and ½ teaspoon **sesame oil.** Toss together 2 ounces **snow peas,** 1 sliced **scallion,** a pinch of **red-pepper flakes,** and ½ teaspoon **sesame oil;** season with **salt** and **pepper.** Place 5 ounces firm **tofu,** cut into thirds, on a rimmed baking sheet. Drizzle with half the sauce; broil 2 minutes. Add snow pea mixture; broil 1 minute. Serve over **rice;** drizzle with remaining sauce.

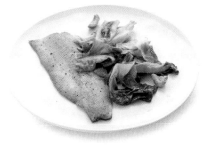

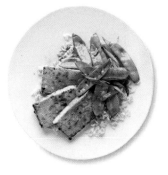

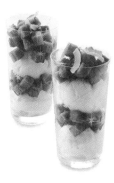

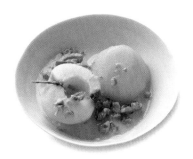

WATERMELON AND COCONUT SORBET PARFAITS

In each parfait glass, layer 2 scoops of **coconut sorbet** with ½ cup cubed **seeded watermelon.** Sprinkle with finely grated **lime** zest and toasted **coconut flakes.**

CINNAMON-POACHED APPLES WITH TOASTED WALNUTS

Bring 3 cups **apple juice,** ½ **cinnamon stick,** and a 1-inch piece of fresh **ginger** (no need to peel) to a boil in a medium saucepan. Add 2 peeled, halved, and cored **apples;** cover with a parchment round and simmer until tender, 8 minutes. Remove apples from liquid and serve, sprinkled with chopped toasted **walnuts.**

HONEY-ROASTED PLUMS

Preheat oven to 400°F. In a 3-quart shallow baking dish, combine ½ tablespoon melted unsalted **butter** and ¼ cup each **honey** and **orange juice.** Arrange 2 large halved, pitted **plums,** cut side down, in dish. Bake until tender, 30 minutes, turning over during final 10 minutes and spooning juices over fruit. Stir together 1½ tablespoons **cream cheese** and ½ teaspoon **milk;** dollop over warm fruit.

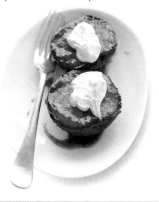

PINEAPPLE WITH GINGER YOGURT SAUCE

Place 1 tablespoon finely grated fresh **ginger** (from a 1-inch piece) in a fine-mesh sieve set over a small bowl. Press with a spoon to release juice (you should have about 2 teaspoons). Discard pulp. Add 1 cup plain low-fat **yogurt** and 3 tablespoons **honey** to bowl and mix to combine. (Sauce can be covered and refrigerated up to 2 days.) Drizzle sauce over **pineapple** wedges and top with toasted sliced **almonds.**

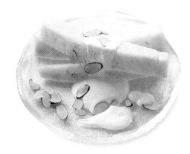

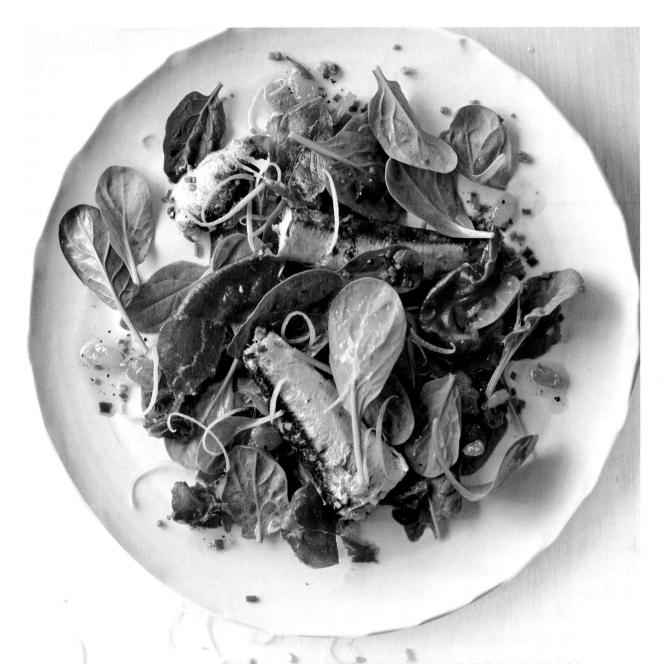

A CAN OF SARDINES KEEPS THE DOCTOR AWAY

"I love sardines—they are so healthy and couldn't be easier
to prepare. Sometimes after a long day I'll get home and just
open a tin of sardines, drizzle a little lemon over the fish, and
know I've had one of the most nutritious things I can eat. Or, I
incorporate them into a spinach salad with golden raisins and
crisped prosciutto, or toss them into pasta dishes."

HOW TO MAKE A BASIC VINAIGRETTE

You will be much more likely to eat a salad every day if you have the components on hand and ready to serve. Get in the habit of prewashing and portioning your greens, and making weekly batches of a basic vinaigrette.

Wash your greens by swishing them in a large bowl filled with cool water. The greens will rise to the surface; the sand and sediment will fall to the bottom of the bowl. Lift the greens from the water and transfer to a salad spinner; spin until very dry. Tear the lettuce into bite-size pieces.

Mixing a salad is a matter of proportion. You'll get the best results with four parts greens to one part dressing, and two to three parts oil to one part acid (vinegar, citrus juice, or a combination of both). Here's an easy, reliable recipe for an everyday salad dressing.

BASIC VINAIGRETTE MAKES ABOUT 1 CUP

- ¼ cup **vinegar** (such as red wine, balsamic, or rice wine) or fresh lemon juice
- 1 teaspoon **Dijon mustard**

  Coarse **salt** (such as sea salt or kosher salt) and freshly ground **pepper**
- ¼ teaspoon **sugar** (optional)
- ½ cup **extra-virgin olive oil**

Whisk together vinegar, mustard, salt, pepper, and sugar in a bowl. (If desired, you may also add other flavorings at this point, such as finely chopped fresh herbs, finely grated citrus zest, minced shallot, or a small amount of crumbled cheese.) Whisking constantly, gradually add oil until emulsified. Refrigerate in an airtight container up to 2 weeks.

HOW TO MAKE A QUICK SOUP

Soups make simple and delicious kitchen-sink meals. Many soup recipes follow the same preparation: sauté vegetables until tender, then add a cooking liquid (water or chicken broth) and heartier ingredients (such as vegetables, whole grains, lentils, or beans), and simmer. When in doubt, you can never go wrong with the classic vegetable soup base of finely chopped onion, carrot, and celery.

This healthful soup makes good use of the pantry and vegetable bin:

LENTIL AND BULGUR SOUP MAKES 4 SERVINGS

- 2 tablespoons **extra-virgin olive oil,** plus more for drizzling
- 1 **small onion,** thinly sliced
- 1 **carrot,** peeled and finely chopped
- 1 **celery stalk,** finely chopped
- 6 cups **water**
- 1 cup green or brown **lentils,** rinsed and picked over
- ½ cup **bulgur wheat**
- 2 to 3 tablespoons **red wine vinegar**

  Coarse **salt** and freshly ground **pepper**

Heat oil in a medium saucepan over medium. Cook the onion, carrot, and celery until tender, stirring occasionally, about 6 minutes. Add the water and lentils, and bring to a boil. Reduce heat, and simmer, partially covered, until lentils are tender but not mushy, about 20 minutes.

Stir in bulgur, and cook, partially covered, until bulgur is tender but still slightly chewy, about 5 minutes. Drizzle with vinegar to taste. Season with salt and pepper. Drizzle with oil, and season with additional pepper.

HOW TO ROAST

Vegetables are a natural choice for roasting. This ever-so-simple method seals ingredients into a satisfying caramelized crust. Toss ingredients (cut vegetables into uniform pieces for even cooking) with oil to lightly coat, then season with salt, pepper, and aromatic spices and herbs (if desired). Place in a single layer on a rimmed sheet pan and cook in a very hot oven, from 400°F to 450°F, until slightly charred and cooked through. As a rule, about 2 tablespoons oil (olive and high-heat oils like safflower or grapeseed work best) per pound of vegetables should suffice. Here's a recipe for roasted vegetables that makes a great light lunch or dinner when paired with cooked whole grains or a green salad. Toss leftovers with pasta or add to a salad to make it more substantial.

ROASTED FALL VEGETABLES MAKES 4 SERVINGS

- 1 pound **butternut squash,** peeled, seeded, and cut into 1½-inch pieces
- 1 pound **red new potatoes,** well scrubbed and quartered
- ½ pound medium **red onions,** peeled and quartered
- ½ pound **carrots,** halved lengthwise, if thick, and cut into 1½-inch lengths
- 2 to 3 **garlic cloves,** peeled and smashed with the flat side of a chef's knife
- 1 tablespoon plus 1½ teaspoons **olive oil**

  Coarse **salt** and freshly ground **pepper**

Preheat oven to 450°F. Divide vegetables and garlic between two rimmed baking sheets (lined with parchment paper, if desired, for easy cleanup). Toss with oil, 1 teaspoon salt, and ¼ teaspoon pepper.

Roast until vegetables are tender and beginning to brown, 40 to 50 minutes, tossing them and rotating sheets from top to bottom halfway through. Serve hot or at room temperature. (To store: Let cool, place in an airtight container, and refrigerate up to 3 days. Pour off any accumulated liquid before using.)

HOW TO STIR-FRY

This technique relies on intense heat to sear proteins and cook vegetables quickly, without adding much oil. Try it for preparing easy one-dish, single-serving, vegetable-rich meals. A wok works best, but if you don't have one, use a cast-iron skillet. The key is to get the pan very hot before adding the oil. When the oil is just about to start smoking, start by searing the meat (if using), then add any spices and other seasonings along with the vegetables. The recipe below calls for snap peas, but practically any vegetable can be swapped in (or used in combination)—asparagus, broccoli, mushrooms, bell peppers, bok choy, and scallions are all good options, but feel free to experiment with whatever you have on hand.

CHICKEN, SNAP PEA, AND PEANUT STIR-FRY SERVES 1

- 1 teaspoon **peanut oil**
- 1 boneless, skinless **chicken breast** half, thinly sliced crosswise
- 1 **garlic clove,** thinly sliced
- ½ **serrano** or **jalapeño chile,** thinly sliced crosswise
- 4 ounces **snow peas** (about 1½ cups), stem ends trimmed
    Coarse salt and freshly ground **pepper**
- 1 tablespoon fresh **lime juice**
- 1 tablespoon chopped **roasted peanuts**
- ¼ cup fresh **basil leaves,** torn (optional)
    Cooked **rice,** for serving

Heat a wok or skillet over medium-high. Add oil; when hot but not smoking, cook chicken until browned, tossing frequently, 2 to 3 minutes.

Add garlic, chile, snow peas, and 2 tablespoons water; cook, tossing, until chicken is opaque throughout, about 3 minutes. Season with salt and pepper; stir in lime juice, peanuts, and basil (if using). Serve immediately with rice.

HOW TO COOK IN PARCHMENT

Steaming food in parchment, or *en papillote*, works well for poultry, sliced vegetables, and delicate fish like sole or halibut. The juices from each ingredient are sealed inside the pouch to flavor the dish and keep it moist as it cooks. To create a half-moon–shaped packet, first place ingredients on one side of a parchment square and fold it in half, pleating around the edges to seal the pouch as you go. Bake in the oven at 375°F until the parchment puffs up, 12 to 15 minutes. Here is a recipe for parchment-steamed fish and vegetables:

SALMON AND ZUCCHINI BAKED IN PARCHMENT SERVES 1

1 small **zucchini,** halved lengthwise and thinly sliced

1 **shallot,** thinly sliced

1 tablespoon unsalted **butter,** cut into pieces

¼ teaspoon **dried dill**

1 **lemon slice,** halved, plus 2 teaspoons fresh **lemon juice**

Coarse **salt** and ground **pepper**

1 skinless **salmon fillet**

Preheat oven to 350°F. Fold a large piece of parchment paper (about 15 by 16 inches) in half to crease it; open and lay it flat.

On one side of crease, mound zucchini; top with shallot, butter, dill, and lemon slices. Season with salt and pepper. Place salmon on top; drizzle with lemon juice, and season with salt and pepper. To close, fold parchment over salmon; make small overlapping pleats to seal the open sides and create a half-moon–shaped packet. Place on a rimmed baking sheet; bake until salmon is opaque throughout, 15 to 17 minutes.

To serve, place the packet on a plate and cut it open; or, alternatively, make a slit in the paper and use a large metal spatula to transfer the contents to a plate.

CONSIDER *your changing needs*

In many ways, eating a healthful diet is even more important as you age than when you were younger. As your metabolism slows, you require less food. Yet your body becomes less efficient at absorbing crucial vitamins, so the calories you consume need to be of the highest quality. Poor nutrition weakens the immune system, making you more susceptible to infections (especially food-borne illnesses), as well as cancer. Thankfully, a nutrient-rich diet can make up for many of these age-related deficits.

In general, if you're eating a varied diet, you're probably meeting your needs for all the key vitamins and minerals critical for reducing infection risk and defending against age-related changes. But the next time you're in for a checkup, have your doctor measure your level of B vitamins. Up to 30 percent of people over 50 may be deficient in this vitamin crucial to healthy brain and nerve function. Conversely, make sure you're not getting too much iron. Premenopausal women need 18 mg a day, but after a woman stops menstruating she only needs 8 mg/day. Men should also watch their iron intake, as buildup of this mineral can stress the heart. Changes in taste and digestion also play a role in nutrition. You'll want to pay attention to these shifts to ensure you get the most out of your diet.

MIND ANY CHANGES IN TASTE

With age, salivary glands slow their activity, and medications may cause further drops in saliva production, resulting in dry mouth and difficulty swallowing. Loss of teeth and ill-fitting dentures can reduce the muscle mass of the chewing muscles and the tongue, compromising the ability to swallow. Taste acuity may also diminish, as the number of taste buds gradually decreases and the remaining buds shrink. Sweet and salty tastes are generally the first to be affected—which can contribute to overconsumption of these flavors. Here's what you can do.

PACE YOURSELF

Make a daily meal plan; regularly scheduled meals boost appetite and digestion. You'll start to produce needed enzymes and digestive juices regularly instead of randomly.[8] Also, take smaller bites and chew thoroughly, both of which help with swallowing problems and promote feelings of fullness. Putting down your utensils as you chew can help you slow your pace and curb overeating.

SUBSTITUTE FOR SALT

Owing to changes in taste, you may find yourself reaching for salt. Too much salt can elevate blood pressure and cause fluid retention. Instead, try citrus juice for brightness, herbs and spices for flavor, or black peppercorns or crushed red pepper flakes for heat.

STAY HYDRATED

As we age, our body loses some of its ability to regulate fluid levels owing to a dulling sense of thirst, so we may get dehydrated more quickly. Stash a glass by every sink so you remember to drink liquids throughout the day. Drink herbal tea rather than caffeinated hot drinks or sodas to avoid the diuretic effect of caffeine. Or start a meal with soup: a broth-based vegetable soup supplies fluid and is a way to increase your vegetable intake.

CONSIDER HOW MEDICATION AFFECTS FOOD INTAKE

Talk to your doctor if your appetite or taste has altered while taking certain medications. Anything from eyedrops to antibiotics and anti-indigestion aids can cause changes in your sense of taste. Your doctor may be able to prescribe an alternative medication.

MONITOR CHANGES IN DIGESTION

Changes in digestive-tract health can be minor but irritating. If you've gained weight, you may experience heartburn. You may begin to have difficulty digesting dairy or raw vegetables. And even if you've been regular all your life, you may experience constipation or other fluctuations in your normal elimination patterns. "Most of the changes that you notice can be easily controlled by lifestyle modifications, such as chewing more thoroughly, drinking more water, and eating smaller, more high-fiber meals," notes Dr. Sita Chokhavatia, an associate professor of gastroenterology at the Mount Sinai School of Medicine. But that doesn't mean you should ignore symptoms. "For instance, if you're accustomed to having a bowel movement daily and you haven't gone for three days, it's worth a call to your doctor."

FILL UP ON FIBER

Consuming more high-fiber fruits and vegetables than saturated fats and red meat keeps you regular, and some studies have shown that it may decrease your risk of colon and rectal cancer. Since it also helps lower blood cholesterol and moderate the rise of blood sugar after a meal, fiber helps reduce your risk of heart disease and diabetes. The Institute of Medicine of the National Academies recommends 21 grams of fiber a day for women 51 and older; 30 grams for men of the same age.

Some excellent sources of fiber include fruits, vegetables, beans, nuts, and whole grains. Ground flaxseed provides about 3 grams of fiber per tablespoon. Its nutty flavor complements many foods: add 1 to 2 tablespoons to pancake batter, oatmeal, smoothies, or yogurt. Some studies have found it decreases inflammation, reduces blood sugar, and also lowers cholesterol.[9]

DRINK MORE WATER

Staying well hydrated accelerates digestion and helps the body break down foods more efficiently. Water also helps the body flush out toxins and waste through urination, perspiration, and bowel movements. If you're not getting enough fluids, you'll likely experience constipation. Follow the tips in "Stay Hydrated," above, for getting enough water.

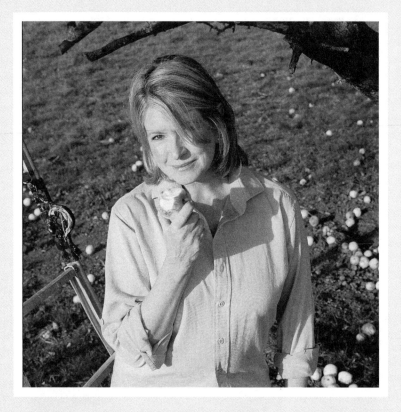

REALLY FRESH SNACKS

I'm not a big snacker. There are no nuts or anything else tucked away in my pocketbook—I'm not a squirrel! But if I walk by something fresh that looks appealing, I'll taste it.

My new favorite: eating an apple right off the tree. While I'm walking or even horseback riding on my farm, I'll reach for an apple on the branch. When the apples are frozen in winter, they're even better! Fruit, particularly when it's in season and purchased fresh from the farmstand, is the healthiest snack you can find—the fiber curbs appetite, and it's full of wonderful vitamins and antioxidants.

EAT RIGHT FOR HEALING

If you've been ill or injured, eating may be the last thing on your mind. But the truth is, you've never needed the powerful healing properties of good food more. After serious illness, injury, or surgery, your pituitary gland releases growth hormone, which boosts metabolism in an attempt to restore order and balance. You can help this process if you do the following.

EAT IN SPITE OF YOUR APPETITE

It's not uncommon to lose your appetite, but to give your body the fuel it needs to heal, stick to a regular meal schedule.

DRINK PLENTY OF CLEAR FLUIDS

There's a reason chicken soup is a cure-all. Broth, miso soup, teas, and apple juice supply nutrients that are easily broken down by the body, so you don't waste precious energy digesting dense, heavy foods while you recuperate.

SUPPLEMENT WITH WHEY

Your healing body needs more protein than usual, and whey is a high-quality, readily available source that your body can easily absorb. Stir whey protein powder (found in health-food stores) into broth or juice.

SPICE IT UP

Certain spices are known for their restorative properties, including easing joint pain and improving circulation. According to Ayurvedic medicine—a system of healing originating in ancient India—spices help stimulate your agni, or inner fire, making you feel more energetic. Here's what a few of these spices can do when consumed in medicinal amounts:

TURMERIC It's the spice that gives curry powder and mustard their deep yellow colors. Rich in antioxidants, turmeric may help fight cancer and contains inflammation-fighting compounds called curcuminoids, which may help prevent Alzheimer's disease, joint inflammation, and carpal tunnel syndrome. It may also help reduce cholesterol and improve certain eye conditions, plus heal skin infections when used topically.

GINGER For centuries, ginger has been used as a digestive tonic, an appetite stimulant, and a treatment for nausea. Two of its active ingredients, gingerol and shogaol, are responsible for the anti-nausea and anti-vomiting effects. The spice shows promise in treating osteoarthritis and rheumatoid arthritis.

CINNAMON From the bark of trees native to Asia, cinnamon may lower blood sugar in people with type 2 diabetes and has antimicrobial properties.

CHILI POWDER AND PAPRIKA Both contain capsaicin, which is used in skin creams to reduce pain, including that due to osteoarthritis. They also have antioxidant and blood-thinning qualities.

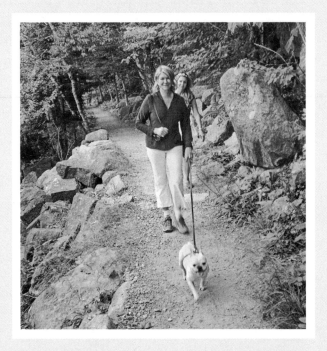

CHAPTER 2

Healthy Fitness

STAY *active every day* 76

INCREASE *your endurance* 83

MAINTAIN *your flexibility* 93

BUILD *your balance* 98

FOCUS *on core strength* 102

STRENGTHEN *for stability* 106

I exercise for an hour every single morning. It's as if I've signed a contract with myself to wake up and get on the treadmill and lift weights. It's nonnegotiable. Do I always feel like working out early in the morning? No. Much of the time I'd rather read a book or return e-mail. But I do it.

All that gym work enables me to lead as active a life as possible. I cycle, I hike, I garden, I ride horseback. I take walks almost every day. Walking always stays interesting because I take a different path every time. Should I walk through the woods or alongside the fields? Stroll out to the garden to see what's sprouting or go over to the apple tree to see whether those eggs in the nest have hatched? Weather adds its own note of variety: a chilly morning will inspire me to stride down to see if the pond has frozen, a sultry summer afternoon is perfect for a stroll under shady trees. If I'm in the city, I take different streets every time and look at the stores, the windows, and the people.

When I'm on a new path, I'm alert, I'm involved, and I am ready to discover and to learn something unexpected. That makes the walk worthwhile, to finish it having gained some new piece of information, some new insight. When I'm outdoors walking, it doesn't feel like exercise. It's moving and participating in the world.

STAY *active every day*

When you were a child, you didn't have to schedule exercise—you just ran outside to play. And whether that meant jumping rope, climbing trees, or racing bicycles, you experienced all of the benefits that exercise has to offer, almost intuitively. Your muscles grew stronger, your lungs became sturdier, and your imagination was stimulated as well. You absorbed fresh air and sunshine, and you knew about every intriguing hollow tree or secret wild raspberry patch in your neighborhood.

Of course, today's schedules are busier, and you probably can't skip and climb quite the way you did as a kid. We have to push ourselves to stay active, or life gets in the way. But that doesn't mean physical activity can't offer those same benefits, opening the door to a more active, satisfying life. Exercise adds years to your life and life to your years, making every day more productive and enjoyable. And even if you've been sedentary for most of your adulthood, it's not too late to start. If you are fit in midlife, you double your chances of living to 85 or older, according to an analysis by cardiologists at the University of Texas Southwestern Medical Center.[1]

What makes exercise such a powerful weapon against aging and disease? "Arteries have walls that contain muscles, so they can dilate or constrict," explains Dr. Jana Klauer, the New York–based physician specializing in nutrition and metabolism. "When you exercise, you strengthen those muscles so they can dilate to allow more blood flow. That means the heart can pump more efficiently."

And that's just the beginning. Exercise also keeps your lungs healthier, counteracting the diminishment of respiratory capacity that often comes with age, and reduces the risk factors for chronic conditions that can shorten the life span: high blood pressure, blood sugar, and cholesterol. "Exercise is an especially effective way to improve health and extend healthy longevity," Dr. Klauer adds. "There's no better medicine I can prescribe!"

This chapter contains lots of tips for designing your own customized workout plan—one that will keep you engaged, challenged, and running outside to play and participate in the world around you for decades to come.

GET MOVING

You don't need to invest in a fancy gym membership or expensive equipment to make a commitment to regular physical activity. When you see fitness as just another component of your daily life, you'll discover so many ways to increase movement throughout each day—parking a little farther away, taking the stairs instead of the elevator, spending an afternoon outside in the garden, or exploring your neighborhood by bicycle.

You'll have more energy, feel less stressed, and sleep better at night—and the more you move, the easier it becomes. Here are a few suggestions for staying active.

SPEND TIME OUTDOORS

The outdoor world truly is your playground, and there's an outdoor activity that's right for everybody. In the warmer months you can rent a rowboat, canoe, or kayak, learn to sail or to ride a horse, play golf or tennis, go tubing on a local river, pick in-season produce at a local farm, or attend an outdoor yoga retreat. When it's colder, consider skiing, snowshoeing, sledding, or ice-skating. Try to spend two afternoons per month playing outside with loved ones. Outdoor exercise challenges the muscles in unexpected ways, and all that fresh air and sunshine can boost your production of vitamin D, a key player in both bone health and mood elevation.

MAKE TIME TO "PLAY"

When you can't get outside, find ways to play indoors. Try Ping-Pong, bowling, bocce ball, or play video games that require you to move or dance in tandem.

Dancing is another invigorating, full body tune-up. Whether you prefer ballroom, belly, clogging, or lindy-hopping, you'll be working your muscles, bones, and joints. You'll also improve your posture, increase your flexibility, and, depending on the intensity, boost your physical stamina. It's a great activity to pick up as you age, because dancing can make you more sure-footed—one study found that adults who took dance lessons weekly cut their risk of falling by half in just three months.[2] And because many dance styles require a partner, it's a built-in opportunity to make new friends and stay engaged with longtime ones.

GET "ACCIDENTAL" EXERCISE

Make a point of doing as many of the following as you can on a daily basis, and you could burn about 200 extra calories per day. None of these activities alone will get you into shape, but when combined, they'll help you stave off weight gain and provide little "movement breaks" throughout your day to stretch your muscles and clear your mind. Remember that even the littlest bit of activity can go a long way toward keeping joints supple and muscles toned.

- Climb stairs instead of taking the elevator.
- Walk up and down moving escalators.
- Park at the far end of a mall parking lot and walk to the entrance.
- Take a stroll around the block at lunchtime or whenever you need to clear your head.
- Clean the house.
- Race yourself to the mailbox.
- Get off the bus a stop early and walk home.
- Swap your car for a bike.
- Pace while you talk on the phone.
- Line-dry your laundry.
- Stand instead of sitting whenever possible.

For extra motivation, wear a pedometer to track how much more you're walking, and challenge yourself to beat your records. Research has shown that taking 10,000 steps a day promotes optimal health. (See www.thewalkingsite.com for more information.) And remember to keep exercise a part of your daily routine even when you travel.

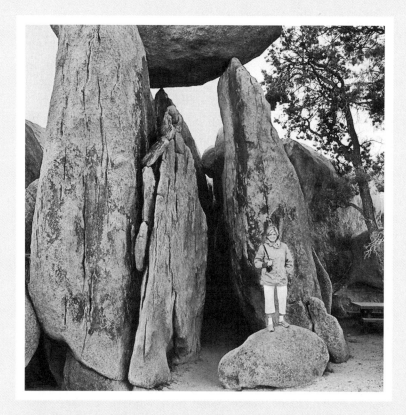

Enjoying a hike in Joshua Tree National Park in 2009.

COMBINE TRAVEL WITH EXERCISE

I love to walk. But when I discovered hiking, it took walking to a whole new level. Suddenly, I found I could combine walking with my passion for traveling. In one sense, it's just walking, but it takes me to new heights, literally. I've hiked all over Acadia National Park in Maine, near where I have my summer home, but it's fun to figure out where else in the world I want to hike. So far I've accomplished a few major hikes, such as Mount Kilimanjaro, the Inca Trail, and Northern Sikkim. They were all so fabulous and memorable. Next I'd love to do some trails in China.

WORK IN THE GARDEN

If you've ever grabbed a trowel and dug in, you know that working in a garden is an invigorating constellation of all forms of fitness—and a great way to work up a very respectable, healthy sweat. Gardening combines endurance (hauling bags of compost, pushing a wheelbarrow), strength (raking, hoeing, turning soil), flexibility (bending and stretching to sow seeds or transplant seedlings), core work (digging, shoveling, pulling weeds), and balance (reaching to tie up vines, pruning, stepping over growing plants). The tasks required in garden upkeep change with the day and the season, so it's a workout that also has built-in variety. This explains why research shows that midlife women who garden regularly tend to have slimmer waists and lower weights than those without a horticultural bent.

Doing work around the garden also tends to be more mentally and emotionally rewarding than trudging away on a treadmill at the gym. This may be because you literally reap what you sow—for the same caloric output as many gym workouts, you'll be rewarded with a bounty of beautiful flowers or delicious produce, in addition to all the health benefits. Research also shows that simply being in—or near!—a green space can be therapeutic: hospital patients with views of gardens tend to recover faster than those with rooms facing the parking lot.[3]

Of course, the more you get outside and exert yourself, the greater the benefits. In fact, gardening for at least 30 minutes per day, five days a week, may be enough to reduce your blood pressure, improve cholesterol levels, and help ward off heart disease and type 2 diabetes.[4] Combine tasks that are strenuous enough to leave you slightly winded (using a push mower or hauling a full wheelbarrow, for example) along with those that require strength and flexibility, for a total body workout that can also help ease arthritis pain.

If you don't have a garden of your own—or room to put one in—investigate helping with community or cooperative garden plots, adopting a friend's garden, volunteering at a botanical garden or nursery, or joining an urban tree-trimmer group.

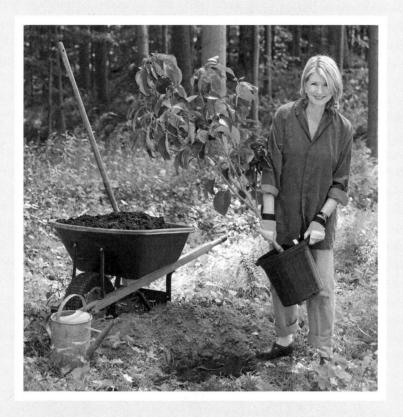

GARDEN YOUR WAY TO BETTER HEALTH

I'm out in my garden every opportunity I have, and it is always very physical. I push wheelbarrows full of dirt, I dig holes to plant, I cultivate on my hands and knees, I reach and stretch to prune, I bend over and squat down—all of that is very, very good for you.

GARDEN SAFETY TIPS

Neither your body nor your flowers will thank you if you injure yourself while exercising your green thumb. Follow these guidelines to prevent accidents:

DRESS FOR THE TASK

Wear gardening gloves, long-sleeve shirts, and pants to protect your skin from branches, thorns, and biting insects. Protect against sun exposure with a wide-brimmed hat and broad-spectrum sunscreen of SPF 15 or higher. Wear goggles when working with chemicals or using tools that generate flying debris. If you're going to kneel for a while, use a foam mat to prevent aching joints.

BEAT THE HEAT

According to the Centers for Disease Control and Prevention, adults over 65 (and children under 4) are particularly prone to heat-related illnesses, including extremely high blood pressure, headaches, rapid pulse, dizziness, nausea, confusion, and even unconsciousness. When working in the heat, drink plenty of liquids; but stay away from alcoholic, sugary, or caffeinated beverages, as these act as diuretics. Take frequent breaks in the shade, and stop working if you experience breathlessness or muscle soreness.

GET A SHOT

About a third of tetanus-related injuries occur in yards and gardens or on farms, so make sure your tetanus vaccination is up to date (experts recommend getting one every ten years). The bacterium that causes the disease resides in the soil and can enter through cuts in the skin, putting gardeners at particular risk.

CHOOSE SMART TOOLS

Look for lightweight tools with handles that are long enough to accommodate all of your fingers so you have a good, strong grip. And beware of marketing hype: pay more attention to how a tool feels in your hand than a label that promises it's "ergonomic."

CARRY WITH CARE

Lifting heavy pots can cause strains and sprains. Whenever you hoist or haul, bend with your knees, as shown below, and keep heavy objects close to your body to avoid straining back muscles. Don't overload wheelbarrows or weed bags. When you're done for the day, prevent soreness by taking a few minutes to stretch.

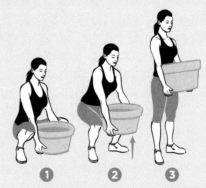

1 **2** **3**

THE PROPER WAY TO LIFT

INCREASE *your endurance*

Think of your endurance level as your life force. This most fundamental form of fitness is literally what propels you through your day and, indeed, through your life. When you have plenty of stamina, you can work and play harder and longer, and truly live life to the fullest. Regular aerobic or cardiovascular exercise increases your endurance level and benefits the circulatory system by working all of the body's major muscles—including the heart, the most important muscle of all. Every step you take, every mile you bike, every lap you swim works to reverse the effects of aging and extend your years of health and activity. Aerobic exercise also boosts brain function. Studies at New York's Columbia University have shown that aerobic exercise improves memory skills, especially the kind that can start to fade in middle age. If you haven't exercised for years but want to begin a new routine, walking is a great way to start.

WALKING

Welcome to the workout routine you'll be able to sustain for a lifetime. Even better, it's an exercise you already know how to do: walking. It's the simplest, safest way to increase your level of physical activity and explore your world. And although it often gets a bad rap as an "easy" workout, walking works the major muscle groups of the body, raises your heart rate, burns calories, and lowers blood pressure—all while imposing only a third of the impact that running does on your joints. Studies have shown that walking can promote better bone strength, fewer heart attacks, and less inflammation. It also lowers your risk of diabetes, improves your outlook, and sharpens your mind.[5] In short, walking is endlessly beneficial.

HOW OFTEN DO I NEED TO WALK?

Pinpointing the appropriate amount of exercise for you has a lot to do with where you're starting out. If you've been sedentary for years, 10 to 15 minutes of walking most days of the week is a good starting point. Once that becomes easy, you can work up to 150 minutes (2½ hours) of walking per week (plus two strength-training sessions—see Strengthen for Stability, page 106), which is the Centers for Disease Control and Prevention (CDC)'s official goal for adults age 45 and older. Don't be daunted if that sounds like a big time commitment—the CDC says it's fine to break your walks into 10-minute chunks. Take a 10-minute walk three times a day, Monday through Friday, and you're set.

Keep in mind that if you're trying to lose weight, you'll need to exercise more overall, in addition to watching your diet. When 50- and 60-year-olds lose weight through diet changes alone, they also lose bone density, muscle mass, strength, and aerobic conditioning—all things you need to preserve as you age. In contrast, people who lose weight via exercise show an increase in both bone mass and muscular strength.[6] Start by adding a walking workout on Sunday and/or Saturday, then work on increasing your weekday walks in 2- to 5-minute increments. (For suggestions on how to incorporate variety into a week's worth of walks, see page 86.)

HOW DO I KNOW IF I NEED TO CHALLENGE MYSELF MORE?

Jot down how long it takes you to walk a quarter mile and then time yourself again every two or three weeks or so; if your time steadily decreases over the course of a few months, you'll know you're building stamina and speed with every workout. If you plateau, try exploring a new route (perhaps with more hills) or varying your workout (see below).

You can also assess the intensity of any workout by using one of personal trainer Mary Tedesco's favorite tools: the Perceived Exertion Scale. Assign a number from 1 to 10 based on a combination of sensations as you're exercising—how you're breathing, if you're breaking a sweat, if your muscles are tiring. The number 1 could mean "extremely easy exertion"; 3 could mean "light exertion"; 5, "somewhat hard exertion"; 7, "hard"; 9, "very hard"; and 10, "extremely hard." If you're pushing yourself to get stronger, try to keep yourself in the 5 to 9 range for most of your workout or challenge yourself with intervals by pushing hard for 5 minutes, then pulling back for 3 minutes, and so on. Don't be afraid to customize the scale to help you best monitor your own progress—and keep yourself honest. Are you slacking off? Pushing too hard? Step it up or ease back accordingly.

Be sure to step back every now and then and assess your overall quality of life. The optimal amount of exercise delivers plenty of feel-good benefits like less stress, more energy, and a better night's sleep. If you're flagging in any of these departments, it might be a sign that you need to be moving more. See Advance Gradually (page 91) for how to increase your overall physical activity without injury.

VARY YOUR EXERCISE ROUTINE

If you do the same workout year-round, you'll get diminishing returns. Since it takes about twelve weeks for your body to hit a plateau, plan on switching your workouts with the seasons, once you've built up some basic cardiovascular fitness through walking. Hike outdoors when the leaves are at their peak in the fall, then switch to swimming at a heated indoor pool in winter, when your body could use that restorative warmth most. Jog your way through the spring, then hop on a bike and cycle all summer. Machines like the elliptical trainer or rower offer other ways to fend off boredom in climate-controlled conditions year-round. Changing your workouts also means you'll be less likely to injure yourself by overtraining.

Even if you'd like to stick with walking, you can vary your routine with props. Toting a walking stick may inspire you to go off-road and do some hiking. Adding Nordic walking poles will get your heart pumping and increase your calorie burn. Shouldering a knapsack provides bone-strengthening resistance—and if it contains lunch, may push you to stay out longer. Ankle weights, arm weights, or squeezable handballs can also make an ordinary walk more challenging.

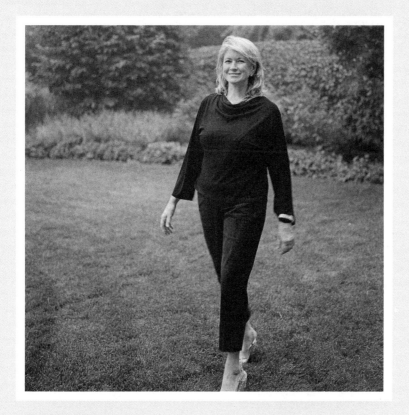

STAND TALL

I'm very conscious of posture in myself and in others. The computer age has made a lot of people more hunched, as we spend more time at our desks. But poor posture not only makes you look older and weaker, it hampers breathing. Personally I'd rather be taller than shorter, and I find that it's very important to have good posture to be tall. I mean, you just look better. So I always remind myself to stand straight with my shoulders back. Try it. If you take a picture of yourself standing normally and standing tall, you'll see the difference.

A WEEK'S WORTH OF WALKS

To demonstrate just how versatile this basic activity is, here is a menu of varied daily walks, each with a different emphasis—try them all, or mix and match to meet your particular needs. You can do any of these walks on a treadmill or in an indoor shopping mall in inclement weather; when it's nice, walk around a park or your neighborhood, or off-road on woodland trails. Even if you don't "need" a certain walk (such as the weight-loss one), it's still a good idea to cycle through all seven types. The payoff for varying your sessions is you'll be using slightly different muscles in different ways—also known as cross-training—and prevent overuse injuries. You'll also be sidestepping burnout. Keeping your mind engaged is the key to sticking with exercise long term.

MONDAY: HEALTHIER-HEART WALK
THE PLAN: AIM FOR THREE 15-MINUTE WALKS, SPACED THROUGHOUT THE DAY.

What the Science Says: Exercise literally flushes the fats (such as unhealthy triglycerides) out of the blood vessels; shorter bouts mean more fat-flushing throughout the day.

The Extras: Speed up your walk to boost the cardiovascular benefits; aim for four 2-minute surges. If you're outdoors or at the mall, pick a landmark—a tree or water fountain—and power up your pace until you reach it. On the treadmill, increase the speed or elevation.

TUESDAY: WEIGHT-LOSS WALK
THE PLAN: AIM FOR ONE 30- TO 40-MINUTE WALK.

What the Science Says: Starting in your forties, your metabolic rate slows 3 to 5 percent per decade, partly owing to muscle loss. To maintain muscle mass and overall firmness, you need to work your muscles using speed, variety, and inclines. Research indicates that interval training (short bursts of more intense activity interspersed with slower-paced recovery periods) burns more fat and calories than maintaining a steady pace.[7]

The Extras: Do 10 to 12 speed or hill intervals. After 2 to 5 minutes of warm-up walking, push the pace to fast for your first 30-second speed interval. Slow down for a 3-minute recovery interval, then push your pace again for 30 seconds, and repeat the recovery interval. Continue this for the rest of the workout. You can also push your pace by walking uphill or up a flight of stairs. (If you're on the treadmill, increase the incline/resistance.)

WEDNESDAY: STRONGER-BONES WALK
THE PLAN: AIM FOR A 20-, 30-, OR 40-MINUTE WALK AT A BRISK PACE.

What the Science Says: Combining the endurance-building power of walking with resistance training strengthens your cardiovascular system; strengthening moves cause muscles to tug on bones, generating new bone growth. If you can get outdoors, do so—walking in sunlight stimulates the body's production of vitamin D, which is essential for calcium absorption.

The Extras: After every 5 or 10 minutes of walking, stop and do some resistance exercises. Try the following:

Push-ups. Do them against a wall or park bench (30 seconds to 1 minute); see diagram below.

Walking lunges. For 30 seconds to 1 minute; see diagram below.

Jumping jacks. For 30 seconds to 1 minute.

Skipping or hopping. Use both legs for 30 seconds.

PUSH-UPS

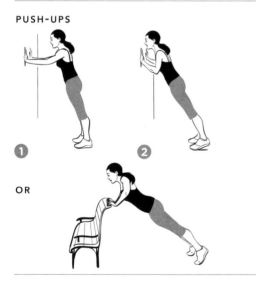

OR

(1) Place your hands at shoulder level in front of you on a wall (or by leaning against a bench). (2) Lower your body toward the wall/bench by bending your arms, keeping back straight. Push back to starting position by straightening out arms. Repeat for 30 seconds to 1 minute.

LUNGES

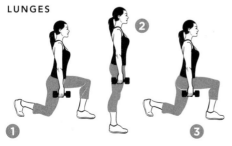

(1) Place one foot in front of the other, two to three feet apart. Square your hips to the front, keeping your back straight and shoulders relaxed and down. Bend the back knee toward the floor; make sure the front knee does not bend past the toes. (2) Straighten both legs. (3) Switch legs. Repeat for 30 seconds to 1 minute.

THURSDAY: BETTER-POSTURE WALK
THE PLAN: AIM FOR A 20- OR 30-MINUTE WALK.

What the Science Says: Lining up your spine correctly reduces wear and tear on the bones, joints, and ligaments of the body, notes Jonathan FitzGordon, a New York City yoga instructor and creator of the FitzGordon Method Core Walking Program (www.corewalking.com). "If you learn to walk aligned, you'll create ease in your body with every step you take," he explains.

The Extras: Every 5 or 10 minutes, focus on these four better-alignment tips as you walk:

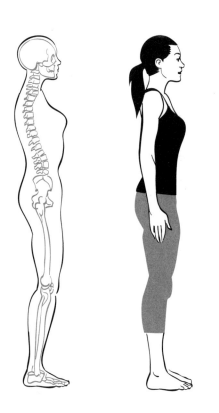

RELAX YOUR BUTTOCKS

To reduce lower back strain and reduce tension, release your glutes as you walk. Let your hips drift back slightly, so they can sway. (Clenched buttocks push the thighbones forward, constricting the hips and lower back.)

LIFT YOUR CROWN AND LEAN FORWARD

Lengthen the spine and the back of your neck to bring your shoulders to the proper position, allowing your spine to unfurl. A jutting head or chin can throw your neck and spine out of alignment.

ENGAGE YOUR CORE

Gently draw your navel in toward your spine to strengthen and stabilize your core muscles. This may be a conscious effort at first, until you train your muscles to maintain this activation. By toning your abdominals, you reduce pressure on the disks between your vertebrae, safeguarding against back injury.

SHORTEN YOUR STRIDE

Overstriding can force knees to hyperextend, which can degrade the joint over time. Take smaller steps; focus your energy forward, keeping hips, knees, and ankles in line.

FRIDAY: LOWER-YOUR-BLOOD-PRESSURE YOGA WALK
THE PLAN: AIM FOR A 40-MINUTE WALK AT A BRISK PACE.

What the Science Says: Those who walk regularly have lower stress levels than those who don't walk at all. Plus, studies show that yoga is a faster, more effective means to lowering blood pressure than listening to classical music.[8]

The Extras: Every 5 or 10 minutes, take a break (or hop off the treadmill) and do one of the three yoga poses below. (If you don't want to pose in public, save these moves for a quiet, private spot after your walk.)

REACH AND FOLD

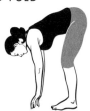

Stand with your arms overhead, touching palms together; hold for 10 seconds. Slowly bend forward from the hips, lowering arms so that fingers reach toward toes. Bend knees slightly if needed in order to reach the floor. Hold for 10 seconds. Return to starting position and repeat twice.

STANDING CAMEL

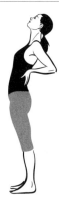

Stand with palms on your lower back, fingertips pointing down; push elbows back and together. Lean back as far as you are comfortable, looking up at the sky. Hold for 15 to 20 seconds. Repeat.

TREE POSE

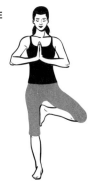

Shift your weight to the right foot, lifting left foot off the ground. Bend your left knee and bring the sole of the foot to the inner right thigh. If you cannot bring the foot to the thigh, simply place it lower on the right leg, but avoid putting foot directly on knee. Press the left foot into the thigh, keeping hips level. Hold. Switch sides and repeat.

SATURDAY: BETTER-BALANCE WALK
THE PLAN: AIM FOR A 30- OR 40-MINUTE WALK AT A BRISK PACE.

What the Science Says: Balance improves with practice, using, for example, the moves detailed at right. Moreover, walking, which involves both the legs and the core, helps strengthen the muscles that surround your joints, boosting your equilibrium.

The Extras: Every 5 or 10 minutes, take a break; if you're on a treadmill, hop off, and do some balancing moves:

Stand on one foot for 20 to 30 seconds. Extra challenge: Do it with your eyes closed—be sure you're on a level surface. Repeat on other foot.

Walk a line or along a curb. In a pinch, walk on a level surface placing the heel of one foot directly in front of the toes of the other on a level surface.

Rise up on toes. Raise up, lower, and rock back on heels. Hold onto a tree, fence, or wall, if needed. Repeat 10 to 15 times.

SUNDAY: MIND-CLEARING WALK
THE PLAN: WALK AT YOUR NORMAL PACE, WHICH HELPS YOU SYNC TO YOUR BODY'S OTHER RHYTHMIC PROCESSES, SUCH AS HEARTBEAT AND BREATHING RATE. AIM FOR AS MUCH TIME AS YOUR SCHEDULE ALLOWS.

What the Science Says: A walk can be a refreshing change of scene, but it can also set the stage for inspired thinking and major mental breakthroughs, says Thom Hartmann, author of *Walking Your Blues Away*. Walking unlocks a full range of your thought power. "When we walk, we stimulate portions of the brain in the right and left hemispheres, giving us access to more areas of our brains than when we're sitting still," he explains.

The Extras: As you're walking, call up the issue or idea for which you need clarity. It can be as richly detailed as a mental image (seeing the finished letter, signed and sealed) or as simple as a question ("What should I say to this person?"). Your mind will inevitably wander; let it. Then, gently guide your thoughts back to your issue or question. Hartmann explains that this interplay between conscious thinking (going over the main points in your mind) and unconscious thinking (daydreaming) brings your whole brain into play and opens you up to inspiration.

FIND YOUR TARGET HEART RATE

Keeping your heart rate in its target range during any exercise will allow you to burn the most fat. Check your pulse to see how many times your heart beats per minute, then track this number over the course of your workouts. As you become more fit, your pulse will go down, so you can see that your workouts are having a positive effect on your heart. Here's a basic formula to calculate your optimal target heart-rate range, so you can determine if your actual heart rate measures up:

- 220 – your current age = maximum heart rate (the highest your heart should be beating per minute during exercise)
- 220 – your current age × .65 = your lower target heart rate limit
- 220 – your current age × .85 = your upper target heart rate limit

ADVANCE GRADUALLY

Once you've adopted an endurance program (walking, jogging, cycling, swimming), it's a good idea to advance gradually so you don't burn out or injure yourself. Aim for this kind of gradual progression:

WEEKS	DURATION	FREQUENCY
1 and 2	20 minutes	3×/week
3 and 4	30 minutes	3×/week
5 and 6	40 minutes	3×/week
7 and 8	50 minutes	3×/week
9 and 10	60 minutes	3×/week
11 and 12	60 minutes	4×/week
13 and 14	60 minutes	5×/week
15 and 16	60 minutes	6×/week
17 and 18	60 minutes	7×/week

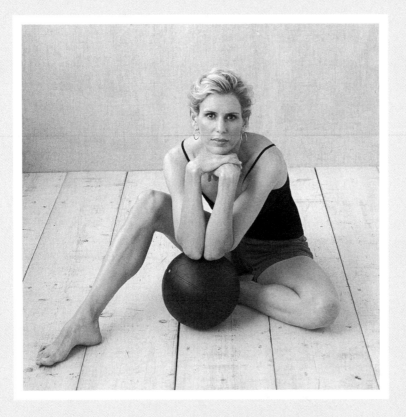

YOGA IS A LIFELONG PRACTICE

I do yoga two to three times a week, particularly around lunchtime. James Murphy, the director of the Iyengar Yoga Institute in New York, comes to the office, and in just 45 minutes we can do a routine that gives me flexibility, balance, and peace of mind. My daughter, Alexis, pictured above, has been practicing yoga for more than 20 years.

With yoga, you can move on to ever-more interesting challenges. Some of my favorite poses are inversions, like headstands or handstands. These improve circulation and at the same time exercise and tone the organs and glandular system to improve overall health and well-being. In addition, they give you a new perspective on the world, literally.

MAINTAIN *your flexibility*

As the years pass, losing range of motion in your joints can create a dangerous cycle. You stretch and move less, and pretty soon your body can't stretch and move as much as it used to, so then you do even less—and your motion becomes progressively more restricted. Poor flexibility also reduces your strength and endurance. And flexibility is just as crucial for your mental well-being. Research shows that taking time to connect with your body, especially through the practice of yoga, can stimulate your brain's neurotransmitters in ways that relieve stress and stave off depression and anxiety.[9] When you slow down, breathe deep, and really listen to your body, you'll be amazed at how much it can tell you—and how much better you didn't even know you could feel!

DO A FLEX TEST Start by assessing your flexibility with the sit-and-reach test. Sit on the floor with your right leg extended in front of you, toes flexed. Position your left foot against your right inner thigh, so that the left leg opens to the side. Reach for your toes. If you can't reach your toes, count the number of inches between your fingertips and your toes as a negative. If you can reach your toes, give yourself a 0. If you can reach past your toes, count by how many inches, as a positive. Repeat on the other side. (One side will probably be more flexible than the other; you'll want to work on the tighter side to become equally flexible.) Now that you have an idea of your reach, repeat the test every couple of months while practicing a flexibility program to monitor your progress.

WARM UP IN THE BATH Taking a long bath or shower before beginning your flexibility routine prepares your muscles for movement just as effectively as warming up with light exercise—and it's much more relaxing. Your muscles can't tell the difference, so if you're feeling more meditative than energetic, go ahead and soak.

GET A MASSAGE As you're gearing up to become more flexible, consider booking a few sessions with a therapist who specializes in sports massage. It may sound like an indulgence, but it can help pinpoint muscle weaknesses and imbalances in your body. And having a chronically tight muscle manipulated can relax it enough that you can regain some range of motion.

JOIN THE CLUB

More and more health clubs are catering their services toward the over-50 crowd, recognizing that older exercisers want to shape up, but not at the cost of injury. Inquire about classes or instructors who cater to older ages; many of the larger national chains (Bally, Wellbridge) have such offerings. Or do a little online research. Try the American Council on Exercise: www.acefitness.org; International Health, Racquet & Sportsclub Association: www.ihrsa.org; and AARP, formerly the American Association of Retired Persons: www.aarp.org.

STRETCH FOR YOUR WHOLE BODY

These six moves will help you maintain range of motion in the critical torque points of your body: upper back, shoulders, chest, lower back, hips, buttocks, and thighs. You can do these on the floor, but they work equally well in bed, so try adding them as a nice wake-up to your morning routine or a quick, soothing wind-down ritual before you go to bed.

TO FLEX AND STRETCH YOUR:	TRY THIS TECHNIQUE:
LOWER BACK, HIPS, AND BUTTOCKS 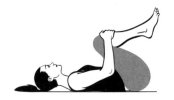	Hug your knees: Lying on your back, pull both knees toward your chest until you feel a comfortable stretch in your back and buttocks. Hold for 15 to 20 seconds. Breathe, release, and repeat.
HAMSTRINGS (BACK OF THE THIGH) 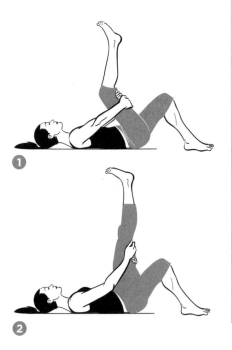	**Get a leg up:** Lie on your back with your left leg bent, foot flat on the floor. (1) Raise your right leg, with knee slightly bent. Support the leg in both hands, clasping behind your thigh. (2) Slowly straighten the leg and walk hands up toward the calf until you feel a stretch in your hamstrings. Hold, breathe, release, and repeat with other leg.

TO FLEX AND STRETCH YOUR:	TRY THIS TECHNIQUE:
SHOULDERS, CHEST, AND UPPER BACK 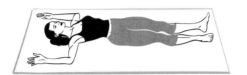	**Open up:** Lie on your back; bend arms and open them to either side of you so elbows align with shoulders like a cactus. Slowly slide arms overhead, keeping in contact with the surface. Keep moving until arms straighten out to stretch your shoulders and chest. Hold, breathe, release, and repeat.
UPPER BACK, SHOULDERS, ARMS 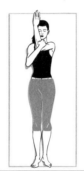	**One-armed reach:** Lie on your back. Grasp your left elbow with your right hand and gently press elbow across the chest toward the opposite shoulder until you feel a comfortable stretch in your upper back. Hold, breathe, release, and repeat with other arm.
CHEST, SHOULDERS, AND MID-BACK 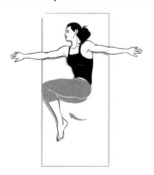	**Two-armed reach:** Lie on your left side with knees bent at a 90-degree angle to the body. Extend your left arm on floor at shoulder height. Reach right arm over on top of left, then slowly open right arm out until it touches the floor behind you and you feel a gentle stretch in your upper and midback. Hold, breathe, release, and repeat on other side.
HIPS, LEGS, AND BUTTOCKS 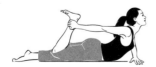	**Body bow:** Lie on your stomach. Bend right knee and grasp right ankle with right hand. Gently pull heel toward buttocks until you feel a stretch in the front of the hip and hamstring. Hold, breathe, release, and repeat with other leg.

STRETCH TO RELAX AND RECHARGE

In addition to limbering up your muscles, stretching can balance your energy, whether you're feeling run-down, sluggish, or keyed up. "Martha uses these four different yoga stretches when she needs to unwind and relax or when she needs to recharge her batteries in the middle of the day," notes James Murphy, the director of the Iyengar Yoga Institute in New York.

TO RELAX AND RECHARGE	TRY THIS TECHNIQUE:
SITTING FOLD 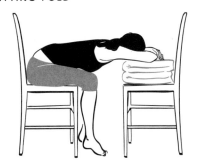	Arrange two chairs facing each other. Sit in a chair with your legs apart, facing the other chair, and extend your body forward until you can rest your arms and head on the opposite chair. If your head isn't supported by the chair, add folded blankets or pillows until your head can rest comfortably. Stay in this position 3 to 5 minutes, observing your breath. This allows the lower back muscles to extend and release and, at the same time, quiets the nervous system.
CHAIR TWIST 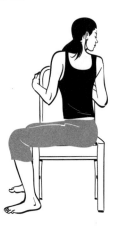	Sit sideways in a sturdy chair so that your legs are parallel to the back of the chair and your right side is nearest the chair back. Grasp the back of the chair with your right hand and twist your trunk to the right. Continue to hold this posture for several breaths. Now switch positions so that your left side is nearest the chair back; grasp the back of the chair and twist to your left. Again, continue the twist for several breaths. "This move wakes up your spine and is great because it frees up all the back muscles from the bottom to the top of your trunk," says Murphy. "By using deeper breath, you access all the muscles of your back, even those smaller ones in between your ribs." This stretch also helps with digestion and promotes health for the lower abdominal organs.

TO RELAX AND RECHARGE	TRY THIS TECHNIQUE:
LEGS UP THE WALL 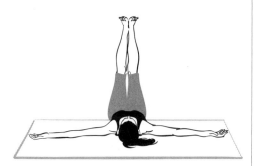	Lie down on the floor and position your hips as close as possible to a wall. Extend both legs straight up the wall, resting them against the wall. Extend both arms at shoulder level along the floor, palms facing up. If your head is tilted back or your neck is uncomfortable, place a folded blanket under your head. Close your eyes and let the back muscles spread and relax onto the floor. Enjoy the relaxation for 5 to 10 minutes, breathing normally. Placing the legs up the wall helps with circulation, relieves tiredness in the legs, and promotes a feeling of well-being.
SHOULDER-ARM EXTENSION 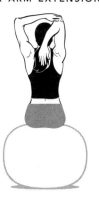	In a chair or on a fitness ball, raise your right arm overhead. Clasp your right arm, just above the elbow, with your left hand. Bend your right elbow and allow your forearm and hand to move down your back. Stay in this position, taking a few normal breaths. Keeping the elbow moving upward, allow the armpit and shoulder areas to stretch and unfold. "Opening the armpit and sides of your chest uplifts the spirits," Murphy says. After holding this position for several breaths, switch arms and repeat on the other side. This can be done whenever you need a mood-booster.

BUILD *your balance*

Better balance reduces your risk of falls—and falls are the most common reason for emergency-room visits among adults 65 and older. But even if you haven't hit your sixties yet, you can take a tumble and end up with an injury that could sideline you from activity for weeks. Developing equilibrium is a complex process, involving coordination among the eyes, tiny liquid-filled tubes in the inner ear (known as the vestibular system), your larger muscles (chiefly the legs and core), and even the nerve endings in your feet. Think of the balance work on these pages as a way of taking out some personal antifall insurance. And remember that balance is not a genetically inherited trait—anyone can improve it with practice. Bear in mind, however, that head colds and balance work don't mix. Congestion can temporarily impair the functioning of your vestibular system. If you find yourself clogged up from a bacterial or viral infection, take a break from your balance routine until the symptoms clear.

SIMPLE STEPS TO IMPROVE YOUR BALANCE

There are two types of balance and balancing exercises: static and dynamic. Static balance entails the ability to maintain your equilibrium while you are stationary. A classic example of a static balance exercise would be standing on one foot. An equally important component of balance is dynamic, which involves your ability to maintain your equilibrium as you move. Good illustrations of this type of balance would be dancing and tai chi. As you'll see, the suggested steps that follow include both aspects of balance.

TREAT YOUR FEET

Supple, strong feet form the foundation of better balance, and a massage can release muscular tension and increase circulation—both of which can make you more sure-footed. So find 5 minutes every few days (or more often, if possible) to give yourself a quick foot massage. It's great to incorporate one into your workout routine's warm-up or cool-down, or while you're watching TV or stretching before bed.

To begin: Knead the bottoms of your feet with both thumbs, working from the heel to the toes. With both hands, massage all around your ankle. Apply gentle pressure to the tops of the feet, working fingers into the fleshy areas between the bones. Finally, grab the foot in both hands and squeeze, as if wringing water from a wet towel.

PRACTICE BALANCE ANYTIME

Whenever you find yourself standing—waiting in line at the bank, in front of the kitchen sink—pick up one foot and try to maintain your equilibrium. Go for duration: stand up during a commercial when you're watching TV and try to stay on one foot for the whole commercial. When you're starting out, make sure you stand near a sturdy support (wall, counter, back of a chair) so you can steady yourself, if needed. The more often you challenge yourself, the more your balance will improve.

SIDE-STEP IT

So-called lateral training develops balance in a dynamic way. You can do specific exercises, such as side-to-side lunges, side shuffles, or stepping (or hopping, for a challenge) over a rolled-up towel. Or, make a point to participate in activities like tennis, volleyball, badminton, and folk dancing, all of which include lots of forward, backward, and sideways moves that continually call on your sense of equilibrium.

TRY TAI CHI

This centuries-old Chinese slow-motion martial art is proven to improve balance. You move continuously, shifting weight from one foot to the other and moving your arms rhythmically, training the muscles in your upper and lower body to function in a more coordinated, balanced fashion. Studies have found that this practice can reduce chronic pain and fatigue, lower blood pressure, and enhance mood.[10] Look for classes at recreation or education centers, YMCAs and YWCAs, and health clubs.

DO ANKLE ALPHABETS

Lift a leg and trace the letters of the alphabet in the air with a foot, first using script, then working up to block letters. This fancy footwork helps your muscles, ligaments, and tendons stay supple, strong, and flexible, all of which aid in balance. A bonus: it decreases fluid accumulation in the tissues, which will keep ankles looking trim and less swollen.

PRACTICE YOUR POSTURE

Program an hourly reminder on your desktop or mobile device to pull your abs in and your shoulders back. Slumping not only makes you look older, it also causes muscle tension, fatigue, and pain. When your body is optimally aligned, you become more balanced.

WALK THE BEAM

Just like a gymnast, you can develop strength and coordination practicing on a balance beam. The Beamfit Beam (beamfit.com) is a foam plank that's low to the ground. At 5 feet long, and only 6 inches wide, performing lunges on this low exercise beam (rather than on the floor) provides plenty of opportunity to improve balance and engage core muscles along the spine and midsection. Barefoot or in sneakers, place one foot in front of the other on the beam, two to three feet apart. Square your hips to the front, keeping your back straight and shoulders relaxed and down. Bend the back knee, toward the beam; make sure the front knee doesn't bend past the toes. Straighten both legs and repeat for a total of 20 lunges. Then switch legs, and repeat 20 times.

WORK YOUR BALANCE MUSCLES

To improve your balance, aim to work in three dimensions: front, back, and to either side. "You need to train your muscles in all directions so that they become uniformly strong and can help prevent a fall," notes Celeste Carlucci, cofounder of Fall Stop . . . Move Strong, an exercise and balance-training program based in New York City.

The older you get, the more purposeful you have to be about working your balance at home so it can come to your rescue in the outside world. These five moves work the major balance muscles: the hip flexors, hip stabilizers, knee flexors and extenders, and the muscles around your ankles. Start with just five repetitions of each move once or twice a day; have a sturdy chair nearby if you need to hold on at first. In just a few sessions, you'll notice a difference. Strengthening these muscles will boost your ability to climb stairs, stand up from an overstuffed chair, and get into and out of a car.

TO BOOST YOUR BALANCE	TRY THIS TECHNIQUE:
MARCH IN PLACE 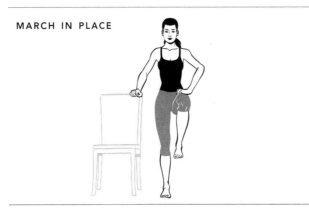	Stand with your right hand on the back of a sturdy chair, then slowly lift your left leg, knee bent, until it forms a right angle (your knee will be aligned with your hip). Lower slowly to the floor and repeat 15 times. Then switch legs (hold the chair with your left hand) for another set of 15 reps.
ONE-LEGGED STAND 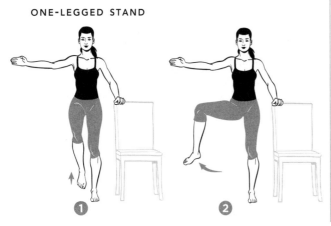	(1) Lightly hold the back of your chair with your left hand and place your weight on your left leg as you extend your right arm out to shoulder height and bend your knee to lift your leg a little and point your right toes toward the floor. (2) Then raise your right leg out to the side, keeping your knee bent and toes pointed. Hold; engage your abdominal muscles for stabilization and don't put too much weight on the chair. Lower your leg and repeat 15 times, then switch to the other side.

TO BOOST YOUR BALANCE	TRY THIS TECHNIQUE:
BACK LUNGE 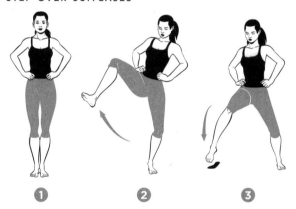	Stand with your feet together, lightly resting your left hand on the back of the chair, then step your right foot back into a lunge. Your right knee should be just above the floor and your left knee should be at a 90-degree angle. Extend your right arm in front of the body, hand flexed, then return to standing. Repeat 15 times, then switch to the other side.
STEP OVER SUITCASES 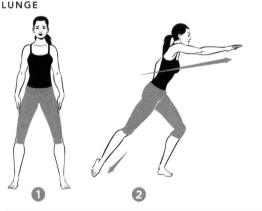	(1) Stand with your feet together, hands on hips. (2) Lift your right foot up, to the side, and (3) down—as if you're stepping over a large suitcase. (Move slowly to maintain your balance!) Repeat 10 times, then switch sides and do 10 reps with your left foot.
SIDE LUNGE	(1) Stand with your feet slightly wider than hip width, arms at your sides. (2) Rotate from your hips to reach your right arm across your body to the left. At the same time, extend the right leg to the right, with your toe pointed. Hold for a count of 2 and repeat on the left; work up to a set of 15 reaches on each side.

FOCUS *on core strength*

Think of your body core as the steering wheel for all your movements—the four muscle groups that make up your core wrap around your abdomen and lower back like a corset, providing strength and support for your organs, as well as promoting flexibility and mobility for your spine. Strengthening these muscles will help prevent back pain, fatigue, and the dreaded tummy paunch.

Core work is something you can add any time you're active, whether you're walking, jogging, cycling, or doing some other favorite exercise. Just make a habit of checking in to see that you're pulling your navel to your spine to activate your core—that's all it takes to add a whole new stabilizing dimension to your workout. And a strong core actually helps you move faster in whatever primary exercise you're doing, because it coordinates the movements of your upper and lower body. You can even work your core when you're not moving—while sitting, standing, driving, or taking the bus. Simply pull your navel into your spine and hold it. Pilates calls the core the "powerhouse," and works it in every possible direction. If your health club offers a Pilates mat class, give it a test drive to get introduced to your core. Look for moves like The Hundred, Rolling Like a Ball, and The Curl-Up—they are all top-notch core strengtheners. Here are other ways to incorporate more core-strengthening moves into your workouts:

TO STRENGTHEN YOUR CORE	TRY THIS TECHNIQUE:
DO YOUR SIT-UPS BACKWARD 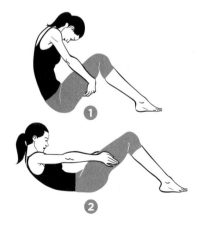	The same old sit-up will feel completely different when you do it in reverse. (1) Start by sitting on a mat with legs together, knees bent, and feet flat on the floor. Position your hands behind your thighs. Draw your navel to your spine and slowly lower so your torso forms a deep "C." (2) Look into your midsection as you lower. Hold, and then slowly return to starting position.

TO STRENGTHEN YOUR CORE	TRY THIS TECHNIQUE:

USE A HULA HOOP

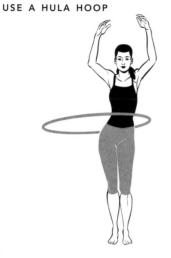

Swiveling your hips to keep a hula hoop in motion around your middle is a great core workout, working all your muscles in 360 degrees. Stand with your feet firmly on the ground and the hula hoop around your waist. Reach down and bring the hoop up against your back, with your hands holding on to each side of the hoop. Throw the hoop to the right (or left) and catch it with your hips, rotating your hips to keep the hoop circling around your waist. Raise your arms up over your head. Aim to keep it going for about 3 minutes.

DO CRUNCHES ON A BALL

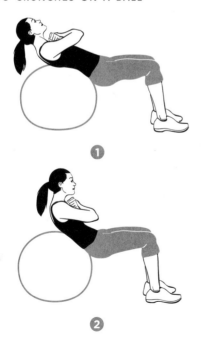

Using a fitness (or Swiss) ball for regular crunches challenges your balance and increases core strength. Make sure the ball is an appropriate size for your height. (1) Sit on the ball and walk your feet out until your back rests against the ball and your knees are at a 90-degree angle. Cross your arms over your chest. (2) Draw your navel to your spine and raise your torso up 45 degrees. Hold, and then slowly return to the starting postition.

TO STRENGTHEN YOUR CORE	**TRY THIS TECHNIQUE:**
HANG AND CURL 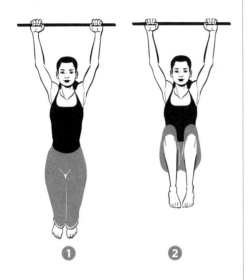	(1) Hang from a pull-up bar (or jungle gym in the park) and (2) slowly try to bring your knees to your chest, curling your lower body by using your abs. This move is especially good to work the lower portion of the core muscles.
WADE THROUGH WATER 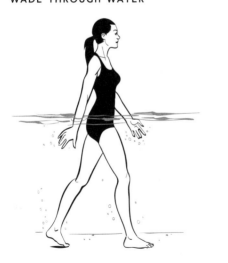	Stride through waist- to chest-deep water in a pool. Walk through the water the same way you would on the ground. Stride with your whole foot on the bottom of the pool, not just your tiptoes. A flotation belt can help keep you upright. Concentrate on tightening your core as you walk along, to give your abs a great workout.

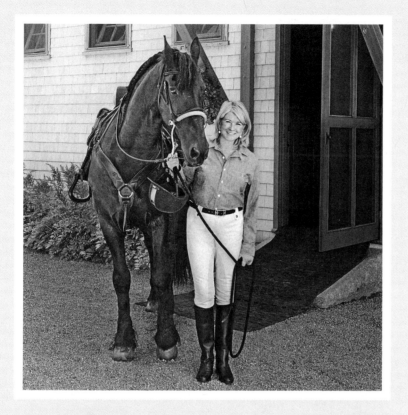

IT'S NEVER TOO LATE TO TAKE UP A NEW SPORT

I took up horseback riding only about ten years ago, and now it's become one of my favorite weekend activities. I get on the horse, and we explore the countryside together. Every time I'm in the saddle, I'm reminded of the importance of my posture and activating my core, because that's how you communicate with your mount.

Be curious about novel things that come along, whether it's a new type of exercise class or a sport that's new to you. Or go back to something you loved in your youth, like ballet or swimming. Just moving is the important thing, and keeping the attitude that you can learn new skills and activities.

STRENGTHEN *for stability*

Much of the loss of muscular strength that we associate with aging is the result of disuse. But research shows that you can improve your strength and even increase your muscle mass, no matter your age, with good old-fashioned weight training.[11] And strength training doesn't just work muscles; it also builds bone mass when your muscles tug on your bones from various angles.

According to researchers at the Brain Research Centre at the University of British Columbia, resistance training may even improve cognitive function, because you have to think about the moves, which creates new connections between brain neurons and, therefore, additional brain circuitry.[12]

PLAN YOUR WORKOUTS

For best results, schedule three to four sessions a week, or do shorter sessions daily, alternating these major muscle groups:

- Biceps/triceps (front and back of arms)
- Pectorals/latissimus dorsi (chest/upper back)
- Deltoids (front and rear shoulders)
- Rectus abdominus/erector spinae (abdomen/lower back)
- Quadriceps/hamstrings (front and back of thighs)
- Tibialis anterior/gastrocnemius and soleus (shins/calves)

CHOOSE YOUR METHOD

Weight machines, such as those found in a gym, are a great choice for beginners. These machines effectively isolate the targeted muscles while keeping you stabilized, so you can experience and recognize how it feels to extend your triceps, or contract your biceps, or curl your hamstrings.

Once you've learned the correct form, include some free-weight moves. Using your body to steady yourself (rather than relying on the machine) sharpens your balance skills. It also burns more calories, since you're engaging more muscles simultaneously.

If you don't like traditional weights, there are plenty of alternatives that will offer resistance training. Try flexible tubing, kettle bells, medicine balls, stretchy latex strips, and household items like soup cans or water bottles with handles. The Pilates Ring, an inexpensive flexible metal circle (see image on page 108), is a great way to add a new form of resistance to a workout. Personal trainer Mary Tedesco puts clients through their paces using the ring—squeezing it between the thighs for an inner-thigh toner, holding it with straight arms in front of the chest and squeezing, standing with the ring against one thigh and pulsing in toward the leg to work the shoulder and back of the arm. "Martha loves the versatility of the ring," says Tedesco. "It's also an easy piece of exercise equipment to pack for a trip."

You can also use your body weight as resistance, as with old-school push-ups, squats, and crunches or in a flowing yoga workout known as *vinyasa*, where you'll transition seamlessly between poses that stretch and strengthen at the same time.

LIFT THE RIGHT WEIGHT

Pick a weight that you think you can lift for 10 to 15 reps, using good form (see page 110). Be honest with yourself: the right weight is the one for which the last few repetitions are hard; the point is to challenge your muscles. Use the guide below to find the proper weight for you.

THE WEIGHT IS . . .	IF YOU . . .	SO TRY . . .
TOO LIGHT	Complete all 10 to 15 reps easily and feel you could have done more. (This is a good sign; it means you're getting stronger.)	Doing a second set with the next heaviest weight.
TOO HEAVY	Start struggling after the fifth repetition.	Stopping in midset and use the next lowest weight to finish your reps.
JUST RIGHT	Can complete all your reps but need to rest after that set.	Taking a short (30-second) rest and doing another set. The goal is to do 3 sets of 10 to 15 reps each.

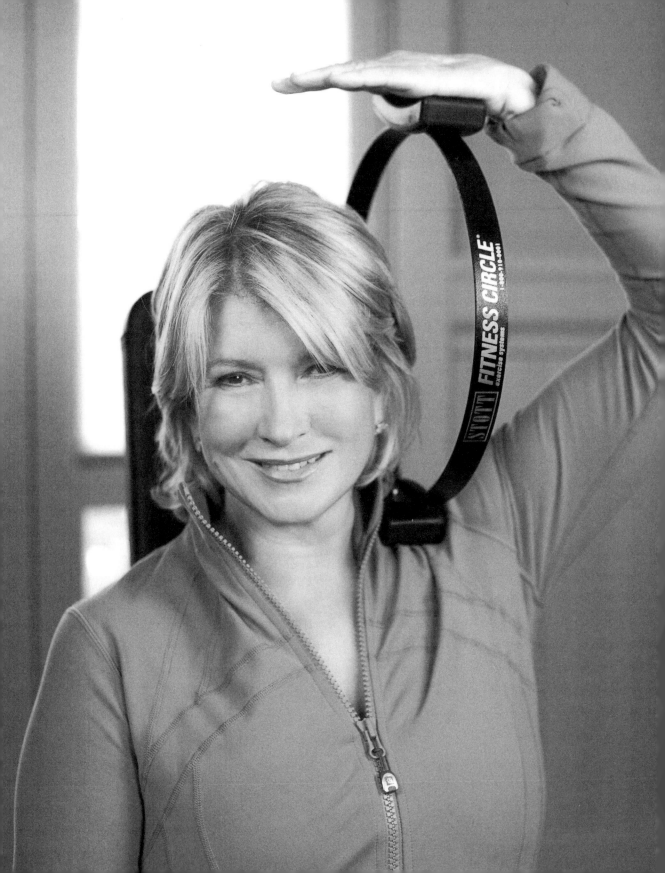

TAKE YOUR WORKOUT WITH YOU

Whenever I travel, I take my Pilates ring, plus a yoga block and strap. With these three tools you can keep up your strength routine in your hotel room or gym. The lightweight metal Pilates ring creates resistance for core work, based on the exercises created by Joseph Pilates. I use it to do leg, arm, and abdominal work—it's wonderfully versatile. With a block and strap, which help with alignment, I can do a yoga flow and be sure I do it safely without an instructor present.

Resistance bands are another excellent prop to take with you on trips. They vary in size and tension, and are excellent stand-ins for weights. (See the exercise-band workouts on pages 112–113.) And, of course, walking is a great way to explore a new city. Be sure to pick up a local map at the airport or at your hotel and then just let yourself wander.

USE GOOD FORM

One benefit of strength training is that it makes you more aware of all your muscles, especially, for women, those of your upper body. As you strength-train, you'll want to maintain good posture so you strengthen muscles evenly and through their entire range of motion. Improved posture helps in the real world, too. Nothing says "old" like a slump. Take a quick body check:

- Ears should be over your shoulders; this prevents the lower jaw thrust, which can weaken and overstretch your neck muscles.
- Shoulder blades should be rolled back and pulled down and together; think of trying to touch your shoulder blades together.
- Navel should be pulled in toward the spine.
- Ankles should be aligned with knees and shoulders.

KNOW WHEN TO CHANGE ROUTINES

If you do the same strength routine over and over, you'll improve—but only up to a point. That doesn't mean you have to toss your routine and start from scratch, though. Instead, make little changes in form and speed to keep challenging your muscles (and producing results). Try some of these switch-it-up variations:

CHANGE YOUR SPEED

The classic way to lift weights is to lift up and lower down using the same amount of time each way. Instead, try powering up quickly and slowly lowering down. Or, lift for a count of 2 and lower to a count of 4.

ADD A MIDPOINT

Pause at a midpoint as you lift or lower. Hold the position for a few seconds, then continue the movement up or down.

VARY THE SETS

Most routines call for three sets of 10 to 15 repetitions, but that formula isn't set in stone. Try doing one giant set, or two or four sets instead of three.

MIX UP THE REPS

Try doing a ladder—a series of reps that increase in number. (For example, from the first set of 12 reps, do a second set of 15 reps and a third set of 18 reps. Or, do a pyramid—a first set of 10 reps, a middle set of 15 reps, and a final set of 10 reps.)

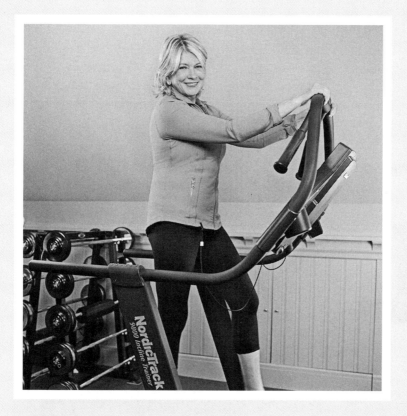

INTERVAL TRAINING

A great way to compress a full-body workout into very little time is to use interval training: 10 minutes on the treadmill, followed immediately by 10 minutes on the rower, then back to 10 minutes on the treadmill. Time flies because you keep switching it and you don't get tired because the treadmill works your lower body while the rower targets your upper body. When I'm done I feel so refreshed and energized, and I have needed only about 30 minutes of exercise.

A CLASSIC STRENGTH CIRCUIT

If you're a beginner, shoot for 10 repetitions of each exercise; and do just one set of reps.
As you get stronger (or if you're more experienced), work up to doing 15 repetitions
of each exercise, and three sets. Note: some of these moves are described using elastic
exercise bands, available at sporting goods stores, but they can also be performed using
your body weight or free weights for resistance.

FOR A STRENGTHENING EXERCISE	TRY THIS TECHNIQUE:
TRICEPS DIPS 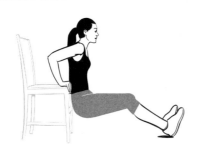	Sit on a sturdy chair or bench and place your palms on the chair/bench surface, close to hips, fingers facing forward, legs stretched out in front of you. Lift your body up off the front edge of the seat by straightening your arms. Slowly lower yourself in front of chair/bench. Keep shoulder blades together and pressed down your back, elbows pointing back. Lower only as far as you feel comfortable. Push yourself up to straight-arm position and repeat.
BACK/SHOULDER PULLS 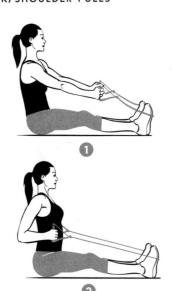	(1) Sit on the floor and extend both legs in front of you. Place heels on the floor so knees are slightly bent. Wrap an exercise band around the soles of both feet, holding both ends in your arms, palms facing toward each other. (2) Keeping your back straight and shoulder blades together, draw the band toward you in a rowing motion and pull your elbows back. Pull your hands toward the sides of your torso, about the level of your belly button. Hold for a count of 2; slowly straighten arms to return to start and repeat.

FOR A STRENGTHENING EXERCISE	TRY THIS TECHNIQUE:

SHOULDER RAISES

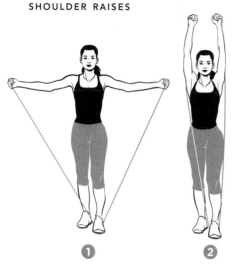

(1) Place your right foot on the center of an exercise band. Hold on to both handles. Position your hands at shoulder level, keeping palms facing forward. (2) Press the band up to the ceiling, straightening both arms overhead. Lower back to starting position and repeat.

BICEPS CURLS

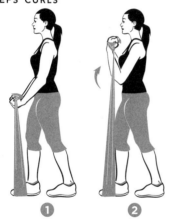

(1) Stand with your right foot on the middle of an elastic exercise band. Stagger your left leg behind you. Hold both ends of the band with your palms facing up. (2) Slowly bend your arms, curling your hands up until they're about 5 inches away from the shoulders. Slowly lower back to start by extending arms. Repeat.

PUSH-UPS

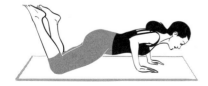

Kneel on a mat. Place your hands directly under your shoulders and activate your abdominals. Keep your back in a straight line from knees to shoulders, and slowly lower your body toward the mat by bending your arms until your chest almost touches the mat, keeping your head up. Repeat. (You can also do push-ups against a wall or bench. See page 87.)

FOR A STRENGTHENING EXERCISE	**TRY THIS TECHNIQUE:**
SQUATS 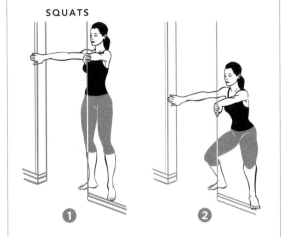	(1) Stand in a doorframe with feet slightly wider than hip-width apart and toes pointing slightly out. (2) Lightly grasping sides of doorframe, bend both knees, sticking your bottom out behind you (imagine you are sitting in a chair) while keeping your upper body upright. Lower yourself only as far as you feel comfortable; use sides for support. Press up from your heels to starting position and repeat.
LUNGES 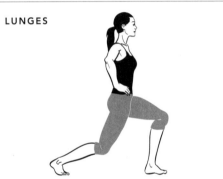	Place your left leg in front of you and stagger your right leg behind you. Place your hands on your hips. Slowly bend both knees to lower your hips toward the floor (your back knee should be 8 to 10 inches from the floor, and your front thigh should be parallel to the floor). Slowly straighten both legs to return to starting position. Repeat.
CALF RAISES 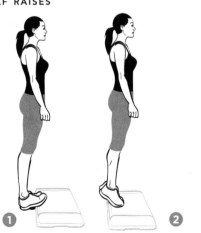	(1) Find an exercise step and stand with the balls of both feet on the edge on the step. Lower both heels toward the floor. (2) Raise your body again by pushing up through the balls of your feet. Hold; repeat. Practice your balance (no holding on) as you do this move.

FOR A STRENGTHENING EXERCISE	TRY THIS TECHNIQUE:
KNEELING LEG EXTENSIONS 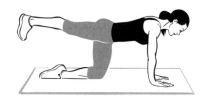	Kneel on a mat and place your hands directly under your shoulders on the mat. Pull in your navel toward your spine. Extend the right leg behind you, leaving the foot flexed. Do not raise your heel higher than the height of your bottom. Bend leg to return to kneeling start. Do all repetitions on one leg before switching to the other leg.
HAMSTRING BRIDGES 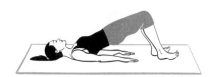	Lie on your back and bend your knees, placing feet flat on a mat. Relax your arms by your sides on a mat. Press your heels into the mat, lifting up your toes, and raise your bottom off the mat. Don't arch your back; try to keep your torso straight from shoulders to hips. Hold for a count of 2 and slowly lower back to mat. Repeat.
ABDOMINAL BRIDGES 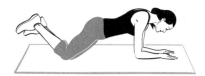	Kneel on a mat and position your forearms on the mat, elbows directly under your shoulders in a push-up position. Raise up your hips so your torso forms a straight line from knees to shoulders. Hold for a count of 10 seconds, then 20 seconds, building up to 60 seconds. Lower back down to starting position and repeat 2 or 3 times.

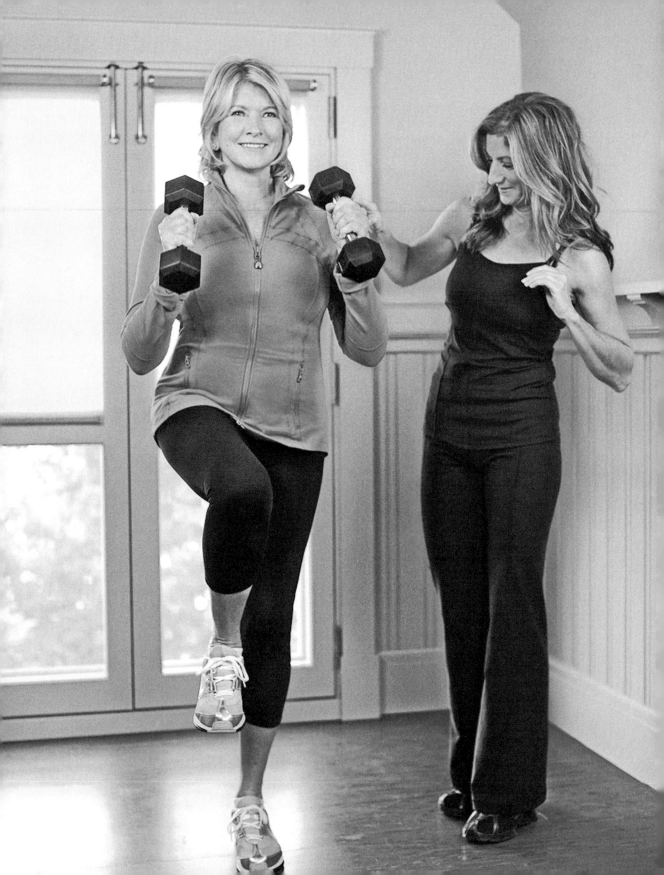

MY FAVORITE WORKOUT

I started lifting weights many years ago, and I've always enjoyed it. I like feeling strong—I can literally feel the improvement after each workout, and I know that at minimum I'm increasing my strength, my bone mass, and maintaining my weight (especially when I'm making up for some delicious indulgence at dinner the night before).

Because I now have good overall strength and am usually pressed for time, Mary, my trainer, has me doing two-in-one moves that are really wonderful. For instance, I'll lie on my back on a bench, holding weights in both hands and arms open perpendicular to the bench. As I bring my hands together in a "fly," I bend one knee to my chest and extend the other leg with each move. That works the chest, legs, and core in one move!

Another one of my favorite moves is the wall-sit. I lean against a big fitness ball that we've positioned on the wall, and I lower into a squat while raising both hands (holding weights) in front of me—then lower my arms as I stand back up. This move also works the whole body.

WORKOUT IN A CHAIR

Yes, it's possible to exercise and get fit even while sitting down—which is great news if you're recovering from illness, injury, or surgery and need to take it easy. But even if you are mobile, you can use chair exercises to squeeze in another workout while you watch television. These six moves, designed by the founders of Fall Stop…Move Strong (www.fallstop.net), show you how to turn an ordinary chair into a workout machine.

FOR A STRENGTHENING EXERCISE	TRY THIS TECHNIQUE:
ABDOMINAL CURL-BACKS 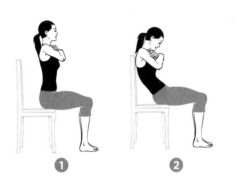	(1) Sit tall with your buttocks on the edge of your chair, and be sure that the arches of your feet are aligned directly underneath your knees. Cross your arms across your chest and pull your navel toward your spine. (2) Slowly lean back until your shoulder blades touch the chair's back, for a count of 4. Once you touch the back of the chair, inhale and return to starting position in 4 counts. Repeat each movement 10 times.
WINDSHIELD WIPERS 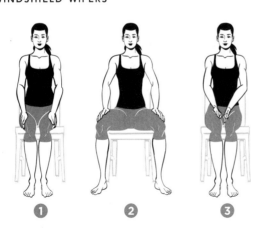	(1) Sit tall with your buttocks on the edge of your chair, legs together, hands on the outside of your knees. Pull your navel toward your spine to engage your abdominal muscles. (2) Open your knees and legs to the sides, resisting with your hands. (3) Move your hands to the inside of your knees and bring knees close together while resisting with hands. Repeat each movement 10 times.

FOR A STRENGTHENING EXERCISE	TRY THIS TECHNIQUE:

CHAIR RAISE

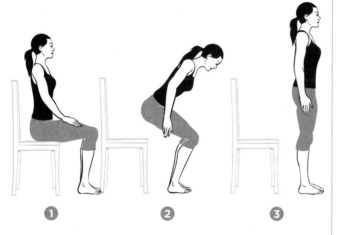

(1) Sit up tall with your feet flat on the floor; rest your hands lightly on your thighs. (2,3) Use your abdominal muscles as you stand slowly into a full upright position, making sure to keep your knees over your toes—don't let legs collapse in—and letting your hands drop to your sides. Then sit back down with control (don't plop!). Work up to a set of 15.

WRIST AND ANKLE ROTATION

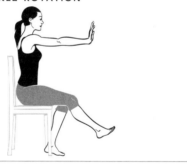

Sit tall in a sturdy chair and raise your right arm and right leg. Repeat each motion 10 times: Rotate hand and foot clockwise; rotate counterclockwise, point and flex, and squeeze. Lower your arm and leg and repeat on the left side.

LEG LIFTS

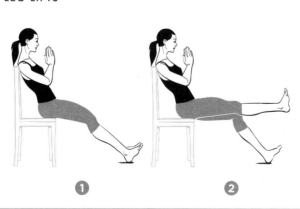

(1) Sit tall with your buttocks on the edge of the chair and rest your upper back against the chair's back, hands above your chest in prayer position. (2) Extend both legs straight in front of you, heels touching the floor, feet flexed. With your navel pulled toward the spine, lift your right leg until it's parallel to the floor (foot remains flexed). Slowly lower leg to floor, and repeat 10 times, then switch to the other side.

FOR A STRENGTHENING EXERCISE	TRY THIS TECHNIQUE:
LEG AND HIP EXTENSION 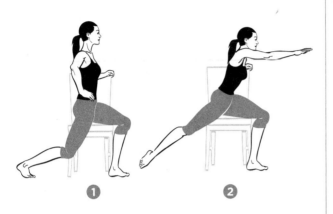	(1) Turn your chair sideways and sit with both of your legs across the chair seat. Then put your weight on your left leg as you extend your right leg behind you. (Grasp the back of the chair with your left arm if you need support.) Gently press your right knee toward the floor and hold for a count of 10. (2) Straighten your right leg and lift your right arm out in front of you; return to the starting position and repeat 15 times, then switch to the other side.
MARTINI STRETCH 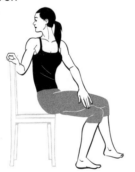	Sitting upright, cross your right leg over your left and turn your upper body to the right. You can place your right hand on the back of the chair and left hand on your right knee to increase the stretch, if needed; hold and take 4 slow, deep breaths. Repeat on the other side.

PUT IT ALL TOGETHER IN A ROUTINE

It's important to mix up whatever you choose to do for exercise. You'll fend off boredom, your body will get a better workout, and you'll be less likely to injure yourself by overtraining. Check out this menu of activity options; each workout is rated on a scale of 1 to 5 (indicated by • marks) in terms of how much it will build each key area of fitness.

Use this list to help you mix and match workouts to meet your needs and create a just-for-you, customized workout plan. Say you love the elliptical machine: it's top-notch for endurance but not as effective as yoga for the core, flexibility, and balance. So, why not do the elliptical two or three times a week and throw in a few yoga sessions? And some weight training for overall strength? Keep adapting your routine to keep it working for you.

WORKOUT	ENDURANCE	STRENGTH	FLEXIBILITY	BALANCE	CORE
AEROBICS	• • • • •	• • •	• • •	• • • •	• • • • •
CYCLING	• • • • •	• • •	•	• • • •	• •
ELLIPTICAL MACHINE	• • • • •	• •	• • •	• • •	• • •
GARDENING	• • •	• • • •	• • •	• • • •	• • • •
HIKING	• • • • •	• • • •	• • •	• • • •	• • • •
PILATES	• •	• • • • •	• • • • •	• • • •	• • • • •
RUNNING	• • • • •	• • •	• •	• • •	• • • •
SKATING (IN-LINE, ICE-, OR ROLLER-)	• • • • •	• • •	• • •	• • • •	• • • • •
SWIMMING	• • • • •	• •	• • • •	• •	• • •
TENNIS	• • • • •	• • •	• • •	• • • •	• • • • •
WALKING	• • • •	• • •	• • •	• • •	• • •
WEIGHT LIFTING	• • •	• • • • •	• • •	• • • •	• • • • •
YOGA	• •	• • • •	• • • • •	• • • • •	• • • • •

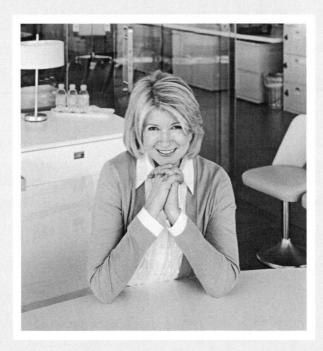

CHAPTER 3

Healthy Brain

CELEBRATE *your brain's golden age* 124

EAT *for a healthier brain* 128

STAY *in shape for a better brain* 129

PREVENT *memory loss* 131

STIMULATE *new brain activity* 138

SLOW DOWN *to power up* 142

My college history professor once told me: "There are no good young historians." I don't know if I believed him at the time, but I have come to realize he was right! Whether it's physiological or just the accumulation of life experience, I think differently now. My process includes more lateral thinking, more synthesizing of different points of view, and more judgment that comes from a larger store of experience and the wisdom of years.

I always encourage others to be prepared. If you often feel as if you don't remember names or can't recall current events or an interesting book you just read, studying up before a party or a meeting is a good idea, because you will have all the facts at your fingertips. You have to work to be a better teacher or conversationalist. But if you do so, people will be impressed by the scope of your knowledge, and your conversations will be more intriguing.

Achieving that level of discipline isn't easy. There's so much coming at us every day, from the media we consume to the people we encounter. As we get older, we're more easily distractible, and we're less able to shut it out. I know that when I have too much input, there's less output from my mind. People say I have a great memory—that I never forget anything. If that's true, it's because I work at it.

CELEBRATE *your brain's golden age*

After age 40, even commonplace memory lapses—like losing your keys or forgetting where you parked your car—can become acts marked by a growing fear. Am I getting old? Am I going downhill fast? Yet these memory glitches are likely no worse than what you experienced at 20, and it's actually better for your brain if you're not so hard on yourself. According to Dr. Cynthia Green, assistant clinical psychiatry professor at the Mount Sinai School of Medicine, blaming your memory at every opportunity can become a self-fulfilling prophecy, as stress affects information retention.

Although we often view memory loss, dementia, and even degenerative diseases like Alzheimer's as synonymous with old age, these conditions aren't inevitable. And we now know that there are certain preventive measures we can take to curb the symptoms even after the onset of these and other brain-health problems.

New science is showing that by exercising the brain regularly, we can actually lower our risk of mental decline.[1] This is because the brain is plastic, meaning that it can change and adapt, producing more cells (known as neurons) and increasing the connections between those cells. Whereas brain researchers used to believe that we lose up to 30 percent of our neurons as we age, now it looks as if we not only hold on to most of those neurons but we can also make new ones if we try.

No one knows exactly why using the brain more is so protective, but one prevailing theory suggests that such activities build up our "cognitive reserve," or neurological stores that delay the appearance of degenerative symptoms. In other words, the more brain cells you have to lose, the more you can use your brain without experiencing a loss of function. Researchers found that older adults who remained intellectually engaged were able to significantly delay the onset of memory loss, even when their brain scans showed pronounced signs of Alzheimer's disease.[2] A brain with strong cognitive reserves can actually fight back against Alzheimer-driven changes, compensating for many age-related decreases in capability. When it comes to your gray matter, there's truth behind the adage "Use it or lose it."

UNDERSTANDING THE MATURE BRAIN

There are certain advantages that the mature brain has over a younger, developing one. Some scientists believe that midlife is our brain's golden age of complex reasoning—studies show that's when we peak in inductive reasoning, spatial orientation, vocabulary, and verbal memory.[3] We also hit our capacity for the brain's "white matter," which coordinates how well the brain regions work together. This means we can integrate new information more quickly and make more efficient associations. As an example, compare your mature judgment to that of a 20-year-old—middle-aged brains are better at recognizing patterns they have internalized from experience, so we make more considered, responsible decisions.

Your brain keeps developing, no matter what your age, and it reflects what you do with it. A host of lifestyle decisions can influence, or even reverse, your rate of decline. Stop worrying about what your brain doesn't do so well anymore and celebrate the stunning powers of your grown-up brain:

- It has developed more powerful systems that can cut through intricacies of complex problems to find concrete answers.

- It more calmly manages emotions and information.

- It has acquired the ability to edit and is more discriminating than in your younger years.

- It has broadened its perspective on the world.

- It has a greater ability to see patterns and connect the dots of disparate events.

- It is more creative.

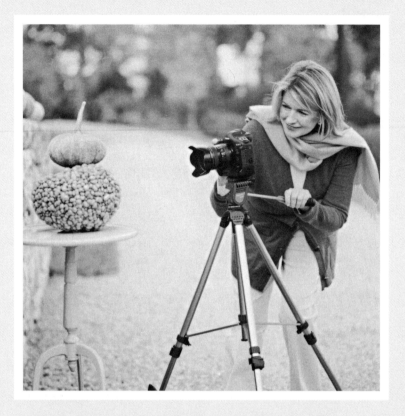

APPRECIATE YOUR CREATIVITY

I am so much more creative these days. I feel my creativity is different from when I was younger; now it is richer and deeper from my life experiences. I want to do more creating in ways that challenge myself, so I have been spending time developing my photography skills, and have also started writing more, which I enjoy now more than ever. I want to get all the stored knowledge out of my brain and into the world. Then, I'll have room to learn new things.

HOW TO FOSTER CREATIVITY

The adult brain is arguably more creative than a younger one because of its superior ability to recognize patterns and to synthesize new information with already embedded knowledge. If it's been many years since you've picked up a pen, brush, or musical instrument, try exposing yourself to new creative stimulants to open up your thinking. For example, you may:

GET OUT MORE

Attend concerts, visit museums, join a theater group and book club. The greater your exposure to creative excellence of all kinds, the more inspired you'll be.

FIND COMMUNITY

Just as a religious congregation can help feed the soul, a group of like-minded creatives can help nurture the imagination. By interacting with others who share similar artistic or creative passions, you'll discover what others are thinking and doing, which should spark your own creativity. Classes are a great place to start. If you like to paint, try taking an art class. If you've always wanted to publish a novel, enroll in a creative writing workshop. There are even customized art programs for seniors, such as Washington D.C.'s Arts for the Aging (www.aftaarts.org) and San Francisco's Institute on Aging (www.ioaging.org). Visit the National Endowment for the Arts website (www.nea.gov) for their Arts in Aging Resource List.

SPEND TIME WITH CHILDREN

If you don't have young kids or grandkids, volunteer in a local school or library. Crafting or drawing alongside children, who take such joy in the pure act of creating, can help jump-start your own out-of-the-box thinking or just take you out of your regular worries without intimidation.

FIND NATURAL INSPIRATION

The emerging field of "eco-therapy" recognizes that spending time in nature can boost mood by reducing the stress hormone cortisol, instill confidence and peace of mind, and inspire creativity. Bring elements of nature (rocks, leaves, shells) home to serve as touchstones to the feelings of calm and open-mindedness that nature brings.

UNPLUG YOURSELF

Turning off the Internet, television, and your smartphone gets rid of the electronic chatter that's become so common in modern life and can help free space for creativity to flourish. Read a book, cook a leisurely meal, or go for a long, solitary walk (see Mind-Clearing Walk, page 90).

JUST GO FOR IT

Many of us feel inhibited to create because of a fear of doing things badly. Don't judge yourself or aim for perfection; simply start somewhere—you'll be amazed at where just a little effort can take you.

EAT *for a healthier brain*

Consider increasing your intake of the following four brain boosters; each has been found to be especially potent for cognitive function. (For more information and instruction on food and nutrition, see Chapter 1.)

OMEGA-RICH FISH

Nearly 40 percent of the fatty acids found in your brain cells' membranes are docosahexanenoic acid, or DHA, a type of omega-3 fatty acid found in cold-water fish such as salmon, tuna, and herring. That's why people who eat fish three times a week (and already have the highest levels of DHA in their bloodstreams) can reduce their risk of dementia by 47 percent, according to the Framingham Heart Study.[4] Fresh is best—canned tuna contains 0.38 grams of DHA while fresh tuna has 1.9 grams. Don't like fish? Take fish oil supplements, also known as omega-3 capsules, or take algal oil capsules, made from algae.

LEAFY GREENS

Long touted for their power to protect against heart disease and certain cancers, vegetables can protect your gray matter as well. At the Rush Institute for Healthy Aging in Chicago, researchers assessed the basic cognitive skills (the ones you need to go about your activities of daily living) of nearly 4,000 men and women aged 65 and over. When they retested this same group six years later, those who ate nearly three helpings of vegetables daily had slowed their cognitive decline by 40 percent versus those who didn't eat as many veggies.[5]

Another study of more than 13,000 participants found that women in their sixties who eat more cruciferous and leafy vegetables (broccoli, cauliflower, spinach, and lettuces) have a lower rate of decline when given a series of learning and memory tests.[6]

DARK CHOCOLATE

Dark chocolate is rich in flavonoids, a class of antioxidants that may protect brain function as we age. In a long-term study, adults over 65 who ate a high-flavonoid diet scored 75 percent better on brain assessments than those who weren't getting enough of this plant-produced compound.[7] Foods with high flavonoid levels are kale, hot peppers, onions, and green tea, so including these in your diet will ensure you're getting an adequate supply—but feel free to top off a meal with a square or two of dark chocolate. Studies suggest that treating yourself to dark chocolate (in moderation) may reduce the risk of stroke by 20 percent, and may also reduce the risk of dying after a stroke. (And, yes, when it comes to chocolate, it's worth getting the really good stuff.)[8]

WATER

Severe dehydration has long been associated with confusion and disorientation; now a small Ohio University study suggests that even mild dehydration can mess with your mental abilities. After measuring hydration levels in healthy older men and women, researchers found that well-hydrated volunteers performed better on memory, attention span, and eye-hand-coordination tests.[9]

Since the nerve cells that control the sensation of thirst become less sensitive with the years, you may be more dehydrated than you feel. Make a habit of sipping water throughout the day, even if you don't feel thirsty.

STAY *in shape for a better brain*

Nothing turns back the clock on mental decline more effectively than a healthy lifestyle. Research overwhelmingly indicates that regular aerobic exercise such as walking can improve memory, sharpen attention, hone concentration, and increase processing speed, all while decreasing your risk for dementia. Vigorous activity causes the brain to release brain-derived neurotrophic factor, which acts as brain fertilizer, increasing the number and the longevity of cells in the hippocampus.

Regular exercise helps improve the flow of oxygen-rich blood to the brain, and also seems to maintain certain short-term memory skills that diminish with age, such as the ability to prioritize, set schedules, and make (and stick to) plans. It's no wonder that a bout of activity can make you feel more focused, attentive, and in control of your daily chores and activities. For specifics on how to build a workout program customized to your needs, turn to Chapter 2. To make sure your plan is as brain-boosting as possible, choose workouts that challenge you with new routines or skills.

PREVENTING HEAD INJURY WHILE YOU EXERCISE

Wear a helmet every time you get on a bicycle, a horse, or a pair of downhill skis or skates. Head injury has been linked to increased risk of Alzheimer's disease, according to the National Institute of Aging as well as University of Pennsylvania researchers. Patients diagnosed with Alzheimer's are nearly ten times more likely to have a history of head trauma, especially one that resulted in loss of consciousness. But while it's common sense, it's tragically not common practice: actress Natasha Richardson died at age 45 from head injuries sustained from a fall during a beginner's skiing lesson; she was not wearing a helmet.

If you do hit your head, call your doctor right away, whether you've lost consciousness or only developed a bump. You don't have to be knocked out in order to sustain a brain injury. Mild Traumatic Brain Injury (MTBI), also known as concussion, is a growing problem in an increasingly active adult population. The consequences of even mild brain injuries may lead to deep and prolonged impairments of the brain.

The U.S. Consumer Product Safety Commission (www.cpsc.gov) has a helpful chart that recommends helmet types for certain activities.

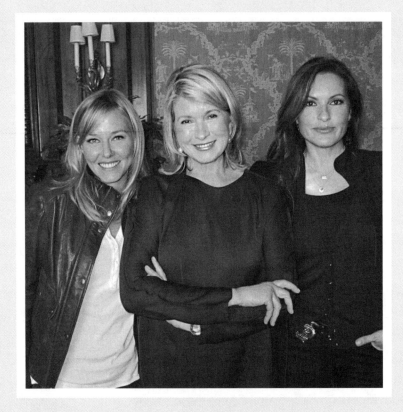

On the set of *Law & Order: SVU* in 2012 with Kelli Giddish (left) and Mariska Hargitay.

CHALLENGE YOUR MEMORY

I am lucky that every day poses challenges that may help me prevent memory loss. For example, I have forced myself to take "acting" assignments like *Law & Order: SVU* (above), even though I am not a trained actor. Spending a day, or two or three, memorizing scripts and acting in sitcoms or serious dramas, although quite frightening to me, helps me, forces me, to do something out of the ordinary—out of the daily routine.

PREVENT *memory loss*

For many of us, memory is the key signifier of brain health. It can also be maddeningly elusive as we age, particularly when we struggle to remember where we put our eyeglasses, the name of the movie we just saw, or whether we took our medication. And it's all too easy to obsess over why we forget rather than focus on why we remember—yet the simple act of dwelling on memory gaps becomes a self-fulfilling prophecy.

The good news is that scientific discoveries about the brain's plasticity have great implications for memory improvement. One of the places where new neuron growth has been shown to occur in the adult brain is the dentate gyrus, located in a strip of the hippocampus, the brain's main memory structure. Neuron growth here has been shown to play a significant role in the formation of new memories. There are many exercises you can employ to boost this type of growth. For example, regular cognitive "brain games" can improve your memory and mental agility.

TIME YOUR TASKS

"An activity or game with a time element helps you think quickly and improves your attention span," says Dr. Cynthia Green, assistant clinical professor of psychiatry at the Mount Sinai School of Medicine. Set a timer for 15 minutes, then play Concentration with a deck of cards (turning over cards to make pairs) or do a crossword puzzle.

PLAY TO YOUR STRENGTHS

We each have a natural tendency to remember either the first or the last—or most recent—facts we've encountered, owing to what are known as the primacy and recency effects. Test yourself by trying to memorize a shopping list, or closing this book and reciting the brain games covered here. Do you remember the first things on a list or the last?

Once you know your individual tendency, you can use your personal strength to shape your memory. Place the most important item on the top or bottom of a list, for example, based on your natural inclination.

ACT LIKE A STUDENT

When you learn something new, quiz yourself. Answering questions requires retrieving information from memory, and that is more useful than merely reviewing the material, say psychologists Jeffrey Karpicke and Janell Blunt of Purdue University. Good questions require you to reconstruct what you know, which itself enhances learning.

This technique works no matter what you're trying to remember, from a person's name to a historical fact or a vocabulary word. Taking pen-on-paper notes or reciting information out loud can also help you retain facts.

PRACTICE WITH POETRY

Committing a poem to memory sharpens our rote-memorization skills, which we used often in school but don't often rely on in real life. Once you've mastered the lines, reciting an entire poem is an impressive party trick. Sign up for the Academy of American Poets' Poem-A-Day program at www.poets.org and get a new poem e-mailed to you every morning.

USE YOUR IMAGINATION

When you visualize, you project that object or event on the screen of your mind. Visualizing an object or upcoming activity in detail—what you'll feel, see, smell, or taste—actively forces more information into additional parts of your brain, creating a larger neural footprint.

Say you're planning a dinner party. Imagine the table settings, smell the food cooking, hear the tinkle of glassware and laughter, look around the table at your assembled guests. Images that contain emotions and personal associations tend to stick better in your memory. If you think about these things in advance, you'll be more likely to put the memory of the event in your permanent memory bank.

DO THINGS DIFFERENTLY

Challenge yourself to do something or consider something in a new way. Some suggestions: write your life story—in seven words; count backwards from one hundred by threes; or reverse your route in the grocery store, starting in the aisle that you usually finish in.

DOODLE

Those quirky little marginalia don't distract you; in fact, making them may help you pay attention, maintain focus, and remember more effectively. A recent study of forty adults listening to a boring phone call found that those subjects who were told to doodle not only did better when quizzed on what they heard during the call but also did 29 percent better than their nondoodling counterparts on a surprise memory test.[10]

REHEARSE AND RESIZE

Memory boosters are basic strategies to help you hold on to the information you need, whether it's a friend's phone number, the name of that person you met at a party, or things you need to buy at the store. Two techniques can help: rehearsing and resizing. To rehearse, go over the information again and again in advance of when you'll need it; repeat "eggs, milk, paper towels," as you drive to the store, for example. Resizing involves breaking down the information into easier-to-retain chunks. You can remember a phone number by thinking of it as three shorter units: area code, exchange, and the remaining four numbers.

SUPPLEMENTING FOR MENTAL CLARITY

If you're feeling tired, sluggish, forgetful, or confused, you may be lacking adequate levels of vitamin B_{12}, a key ingredient necessary to make new red blood cells and DNA, and to keep the nervous system functioning well. You're also more likely to be deficient in this vitamin if you take acid-blocking medications, don't eat meat or dairy products (see page 36 for more sources of B_{12}), or take the diabetes drug Metformin. If you're experiencing any of the above symptoms, see your doctor for a blood test. Taking supplements under a doctor's supervision can help you feel sharper in a matter of weeks.

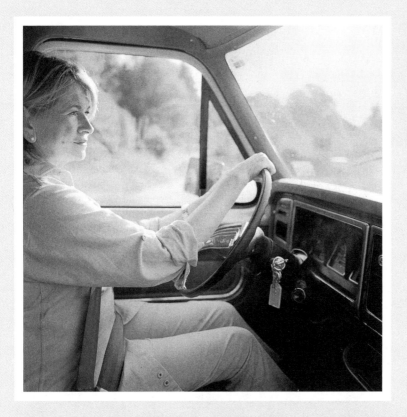

TAKE A DIFFERENT ROUTE EVERY DAY

I almost never take the same route twice. I follow different paths through the woods or around the farm, and in the city, I wander down various streets to peek in on new restaurants or shops. I take new routes coming into the city so there's always something novel and interesting to look at—new architecture, a field, or a reservoir I hadn't seen before. It helps the brain to always keep things interesting! And you'll never be bored.

MEMORY MYTHS

Understanding how memories are formed may give you a greater feeling of mastery over your recall.

MYTH #1

MEMORY IS AN ORGAN
We often talk about memory as if it were a single structure. Not so. Memory is an abstract process. There is no single part of the brain where all remembering occurs.

MYTH #2

THERE IS A SECRET TO GOOD MEMORY
Memory consists of at least three different processing systems (sensory, short-term, and long-term), so there is no single tool or strategy for attaining a good memory. Improving memory is just like developing any other skill: you have to take the time to learn the techniques and practice them.

MYTH #3

MEMORY IS LIKE A MUSCLE
While it is true that practicing memorization can help improve memory, just as lifting weights builds muscles, what you do during practice is more important than the length of time spent practicing. Use the brain games on pages 131–132 to help you hone your best memory-boosting strategy.

MYTH #4

AT A CERTAIN AGE, YOU'RE TOO OLD TO IMPROVE YOUR MEMORY
On the contrary, stop learning new tricks and you will quickly become the proverbial old dog. New research has shown that declines in mental abilities occur later in life than formerly believed. And all memory skills do not decline equally; visual and spatial skills decrease in most people from their twenties to their sixties, but verbal skills (such as the memory for names, stories, words, and numbers) show little decline through the years. A rich life experience and broad knowledge base helps older adults perform some mental tasks at the same or higher speeds as those many years younger.

MYTH #5

A TRAINED MEMORY NEVER FORGETS
It's unrealistic to expect that you will never forget anything again if you work to improve your memory. The advantage of a well-trained memory is that you can remember what you want to remember—but you don't necessarily want to remember everything. Memory training helps you store information in your brain in such a way that you are more likely to find it when you need it (such as when doing a crossword puzzle or having a conversation).

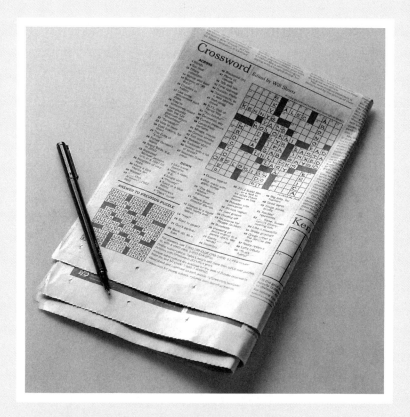

DO BRAIN CALISTHENICS

I've always loved challenging my brain with crossword puzzles and other mental exercises. I was on a plane recently watching a woman across the aisle. Apparently she found brain calisthenics very therapeutic, too—she played solitaire and Scrabble on her iPad and did a crossword puzzle, among other things. She was an inspiration, and I took out my iPad and played a game of Scrabble and did a couple KenKens and a difficult sudoku. Try it!

MEDICATIONS THAT IMPAIR MEMORY

If you're taking one of the drugs below and feel that you are having difficulty with your memory, consult your physician, as these medications have been shown to affect memory. "Each of us has different tolerance levels to different substances," says Dr. Dennis Popeo, a psychiatrist at New York University's Langone Medical Center. "A simple adjustment in your prescription may improve this side effect."

TYPE OF DRUG	GENERIC NAME	BRAND NAME
ANALGESICS	meperidine	Codeine, Demerol, Fiorinal
ANTIANXIETY DRUGS	alprazolam	Xanax
	diazepam	Valium
	lorazepam	Ativan
	oxazepam	Serax
	temazepam	Restoril
	triazolam	Halcion
ANTIBIOTICS	cephalexin	Keflex
	ciprofloxacin	Cipro
	metronidazone	Flagyl
ANTIDEPRESSANTS	amitriptyline	Elavil
	imipramine	Tofranil
ANTIHISTAMINE	diphenhydramine	Benadryl
ANTIHYPERTENSIVES	atenolol	Tenormin
	hydrochlorothiazide	Dyazide
	lotensin	Benazepril
	metoprolol	Toprol

TYPE OF DRUG	GENERIC NAME	BRAND NAME
ANTINAUSEA DRUGS	hydroxyzine	Atarax
	meclizine	Antivert
	metoclopramide	Reglan
	prochlorperazine	Compazine
ANTIPSYCHOTICS	chlorpromazine	Thorazine
	haloperidol	Haldol
	thioridazine	Mellaril
ANTIULCER DRUGS	cimetidine	Tagamet
	ranitidine	Zantac
DECONGESTANT	pseudophedrine	Sudafed
HORMONES	levothyroxine sodium	Synthroid
PAIN DRUGS	acetominophen and hydrocodone	Vicodin
	meperidine	Codeine, Demerol, Fiornal
PARKINSON'S DRUG	amantadine hydrochloride	Symmetrel
SEIZURE MEDICATIONS	carbamazepine	Tegretol
	gabapentin	Neurontin
	valproic acid	Depakote
SLEEP AID	zolpidem	Ambien
STEROID	prednisone	Prednisone

STIMULATE *new brain activity*

Just as picking a new route to walk or drive can energize your brain, opening your mind to different points of view and novel experiences can wake up the brain's synapses, fostering fresh associations and a richer understanding of the world.

CHALLENGE YOUR USUAL THINKING

Your brain has developed pathways of interconnected neurons that help you recognize vocabulary or a politician's sound bite, but if you always use the same well-worn routes to process the same kind of information, your brain receives less stimulation and is less likely to spur the development of new neuronal connections. So, if you usually read fiction, pick up nonfiction. Swap military history for social history.

Similarly, do you watch TV, listen to talk radio, or read a newspaper and simply parrot the information? If so, challenge yourself to consider the information with a more critical mind-set. Analyze those points of view, ask questions, and form your own opinions. Or read a book that challenges some long-held assumptions. You don't have to change your mind, but you may open it up—and your neurons will be all the stronger for it.

You can even try little tricks to challenge your brain's flexibility and routine. Wear your watch upside down or on your other wrist. Or, brush your teeth with the wrong hand. It forces your brain to think out of its comfort zone.[11]

LEARN A NEW LANGUAGE

Speaking two or more languages helps develop the skills to better cope with the symptoms of dementia and other memory-robbing diseases, and it increases your cognitive reserve—those extra brainpower stores that slow cognitive decline. Consider learning something new, studying the language your grandparents spoke, tuning in to a foreign radio station, or giving sign language a try. "We still don't know whether it is beneficial for people to learn more than one language if you don't speak it fluently or every day, but learning a language is nevertheless a good way to exercise your brain," says Dr. Cynthia Green of Mount Sinai School of Medicine.

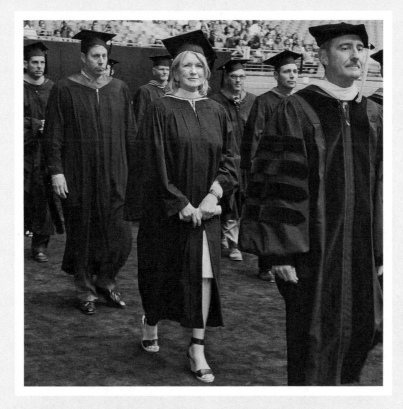

I was honored to speak before more than 2,000 graduates at the commencement ceremony of the University of Phoenix in June 2012.

PURSUE LIFETIME LEARNING

Studying and reading are so important and help you stay relevant. Learning on a daily basis shouldn't feel like a penance or a dreaded task but, rather, a pleasure and a joy. Seek out online courses and lectures. One website that is always full of fascinating information is ted.com. TED stands for Technology, Entertainment, and Design and is a series of conferences founded by Richard Saul Wurman. You can download lectures—most of them 18 minutes or less—for free, from some of the most innovative thinkers in the world. Once you learn something new, share it. Talk to people about what you've learned or what you think. Mutual engagement is key.

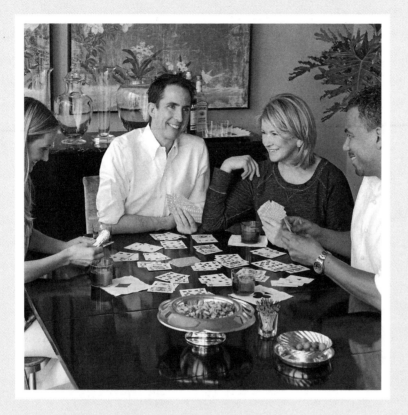

PLAY GAMES SOCIALLY

I am not a big social game player, but the value of knowing a fun card game or word or numbers game to play when there is downtime is very beneficial. I like cards but have really never had a lot of that "downtime" to engage in poker or bridge or even canasta. I recently learned an easy card game called Gozo that can be played by up to five people, and uses two decks of cards. (You can find instructions easily online.) It is a lot of fun and very engaging. I do promise, however, to really learn both poker and bridge, and I also promise to one day have some of that elusive downtime we all dream about.

EXPAND YOUR VOCABULARY

The ability to acquire new words is one of your most enduring cognitive skills. Studies show that you can continue to increase your word power when you're 85 or older.[12] And building your verbal repertoire is a great prep for activities such as word games, writing, and other intellectual challenges.

FORGE YOUR OWN PATH

Take a trip. Whether it's to another part of town or a different part of the world, exploring and adapting to new locations forces you to pay more attention to your environment. You'll stimulate your brain by making decisions, planning your day, and deciding where and what to eat in that novel setting. Indeed, London taxi drivers have larger hippocampi (regions of the brain involved in integrating spatial formulation) than London bus drivers, according to a 2006 study. That's probably because taxi drivers have to navigate changing destinations, while bus drivers follow a set route. Try taking off in a new direction the next time you're running errands or going for a walk—doing so has the same brain-boosting effects.

BE SOCIAL

Conversation requires skills such as cue recognition, memory, attention, and control—all processes that are also involved in many cognitive functions. "Research has shown that those who report higher levels of social engagement have an associated reduced risk for memory loss and dementia," says Dr. Cynthia Green. "You really can't be social without staying focused, thinking quickly, and keeping your mind nimble. Staying social also exposes us to different experiences or ways of thinking, which is great for our intellectual engagement."

GO BACK TO SCHOOL

If you've longed to study Renaissance art or American history, audit classes at a local university. Don't want to pay tuition? Take a course online, where there are many free e-learning opportunities. Open Culture (www.openculture.com) offers more than 450 online courses, audiobooks, and foreign language courses. Also explore university websites: UC Berkeley, Harvard, MIT, and the London School of Economics allow free access to lectures. Or, check out nobelprize.org/mediaplayer to watch lectures about Nobel prize winners.

SLOW DOWN *to power up*

Whether you're reading, practicing brain games, or working on a new project, make sure to allow for frequent breaks. If you balance all your brain-boosting activities with some downtime, your brain will benefit further. Rest and relaxation techniques feed the parasympathetic nervous system, reducing the stress hormone cortisol, which suppresses memory and clear thinking.

TAKE A NAP

Napping may help consolidate new facts into memory and actually make you smarter, say University of California, Berkeley, researchers who have found that nappers outperform their wide-awake counterparts on tests. This may be because sleep helps to clear out the hippocampus, moving new facts to the brain's long-term storage regions, and making room in the hippocampus to absorb more new information.

The older you are, the shorter your naps should be: 20 minutes between 1 to 3 p.m. is ideal for most adults—enough to boost your brain without sabotaging your nighttime sleep.

MEET YOUR SLEEP QUOTA

Consistently getting enough uninterrupted sleep has been linked with a stronger immune system, better memory, and increased learning abilities. In fact, studies show that people have 20 to 30 percent better recall of what they learned during a piano lesson if they are tested after a full eight hours of sleep than if they are tested right after the piano lesson. Sleep may even affect emotional function, as some researchers now believe that chronic sleep deprivation may actually lead to depression, rather than depression causing lack of sleep, as previously thought.

Sleep's connection to creativity is also a subject of scientific exploration. "Sleep, particularly dreaming, helps fuse things that don't seem to have any connection," says Matthew Walker, assistant professor of psychology at the University of California, Berkeley. Like good cooking, when it comes to memory, it's not enough to just chop up the ingredients and put them together. The brain needs time to let things marinate.

TAKE A BREAK TO MEDITATE

From a brain-health perspective, meditation offers many benefits. It can build concentration and attention, because it trains you to hold your focus. It can also help you more effectively manage stress, which can detract from daily memory performance.[13] To get started, set aside 5 minutes to be in a quiet spot, at a time when you will not be interrupted. Get comfortably seated (either on the floor or in a chair). Now, simply be there, in that moment, noticing the rise and fall of your breath. As thoughts come into your mind, just let them go. If you need help doing that, just say to yourself "everything passes" and let the thought go.[14]

When you focus on your breathing during meditation or yoga, you're paying attention to the internal sensations of your body. That stimulates the insular cortex or insula, a prune-size structure deep in the brain that is involved in sensing emotions. Some studies have shown that as you regularly activate the insula (by focusing on your breath), the neurons make more connections in this area, thickening the insula. The upshot is that you become more in touch with yourself and with the feelings of others, since the insula is crucial for empathy. The ability to view a situation through multiple perspectives builds a more flexible, resilient brain.[15]

A common obstacle for beginners interested in starting a meditation practice is the time commitment. Fortunately, a little goes a long way. You don't have to meditate for an hour a day. You can get big benefits from as little as 5 to 8 minutes a day.[16] Check out www.gosit.org for a list of centers and classes near you.

REVIEW AND REFLECT

These techniques can help consolidate learning into your long-term memory.

REVIEW NEW INFORMATION

Just moments after a question is posed, a passage is read, or directions are given, take enough time to think about what has taken place, process the information, and respond, if necessary. Then periodically review it, so you have the chance to revisit, clarify, and commit your learning to memory. By eventually increasing the time between such reviews, you can strengthen long-term neural networks and retain more information.

REFLECT

True reflection is a response to the actual material, as well as thinking about how you learn. "You empower yourself when you take the time for reflection," says Dr. Rick Hanson, author of *The Buddha's Brain*, "because the more you understand about how you learn, the better you become at learning."

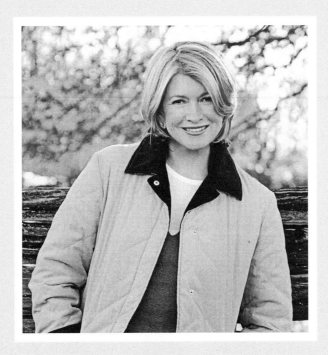

CHAPTER 4

Healthy Outlook

BE OPTIMISTIC *about aging* 146

MAINTAIN *a sense of purpose* 151

STRENGTHEN *social connections* 162

EMBRACE *technology* 166

CULTIVATE *resilience* 168

BEGIN *a series of rituals* 176

FIND *your perspective* 178

I rarely think about how old I am or how old anyone else is—age is just a number. What matters most to me is how engaged, curious, and interesting a person is. I've watched certain people age and admired their approach.

Take my friend David Rockefeller. He's 97, but you would never know it because he is so full of ideas. His closest associates are fifty years his junior and, as a result, his conversation and interests have stayed totally relevant and modern. Similarly, record producer Clive Davis bucks the limitations of age—he hangs out with rap stars, which is admittedly unusual for someone of his generation, but I think that by understanding their language and their poetry, he is totally in tune with those who are probably two generations younger.

I also find I spend time with younger people as well as my peers. I like to socialize with my family members and colleagues because they inspire me to be more adventurous and curious—and can keep up with me on hikes! And now, hanging out with my granddaughter, Jude (born in 2011), and my grandson, Truman (born in 2012), is certainly going to teach me a lot of new things. But age really comes down to spirit—the age you feel you are inside, no matter how old you are outside.

The hallmark of successful aging is getting what you want out of life and doing the things you love to do regardless of age. Whether we are 20 or 80, life can be meaningful, purposeful, and beautiful as long as we have the right guidance and the right solutions to make it so. It's never too early to start and never too late to begin.

BE OPTIMISTIC *about aging*

Consider it a silver lining of our graying nation—baby boomers are redefining the meaning of growing older. Our generation is living longer, enjoying better health, and experiencing more financial security than any that's come before. We're reinterpreting retirement, opting to continue fulfilling careers while still carving out time for travel and family. Boomers have embraced alternative forms of health care and expanded our religious scope to include Eastern philosophies and new spiritual paths. For many of us, we're just hitting our stride. After all, who came up with "50 is the new 30," anyway?

At the same time, taking a positive view of aging is no easy task, since the paradigm is clouded by so many negatives: loss of mobility, loss of memory, loss of loved ones, loss of physical functioning, loss of social value. "Mainly, what we perceive about aging is a projection of our own fears," says geriatric psychiatrist Dr. Marc Agronin, author of *How We Age*. And even we are not immune from the ageist attitude of our youth-obsessed culture. "To an eighteen-year-old, fifty-year-olds may seem ancient, but at fifty, we are as apt to say the same about eighty-year-olds," he observes.

Just as we consider how to improve our experience of aging through diet, exercise, and cognitive training, we need to work on our attitude. We must figure out how to reframe our very notion of what it means to age, and to think of it not as dying slowly, as cynics and curmudgeons would have us believe, but as living fully. Aging can be rich with new experiences and discoveries, great joys, new friends and family members, new ways of being of value to community and society, and, for an increasing number of retirement-age workers, new careers.

For the next few years or decades, focusing on living fully, and finding happiness doing so, will be our central mission. Those with a high degree of "self-efficacy"—the ability to look at challenges as tasks to master, and with a strong sense of one's ability to succeed—will thrive as a result. Also important are the abilities to stay positive, purposeful, socially connected, and resilient.

Here are strategies to help you embrace the next phase of your life with a healthy perspective. The payoff for you, as well as for your loved ones, will be immeasurable.

KEEP A POSITIVE PERSPECTIVE

Research shows that those who feel young and are satisfied with their own experience of aging enjoy positive well-being late in life. They also live longer and stay healthier than folks who have negative impressions of aging.[1] Just what are these seniors doing so right?

A positive perspective may result in greater physical and mental well-being by promoting a healthy lifestyle, which in turn reinforces general vitality. For example, you may decide to wear sunscreen daily to save yourself from premature wrinkling—you want to look young because you feel young. Once you make this a habit, you feel great and start making other beneficial changes, such as exercising regularly and eating less sugar. Thus, optimism begets both well-being and health.

Striving for equanimity is important because the alternative may age you faster. Over the past decade, researchers in the field of positive psychology have made great strides studying the effect of state of mind on the body. It turns out that a sense of mental positivity and resilience can help you approach and overcome life's obstacles in a productive way. These qualities (which can be developed!) can impact how you face everything, from the sniffles to a major crisis like being diagnosed with cancer or heart disease. Optimists are less likely to have heart disease or to die, say researchers at the University of Pittsburgh's School of Medicine, who assessed the health histories of more than 100,000 women who were part of the Women's Health Initiative.[2]

Even just dwelling in negativity temporarily may take a toll on your body. In the Wisconsin Longitudinal Study, women who were asked to write about a negative life experience generated fewer antibodies in response to a flu shot than those who wrote about the happiest moments in their lives, indicating the level of influence your mental state has on your immune system.

In part, developing this optimism means letting go of fear and not sweating the small stuff. "You have to be able to be rational about aging and not let your emotions get the better of you," says psychiatrist Dennis Popeo. According to him, "A big part of growing older is getting to the point of accepting things as they are, changing what is possible, and being okay with the rest of it."

START AN AFFIRMATION FILE

Anytime you get outside approval—a note from a coworker or family member about something positive you did—save it in a special file. Any other accolades—merit awards, perfect attendance records, races completed, pounds lost, old grade-school report cards, letters of recommendation—go in this file. Then, on days when you wonder about your worth to those in your life, you can show yourself just how talented and accomplished you are.

CELEBRATE YOUR MASTER STATUS

As athletes age, they graduate to the master's level of competition. That has a nice ring to it: as a master, you have acquired a repertoire of skills and capabilities beyond the grasp of youth. In your passage through the years, you focused on what was important, discarding what was not helpful. Consider what you've mastered so far—cooking well, fulfilling various leadership roles, playing piano, coaching a team, growing vegetables—and how you'd like to continue to use and build on these skills in the coming years.

LIVE ACCORDING TO YOUR OWN SCRIPT

Here's another exercise: Think of yourself as an actor. When you were younger, perhaps you needed a script; maybe you accepted the role assigned to you. Now that you're older, it's different. You wrote the play; this is your script. You aren't playing a role; you are playing you. All those years in preparation, all that time in rehearsal, all that hard work is finally paying off. It's time for you to take the stage.

Make no mistake: you grow and gain self-confidence when you take a risk. With age, it becomes easier to open yourself up to new experiences because the stakes are low. You've done what you've done; your kids are who they are; your career was what it was. You don't have to worry about whether a certain choice will define you. You are defined. It's your prerogative to do what you want—to leave a class you don't enjoy, to stop reading a book that's boring, to change because you want to change. If you try something new and totally fail, you can always say, "I just wanted to see what would happen." You don't have anything to prove to anyone except yourself.

Instead of using your age as an excuse, try using it as an incentive. Reframe why questions as why not?: Instead of "Why sign up for that online class?" ask "Why not sign up for that class?" You can make new discoveries and allow new paths to unfold.

EMBRACE THE UPSIDE OF "OLDER AND WISER"

Far from being "all downhill from here," there are many cognitive and emotional advantages—significant uphills and impressive peaks—that we can reach through middle age and beyond. Chapter 3 covered the ways in which the brain keeps generating new connections over time, boosting memory and judgment, but broadly speaking, our maturity brings numerous emotional and psychological rewards as well. Dr. Cynthia Green, at the Mount Sinai School of Medicine, offers the following list of great gains we can look forward to:

DEPTH OF KNOWLEDGE

Older people who have been active learners have a greater store of knowledge. "The more years under your belt, the greater your vocabulary, to give one specific example," says Dr. Green. "You can increase your working vocabulary until at least age eighty-five." Reading comprehension and problem-solving skills also deepen and increase with the passing years. Both are examples of so-called crystallized intelligence, which is fact-based and accumulates with greater experience, learning, and skills.

EXPERIENTIAL WISDOM

The Greek philosopher Aristotle defined wisdom as deep understanding tempered by control of emotional reactions. Look at the example of U.S. Airways Captain Chesley "Sully" Sullenberger, who executed an emergency landing on the Hudson River in New York City in January 2009, saving all 155 passengers aboard. It wasn't only his skills as a veteran pilot that saw him through, it was his cumulative life experience. Wisdom is about knowing what to do with knowledge—and good judgment comes with age. As Sully writes in his book *Highest Duty: My Search for What Really Matters*, "We need to try to do the right thing every time, to perform at our best, because we never know what moment in our lives we'll be judged on."

COMPOSURE PSYCHOLOGISTS

Older people are more emotionally balanced and are in a better position to solve highly emotional problems. We have more life experience and thus more precedents to draw upon; we're also better at anticipating the consequences. "Ultimately," says Dr. Green, "it translates into longer, more productive thinkers who potentially offer more benefits than problems to society."

OVERALL HAPPINESS

With the passing years, most of us trend toward greater happiness, according to a twelve-year study of Americans ages 18 to 85.[3] While teenagers and young adults report more anxiety, frustration, and disappointment over things like career goals, salaries, love, and success, older people have made peace with their lives' accomplishments and failures. As we age and gather life experience, many of us increase our emotional health and resilience, note Stanford University researchers. That adds up to happiness.

REPHRASE YOURSELF

Negative perceptions can be dangerously self-fulfilling. Indeed, according to the Ohio Longitudinal Study of Aging and Retirement, people with positive perceptions of aging tended to live nearly eight years longer than those with negative associations. When it comes to longevity, perception trumps loneliness, physical capacity, and even socioeconomic status. So, try to maintain a positive attitude toward the rest of your life; on some level, your subconscious is listening to even offhand remarks.

IF YOU FIND YOURSELF SAYING...	TRY SUBSTITUTING...
"I'm decrepit."	"I am older, but I'm still trying."
"It's all downhill from here."	"As I get older, things are better than I might have thought they'd be."
"All these aches and pains make me feel old."	"In spite of a little ache or pain, it's going to be a good day."
"I'm slowing down."	"I have more time to notice details and nuances."
"I must be senile."	"My memory, although imperfect, works pretty well when I'm organized and I pay attention."
"I look so old."	"I feel young at heart."
"No one notices me because I'm old."	"I need to be more assertive." or "I can make my needs known."
"I'm too old to..."	"I'd like to try this..."
"Things keep getting worse as I get older."	"I have as much pep and curiosity as I did last year."
"Oh no! I forgot her name. I'm losing it!"	"I was never very good at remembering names."

MAINTAIN *a sense of purpose*

In her book *Composing a Further Life: The Age of Active Wisdom,* Mary Catherine Bateson, the cultural anthropologist (and daughter of Margaret Mead), envisioned a new life phase: Adulthood II. She saw this as a time when one chapter of adult life closes and another begins. It doesn't start at a particular age, but it is generally the stage marked by children leaving home, retirement, or the death of/divorce from a longtime spouse. These are the golden years, says Bateson, a period of renewed vitality and energy. What you do with those years is up to you: some may want to hone an undeveloped talent or build a legacy, others might want to focus on giving back. Approach your second adulthood with an invigorated sense of discovery and freedom.

Use your accumulated wisdom, courage, insight, and energy to propel yourself into a new adventure. On the Japanese island of Okinawa, where residents routinely live to 100, they use the word *ikigai,* which connotes a sense of purpose—in other words, a reason to get out of bed each day. This sense of purpose, an agenda to engage your day, does not have to be grandiose. It may be as modest as weeding the garden or keeping in touch with the grandchildren. What's important is that it has the unvarying gravitational pull to keep you engaged and active each day.

STRIVE TO BE CONSCIENTIOUS

Being diligent, responsible, hardworking, organized, and self-disciplined—all aspects of what researchers characterize as conscientiousness—increases your quality of life, according to a study at the Rush University Medical Center in Chicago. Those who were identified as exceptionally conscientious reduced their risk of developing Alzheimer's symptoms by a whopping 89 percent, compared with those who were less conscientious.

Now, you might think it's too late to change your tendencies, that your personality was formed long ago and influenced by your genes. But conscientiousness is one personality trait that you can actively cultivate. A Stanford University study of more than 130,000 people ages 21 to 60 found that while most showed the greatest gain in conscientiousness during the years before they turned 20, they tended to increase their capacity for the trait throughout their lives.

Expanding your capacity for conscientiousness is a matter of daily practice. Researchers have identified the top behaviors associated with this trait: being clean and tidy, working hard, following the rules of social decorum, being disciplined, setting goals, and being organized and prepared.[4] It sounds obvious, but paying attention to the small stuff pays off in a big way. "For an older person who wants to improve his or her conscientiousness, it really comes down to maintaining these behaviors and not letting things slide because you're no longer working or you're sick or simply because you're old," says geriatric psychiatrist Dr. Dennis Popeo, of New York University's Langone Medical Center.

KEEP YOUR CURRENT SYSTEMS GOING

Whether you prefer to keep paper records or store everything on your computer, organize your bills and important documents, alphabetize or organize your recipes, and keep a datebook of appointments and social outings. Do as much housecleaning as you can (or want to); if you've delegated the task, then give yourself the job of keeping your desk neat and organizing bookshelves, drawers, or closets. Finish what you start. Make a to-do list and complete it. Keep memberships, insurance policies, and licenses up to date. Take your medications, exercise regularly, and schedule regular doctor's appointments.

PAY ATTENTION TO YOUR SOCIAL LIFE

Resist the vague platitudes and be more definitive. Don't just say casually, "Let's get together." Get out your datebook and plan a time to meet. Show up for that meeting punctually. Set yourself a goal to be social at least twice a week, whether it's going to a book group, taking a walk with a friend, or going to church or temple services.

Vanity can be a good thing. Make an effort to look your best. Polish your shoes, keep your clothing in good repair, get regular haircuts, choose an outfit to wear even if you're not going out. Remember to honor social commitments.

It's easy to get complacent, but take a stand against it, whether you are considering ducking out of an obligation, canceling plans at the last minute, or waffling on whether you'll exercise or go to your place of worship this weekend.

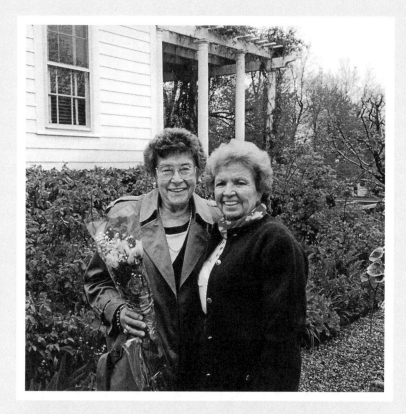

My mother, Martha Kostyra, with her friend, artist Camille Haner, in Westport, Connecticut, in 2000.

MEETING MY MOTHER'S FRIENDS

When my mother died, I was astonished by how many people came to her funeral. It was standing-room-only in this large Catholic church in Weston, Connecticut. Honestly, I had no idea how many friends she had! I knew that she kept busy; she was always writing letters, calling to catch up, offering to drive someone to do errands or see the doctor. But I saw that she was so extremely connected to the people in her town. Talking to these friends after the service was such a lovely, moving experience. They each offered me some little reminiscence of my mom—stories, insights, and memories. We all need to work harder on social skills—visiting, remembering birthdays, taking trips together—with both friends and family.

DON'T RETIRE: RE-CAREER

When asked her secret to longevity, one nonagenarian replied, "It's four easy words—never, never, never retire. Keep going, keep moving, keep thinking, keep living." Being involved in meaningful work is one of the best things you can do for successful brain and body aging, says Dr. Dennis Popeo. "It's 'medicine' in the best sense of the word. Working offers an older person the benefits of social engagement and purpose."

Working may also stave off cognitive decline, according to the National Institute on Aging. Their surveys show that retirees don't perform as well on cognitive tests as those who are still working, and global research supports this: in the United States and Denmark, where workers stay employed longer, people score highest on cognitive tests. So far, researchers can't pinpoint the aspect of "working" that benefits brain function, whether it's social interaction or the physical aspects of a job, but whatever the longevity secret of employment, it's working!

Even if you do choose or have to retire, it's important to make an extra effort to stay intellectually engaged. Consider consulting part time or doing pro bono work. If you do wish to stay employed, bear in mind that finding your new role in the workforce can be challenging. AARP, formerly the American Association of Retired Persons, has taken up this crusade, working with large companies to promote the hiring of older workers. See www.aarp.org/work/job-hunting.

TRY VOLUNTEERING

Working on a volunteer basis or as an intern are two ways to try on a new career for size. Ask to fill in for someone on maternity/paternity or sick leave; this is called *locum tenens*, Latin for "place holder," when someone temporarily fulfills the duties of another.

SEGUE TO A NEW CAREER

Re-careering may involve refining or renovating your skill set. Or you might try something completely different—an interest or a hobby that you want to focus on for this new phase of your life. One woman turned a lifelong love of birds into work as a wildlife rehabilitator. After taking classes and getting a state license to handle wildlife, she rescues ospreys and other raptors.

LOOK FOR NEW OPPORTUNITIES

Start with your own expertise, whether it's your vocation or avocation. If you've always loved art, for instance, channel that passion and knowledge into being a docent for a museum. If you had a career as a tradesman, ask home improvement centers if they are hiring people with your skill set.

"Never before have so many people had so much knowledge and so much time to use it" is the belief of www.encore.org, a website that helps middle-aged and older adults transition into second careers that help the greater good. It maintains listings of resources that include programs, people, and preparation for a later-life career. Look for opportunities around you: ask to shadow someone who's doing a job you're interested in.

GIVE BACK

A meaningful life often goes hand in hand with making a difference in the world, giving freely of our time, our knowledge, and our talent. People volunteer for many reasons, but almost everyone reports a deep sense of satisfaction and accomplishment from the experience, a sort of "helper's high." And volunteering yields even more benefits the older you get. Those over 60 experienced greater increases in physical and mental health than did younger volunteers.[5]

SHARE YOUR KNOWLEDGE

Passing on our wisdom isn't just good parenting or mentoring, it may actually help us live longer. This "Grandmother Hypothesis" is a theory to explain the existence of menopause and how a long postfertile period could confer an evolutionary advantage. As we pass on our culture and wisdom, we retain value long past the age of reproduction. Indeed, studies conducted with elephants, apes, and other primates show that when matriarchs live longer, their clan enjoys a higher infant survival rate, but only on the maternal side. It's a virtuous cycle: the more culture we have to pass on, the more value we have, and the longer we live.

So share your talents. Teach a class at your local community center. Many craft stores have communal tables where crafters can gather and work together (think knitting or ceramics); offer to teach a small group a new stitch or a potting technique.

Become a foster grandparent or mentor a child. Coach a team. Did you know that many nursing homes now have video-game leagues for bowling or tennis? If you've got some gaming expertise, pass it on! When you share your time and your talents, you not only help someone else, you help yourself in the process.

Or try teaching. Experience Corps (experiencecorps.org), a nonprofit volunteer program that places tutors in schools, provides an opportunity for adults age 55 and older to serve as tutors and mentors to students in urban public elementary schools and afterschool programs. Participants have reported that the experience raised their self-esteem, increased their circle of friends, and improved their lives overall.

Help a friend, family member, or college student get organized with tasks like starting a filing system or using online bill pay. Volunteer to do the books at your church or golf club. Help a friend catch up on correspondence. Being a mentor and passing on your wisdom not only helps someone else, but also solidifies for you why these conscientious behaviors are so important.

EMBRACE A HOBBY—OR A FEW

Your love of crochet, World War II memorabilia, or jewelry-making isn't "just" a hobby. Research shows that pursuing your passion can add eight hours of joy—defined as a deep sense of satisfaction, gratification, and accomplishment—to your week.[6] Hobbies lead to continued learning and mastery, become a means of self-expression, and tap into your core values.

Researchers have also found that those who pursue a hobby and keep it up in later years have better moods, fewer bouts with depression, less stress, and better immune function.[7] According to a large Japanese study, those who don't engage in hobbies may even be at greater risk for chronic health problems.

EXPLORE YOUR PASSION

Start by pinpointing what interests you: gardening, opera, Renaissance art, collecting, antiquing, poetry. Chances are, there's a group of like-minded others who have formed a local or online community for that interest or hobby that can help you in your pursuit of pleasure. Simply Google [your interest] plus "groups," "interest groups," or "associations." You'll find a list of links that will supply information and inspiration for finding direction, taking classes, and exploring new opportunities. If you want to deepen your knowledge of sewing, scrapbooking, or making keepsakes, ornaments, and other crafts, check out books on the topic, or watch instructional videos online.

BREAK THROUGH BARRIERS

Don't let a perceived lack of talent stop you from embarking on an artistic pursuit, whether it's a brand-new interest or something you did in your youth. Yes, you may have disappointed your piano teacher, been told just to mouth the words by a choral director, or never won an award in art—but who's judging you now? If you love music, singing, or art, give it another try as an adult. Or, call your local community college, arts society, or recreation center to find resources for private instruction or group lessons. You can also find a list of arts programs for seniors at the National Endowment for the Arts website (www.nea.gov) for its Arts in Aging Resource List.

JOIN THE CLUB

Picking up a new hobby needn't be a solo act. Research shows that you'll gain added benefits by bringing along a friend. "Social connections and having fun are key to mental and physical health," says Stanford University psychologist Kelly McGonigal, Ph.D. "They protect you from heart disease, stress, depression, and even colds." If hiking is a favorite, find like-minded adventurers through Sierra Club's local outings (www.sierraclub.org/outings). Or if your interest leans toward outdoor photography, gardening, or bird-watching, consider starting your own group. Connect with others who share your passion, no matter how obscure, at www.meetup.com. The website brings together hobbyists in communities across the country.

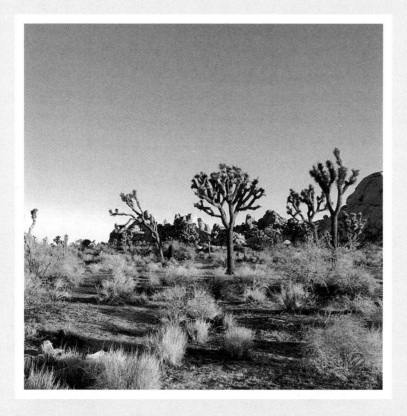

CREATE A BUCKET LIST

Keeping a list of things you want to do or feel you must do during your lifetime—and then checking them off before you kick the bucket—is a really good thing. That's why movies like *The Bucket List* resonate with so many of us. It certainly resonated with me. While on a photo shoot in Palm Springs, California, it was important to me to visit Joshua Tree National Park (above). Known for its incredible rock formations and its extraordinary vegetative wonders, it had long been on my "bucket list." It was well worth the early 4 a.m. departure and the long drive into the desert. It is one of those places I will never forget.

SEE THE WORLD

All the reasons that made travel so great when you were younger—gaining new perspectives, challenging old assumptions, broadening your worldview—still apply in later years. Further, researchers at the University of Arkansas cite travel as a factor in longevity, principally because it involves social connection.

When it comes to planning a trip, individual preferences are as diverse as destinations. You may like the company of many different generations; others may prefer to travel with a more homogeneous age group. Some businesses specialize in elder travel. ElderTreks (www.eldertreks.com) is an adventure-travel company for people age 50 and over. The Society for Accessible Travel and Hospitality (www.sath.org) offers referrals to travel agents who can handle most special needs. Accessible Travel and Leisure (www.accessibletravel.co.uk) specializes in barrier-free vacations for those who have trouble getting around. Or perhaps you want to choose travel mates with whom you've shared an experience, such as college friends. Many universities offer educational travel trips as well as simple pleasure excursions. Genealogical tourism, or traveling to explore your family history, is also a growing trend among boomers, perhaps because our generation prefers to travel for personal enrichment rather than simply to escape.

TRAVEL FOR YOUR HEALTH

Beyond providing a necessary mental break, mounting evidence shows that vacations are important to your physical health. Information from the Framingham Heart Study found that women who took at least two vacations a year were less likely to develop coronary heart disease or have a heart attack than those who took a vacation only every six years or less. These findings have been substantiated in follow-up research. Another study by researchers at the State University of New York and the University of Pittsburgh focused on middle-aged men at high risk for coronary heart disease. They found that those who did not take a vacation every year had a 21 percent higher risk of death from all causes and were 32 percent more likely to die of a heart attack.

SHARE YOUR HOME WITH A PET

Pets can be a lot of work, but they also offer aging owners multiple wellness benefits. Here's what adopting a dog, cat, or other furry friend can do for you:

PETS HELP YOU LIVE LONGER

Research shows that hanging out with domestic animals reduces blood pressure, cholesterol levels, and triglyceride levels—all of which promote longevity, especially if you have a history of heart disease or heart attacks. Pets also reduce our stress levels.

PETS GET YOU MOVING

People who own dogs are 69 percent more likely to get in leisure-time physical activity than non–dog owners, according to a study of six thousand people published in the *Journal of Physical Activity and Health*.

PETS PREVENT LONELINESS AND DEPRESSION

Over half of all pet owners consider their animals to be companions, not property—and 97 percent of us talk to our pets. As part of their medical screening, some health insurance companies even ask clients over age 75 if they have a pet.

IF YOU'RE ALLERGIC TO PETS

Keep in mind that some people are highly allergic to pet dander. If this is the case, invest in a dog bed or other pet-specific bedding so your animals don't sleep with you, and consider limiting them to kitchens, dens, and other areas of the house without a lot of soft furnishings, which are pet-dander magnets. Add a HEPA filter to central air conditioning and central heating to remove pet allergens from the air (see page 294). You can also try bathing pets once a week in plain water or wiping them down with a damp cloth to keep dander from spreading.

If you aren't able to keep a pet where you live, consider volunteering with a local animal shelter, or contact Pet Partners to find out about volunteering at a pet therapy program in your area or for a home visit (www.petpartners.org).

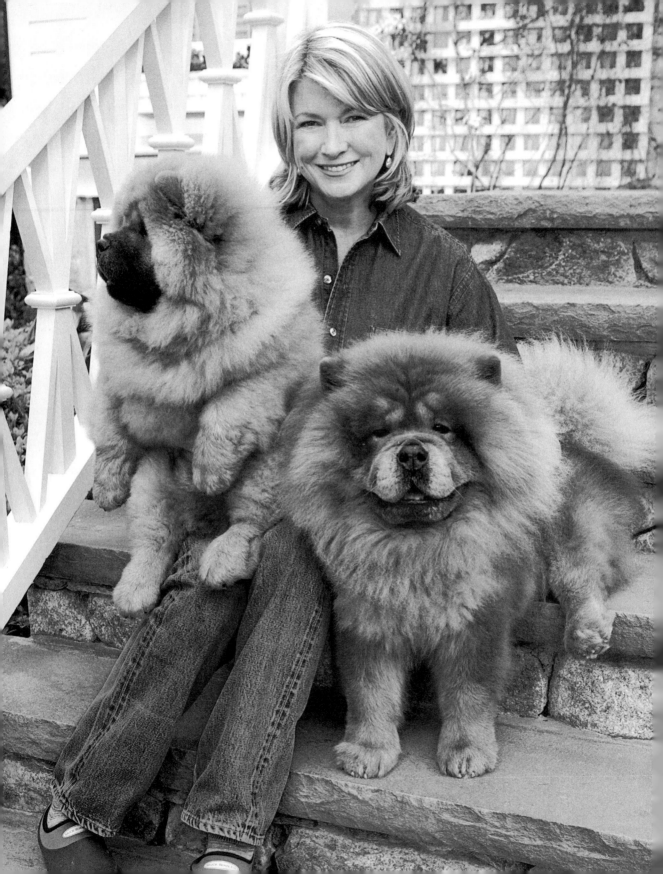

PETS ARE GOOD FOR YOUR HEALTH

Everyone knows of my love for domestic animals and my feelings about their importance to a life well lived. I got my first dog, a beautiful Keeshond female, in 1969, and my first cat, a longhaired kitten, shortly before that. Today I share my home with three dogs (two French bulldogs and a chow chow), five Himalayan cats, and twenty-five red canaries. (I'm pictured opposite with Paw Paw, my beloved chow who passed away in 2008, and Genghis Khan, or G.K. for short.) Pets have always been important members of my family no matter where I've lived, and nearly all have enjoyed healthy, long lives.

Both cats and dogs can be playful and energetic when you need a lift, and can be eager for cuddling, conversation, and love when you crave companionship. I treat them like little children—I talk to them, reprimand them gently, and spoil them. I often go for long walks with my Frenchies, Francesca and Sharkey. They are very active dogs who enjoy outdoor activities as much as I do. Cats are less demanding of attention but no less rewarding. Birds like to sing or chatter, and they love interaction. They make lively and vocal housemates. I believe the secret to good pet ownership is choosing a compatible breed and taking the time to train, nurture, and care for that pet very well.

STRENGTHEN *social connections*

How many people do you consider to be part of your social circle—family, friends, coworkers? The size of the average adult's network is roughly 150 people, give or take a few. According to evolutionary biologist Robin Dunbar, this impressive number is possible thanks to the prefrontal cortex, your brain's biggest area, which processes social information, such as the moods and personalities of others. We make so many personal connections because we're so good at processing the nuances of social interactions. And this ability protects our brain as we age because social interaction helps establish our "cognitive reserve," that sort of savings account for the mind that allows your brain to keep functioning optimally. Staying social also limits the sense of isolation that may come with later years, as friends move away, family members grow up, or loved ones die.

Maintaining social connections can be accomplished through volunteering, entertaining, gathering in book or other discussion clubs, or even playing games. Research has shown that staying social protects against blue moods, inertia, depression, loneliness, and anxiety. If you've lost touch with friends or extended family over the years, now's the time to rebuild your network.

STAY CONNECTED TO FAMILY

Families used to put down roots in a community and stay for generations, but this is far less likely to happen now. Moving for work has become the norm, so families, no matter how close, are often geographically far flung. But that makes homecomings all the sweeter. And in between reunions, technology has made it easier than ever to stay in touch: the video computer chat service Skype is a simple and inexpensive way to virtually visit family members around the globe. And more and more families are setting up social-network pages so they can upload photos and exchange messages. Older generations may keep the family photograph albums, videos, and archives of family letters, but digital technology lets you share this memorabilia with the whole family, wherever they may be.

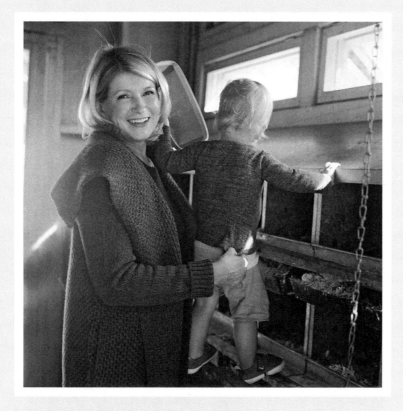

Gathering eggs from the chickens on my farm with my granddaughter, Jude, in 2012.

FIND TIME FOR FAMILY

I am a legendary workaholic and have often found myself sacrificing time with friends and family for work-related activities. However, all that has changed since my two grandchildren were born, and I try to make time, good time, to spend with them as often as I can. The time I spend with them, or with my nieces and nephews and godchildren, is rejuvenating, energizing, and greatly enjoyable. And I am finding that the connection with them creates connections with other young people.

STAY CONNECTED TO COMMUNITY

Getting involved—with a civic group, a place of worship, a club, or even a block or apartment association—can increase your longevity. Research has found that men and women who participated in such community activities were found to have a significantly longer life expectancy than those who didn't.[8]

GO TO YOUR HOUSE OF WORSHIP

Even if you're not particularly religious, many religious institutions have community outreach programs that can be valuable resources. You can volunteer at a food pantry, sign up for Habitat for Humanity, keep a senior citizen company, or help organize a rummage sale.

BEAUTIFY YOUR NEIGHBORHOOD

Find a local garden club or conservancy at a public park that needs volunteers to help keep up the plantings. In large cities, neighborhood groups offer "urban ranger" activities, such as pruning sidewalk trees and weeding public planters.

FIND A FRATERNAL ORGANIZATION

Groups like the Rotary Club, the Knights of Columbus, and Masonic Lodges offer frequent get-togethers and social activities, as well as possibilities for volunteering, mentoring, or otherwise getting involved.

USE YOUR SKILLS

With a lifetime of experience under your belt, consider volunteering at organizations that could use your knowledge. SCORE connects mentors with startups and small businesses (www.score.org). Whatever your skill set, there's likely someone who would appreciate your insights.

FIGHT THE URGE TO BECOME A RECLUSE

As we age, physical and emotional loss can contribute to feelings of isolation. Diminishing hearing, sight, and functional ability keep many elderly people from interacting with others. The inevitable losses of friends and spouses can contribute to a deep sense of solitude that makes the elderly reclusive. "People who don't have socialization become depressed," says Sheila Barton, social worker at the Martha Stewart Center for Living. "We need social contact. It's the way we're constructed. If people remain socially active, they live longer, and they're happier." Barton recommends the following for staying connected:

Own Your Age. Many people avoid telling others their age because they don't want to be seen as old. Yet with life experience comes wisdom, humor, and character. Try to find others who enjoy intellectual conversation and can relate to your life experiences. Research has shown connections between depression and cognitive loss, so when you improve your mood and you interact with others, you keep your intelligence sharp!

Keep a Routine. "When someone is reclusive, they don't have routines, so people don't see or notice them," says Barton. Staying connected with community, in the ways outlined above, can help build these routines into daily life.

EXPAND YOUR SOCIAL CIRCLE

Be sure to look beyond family as you consider the people who compose your social networks. Studies show that people who maintain a reasonable number of nonfamily supports, especially one or two individuals they consider to be close confidants, are likely to live longer.

FIND FORMER FRIENDS

Young adults may spend decades avoiding reunions, but as the years go by, people often develop an honest desire to reconnect and exchange life stories. Reuniting provides an opportunity to renew a bond as you reminisce about times spent together, and importantly, reconcile who you once were with who you have become. If you can't physically attend a school reunion, the Internet makes it easy to reconnect with schoolmates. Check college alumni association pages, the website www.classmates.com, or online phone books. Likewise, many neighborhoods, particularly urban enclaves, have developed social networks and newsletters to encourage connection among people who grew up together during a certain era. You can also try locating people through the Social Security Administration for a small fee. If you give the agency a name and a year of birth, officials will forward your contact information.

TAKE UP A COMPANION SPORT

Bowling, golf, Ping-Pong, doubles tennis, and bocce ball all require partners, which will help you form social connections and reinforce your commitment to the sport.

EXERCISE WITH A GROUP

Signing up for a gym membership or yoga class with a friend and agreeing to exercise together can be a good way to reinforce both physical activity and social interaction. If you don't have a partner, many facilities will match you with someone of similar skill level.

TRY A SOCIAL GAME

Sitting around a table playing bridge (forget its fuddy-duddy reputation—Bill Gates and Warren Buffett play!), mah-jongg, chess, poker, or checkers engages your brain and keeps you socially connected. These games stimulate several senses: you have to listen to bids, remember what's been played, communicate with your partner, and plot your next move. These games also promote continued learning: you learn with each round played and new tactic acquired.

BOND THROUGH HOBBIES

Plan crafting nights with friends or spend time at the communal tables at craft-specialty stores. Look into an open night at a local nursery or woodworking or pottery store, or join a food co-op or CSA (community-supported agriculture). If you can't find a preexisting organization you'd like to join, start one. Whatever your interest, be it winetasting, beer making, puzzle solving, current events, books, or movies, chances are you can find a few like-minded souls to form a club. Talk to friends or post a flyer at a local bookstore or on a virtual billboard.

START NEW TRADITIONS

Holidays or other annual events (the cherry blossoms in spring, the Oscars, or the Super Bowl) are opportunities to plan for the future, stay connected with friends, and enjoy a fun afternoon or evening together. It doesn't have to be elaborate, just a heartfelt commitment to get together on a particular date.

EMBRACE *technology*

As we age, it's essential to stay relevant—not just for our cognitive well-being but also because we still have an important role to play in society. Today all business and communication is conducted using high-tech tools, and it's hard to remain plugged in to our evolving culture without literally plugging in. The digital age has speeded things up in ways that may feel uncomfortable, but it can also be harnessed to make life more efficient, from managing your own affairs to staying in touch with others. Just accessing entertainment, information, and directions has become so much easier.

If you're not ready to commit, there are plenty of stores that let you try out new technologies before purchasing them; many even offer workshops on how to use them, too. Check your local library as well. Don't let a sense that you won't be able to figure it out hold you back—you will be amazed at how intuitive and useful these tools can be.

BUILD YOUR VIRTUAL SOCIAL NETWORKS

Studies show that those who use the Internet have larger social networks—and that adults age 74 and older are the fastest growing age group on social networking sites![9] This is good news because Internet use among seniors is associated with a 20 percent lower rate of depression, according to the Phoenix Center for Advanced Legal and Economic Public Policy Studies, a think tank. Facebook and Google+ are intuitive and easy to use—and probably everybody you know (or could hope to meet!) is already on there. If you're still working, LinkedIn is a good resource for finding and connecting with professional colleagues.

GET TECHNICAL HELP

If you need assistance with your computer or Internet-surfing skills, try asking for guidance from a tech-savvy teen or check out one of these resources. At www.eldercare.gov, you'll find referrals to agencies with senior tech-training programs in your area. Seniornet.com offers basic computer classes at locations across the country. And www.oats.org offers resources for tech education, as well as links to senior blogs and online communities. TheProjectGoal.org offers resources that promote Internet use by older adults.

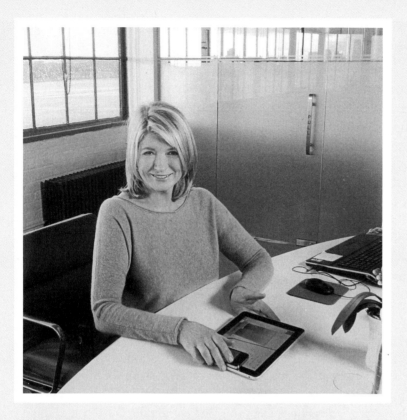

KEEP UP WITH TECHNOLOGY

I have always been a very early adopter. I bought my first computer, the original IBM PC, back in 1982, because I wanted to understand what it was and what it could do for me. So when somebody tells me, "I don't have a smartphone," or "I don't own a computer," I don't know what that person is thinking. I encourage my friends to try everything—new social media, tablet technologies like the iPad—because, first of all, I think it's all interesting, and second, because I think it's useful and relevant to our lives.

CULTIVATE *resilience*

For years, the conventional view was that our ability to rebound from tragedy or crisis was the product of lucky genes, but grief and bereavement experts have discovered that this capacity can be developed. In fact, some research has shown that your capacity for resilience increases with age, simply because you have more experience under your belt.[10]

Resilience is not so much a specific personality trait as a collection of behaviors, thoughts, and actions. These include a basic sense of optimism, a "moral compass" or unshakable set of beliefs, a sense of purpose in life, strong social support, faith or a sense of spirituality, and good humor. Resilience can be your protection against the speed bumps of aging: depression, anxiety, and grief. It doesn't guarantee immunity from these negative emotions, but it can help you recover more quickly.

LEARN TO COPE WITH STRESS

Chronic stress and anxiety have the opposite effect of exercise on the brain: they kill neurons and prevent the creation of new ones, according to Dr. Dennis Popeo, a psychiatrist at New York University's Langone Medical Center. During stressful times, the body releases glucocorticoids, hormones that can damage cells in the hippocampus. That's probably why you may not retain new information or adapt to novel situations when you're stressed or depressed. In many ways, optimism and happiness are like muscles—you have to train them and work them consistently.

As the years pass, your body becomes more vulnerable to stress hormones. An illness, such as a flu or cold, that may have merely slowed you down in earlier years may instead result in short-term disability or long-term dependence. The older you get, the more important it is to get a grip on stress.

Fortunately, tried-and-true stress relievers—meditation, deep breathing, yoga, progressive relaxation—are effective no matter how old you are. But you have to commit to practicing them on a regular basis. Can't see yourself meditating for 20 minutes a day? Start smaller: try meditating for 5 minutes a day and assess your stress levels after a week. If meditation isn't working, sit in a quiet place and try 4-square breathing. Breathe in for a count of 4, hold for 4, breathe out for a count of 4, hold for a count of 4. Repeat. Or you may find a combination of techniques—a twice-weekly yoga class and progressive relaxation before you go to sleep—stems your stress response.

REWIRE YOUR BRAIN TO REDUCE STRESS

Your mind has incredible influence over your body, and stress can have a significant impact on overall health. When we feel anxious, the brain triggers hormones such as cortisol, which flood the body and contribute to physical issues such as inflammation, weakened immunity, and high blood pressure. In the long run, these can influence seemingly unrelated outcomes including heart disease and cancer.

Your brain has three components: the hindbrain, which focuses on activities of basic survival, such as breathing; the limbic system, which supports emotions; and the cerebral cortex, which interprets events. These regions are intertwined. When you experience an event as a stressor, the hindbrain activates a stress reaction. This can increase the heart rate and blood pressure, and cause other physical manifestations of anxiety that can eventually lead to disease. The limbic system associates the stressor with the physical feelings of anxiety and fear. We then "realize," in the cortex, that the initial event is a stressor, and we learn to avoid that event, or others like it. This sequence of events can be modified. By consciously shifting your perception and interpretation of events, you can alter your reactions, rewiring their impact on your body.

ACCENTUATE THE POSITIVE

Most of life is full of neutral and positive moments, and negatives are relatively rare. However, owing to what scientists have dubbed the "negativity bias" of the brain, we tend to focus on and record mainly negative experiences, while neutral and positive moments are more ephemeral and less apt to register in memory, according to Rick Hanson, author of *The Buddha's Brain: The Practical Neuroscience of Happiness, Love, and Wisdom.* To stay positive, you need to build up positive memories, which in turn can enhance your brain's plasticity.

Here's Rick Hanson's three-step process:

1. Turn positive events into positive experiences. All kinds of good things happen in your daily life that you hardly notice at all. Someone pays you a compliment—you barely pay attention to it, or you deflect it. Instead, take time to recognize every positive moment and experience it.

2. Savor positive experiences. Once you get used to recognizing these types of experiences, take it a step further and relish each good moment: hold on to it for 20 or 30 seconds, and allow yourself to really feel it in your body. The longer you hold these moments in your awareness, the more neurons fire simultaneously so they start wiring together to form a memory.

3. Consider how the experience is sinking into you and becoming a part of you. In other words, help weave it into the fabric of your brain and yourself.

PRACTICE MINDFULNESS

Techniques such as mindfulness meditation are particularly effective in retraining your thought patterns. Mindfulness means paying attention to your current task or setting. Practice during an activity that's part of your daily routine—say, brushing your teeth. As you brush, tune in with all your senses: note the taste and scent of the toothpaste, listen to water gurgle down the drain, notice the light coming in the window. When other thoughts intrude, notice them, then turn your attention back to the moment. The distraction of outside thoughts is likely to happen frequently. Don't judge yourself or become upset; simply notice them and return to your task.

You can employ mindfulness as you make your bed, walk to get the mail, or do an errand. Studies have shown that this form of meditation can decrease anxiety and stress and help you develop a more positive outlook.

FIND FRESH PERSPECTIVE

Have you ever felt you can't concentrate because of all the noise and distracting thoughts in your head? Dr. Cynthia Greene, assistant clinical professor of psychiatry at the Mount Sinai School of Medicine, recommends this exercise to get out of your head, which begins by taking a 5-minute walk in a familiar place. "Instead of letting your thoughts run away with you, focus on your surroundings," she urges. At the end of the walk, jot down five new things that you've never noticed before. This technique is a good way to train your attention "endurance" and reduce stress at the same time.

LIVE TO LAUGH

When your grandmother told you "laughter is the best medicine," she was absolutely right. Some research suggests that humorless, reserved personality types have higher rates of heart disease than their more easily amused counterparts.[11] When we laugh, we loosen our grip on how things "must be" or how we want them to be. Poking fun at ourselves allows us to step away from our egos. We feel physically lighter (laughter releases endorphins), and we open up to more readily accept wisdom.

For help in the humor department, rent comedies, watch stand-up routines, call your funniest friend, and do whatever else it takes to elicit belly laughs. Try to laugh at yourself, too—spilling the milk or losing your keys can all be opportunities to smile instead of stress. Still having trouble letting go? Fake it till you make it: It may sound odd, but even pretending to laugh or forcing a smile can lead to real laughter.

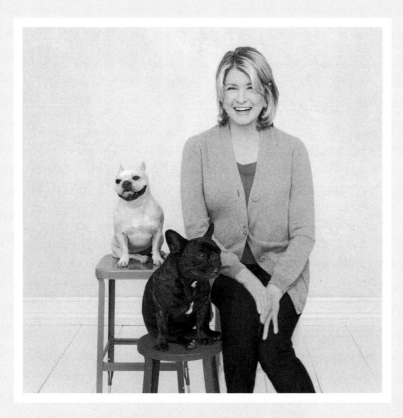

THE POWER OF LAUGHTER

My daughter told me about a man in India, Dr. Madan Kataria, who wakes up hundreds of thousands of people on the radio with a laughter program. What a wonderful way to start the day by infectiously instilling in such a vast audience joy and humor. To laugh is restorative and proven to increase a sense of well-being and a sense of calm in even the most chaotic environment. Finding humor in the action of a child or pet, or in a newspaper article, can provide a fresh outlook and a helpful distraction. Watching a favorite late-night comedian—mine are David Letterman, Jon Stewart, and Jimmy Kimmel—can certainly add a different perspective and a light-heartedness we all need.

LEARN TO WORRY WELL

Worry is not in itself good or bad—it's simply a function of your mind, says author Rick Hanson. How you worry is what matters, and unproductive or "bad worry" is just plain bad for you.

Let's say you've been diagnosed with high blood pressure or pre-diabetes. Instead of taking action, you indulge in catastrophic thoughts about the things that can go wrong now that you've been diagnosed: your insurance will go up; you won't be able to do the activities you currently enjoy; you might end up in a wheelchair. You cycle through these possible outcomes, imagining them vividly and repeatedly, without taking any action. Over time, this kind of bad worry triggers anxiety, which in turn triggers out-of-control stress, which leaves you feeling worse than ever, and puts you at greater risk for more health problems ranging from insomnia to eating disorders to heart disease. On the other hand, productive worry, or "good worry," helps you solve problems and achieve peace of mind. Take the same scenario. You feel a jolt of fear upon hearing the news from your doctor. But this time, you put your worry skills to work for you. First, you distinguish between what you can't control (your diagnosis) and what you can control (the progression of your condition). Second, you identify the root cause of your fear: you lack the knowledge necessary to lose the extra weight, which would ameliorate your high blood pressure or pre-diabetic blood sugar level. Third, you identify resources for solving this problem: you'll read about healthy weight loss and ask your friends, nutritionist, or doctor for advice. See the difference? Practice good worry, not bad.

If nothing seems to stick, consider making an appointment with a cognitive therapist to help you gain insight into your thought processes and how to manage them. Regular activity, healthy eating, and laughter (see page 171) also help you navigate the stress rapids in the river of life. Find the time to do something you feel passionate about on a regular basis. Recognize that you can modify these activities to accommodate your age and ability. If cooking elaborate soup-to-nuts dinners made you feel good in the past, making just an impressive main course and filling in with simpler (or purchased) side dishes may elicit the same satisfaction.

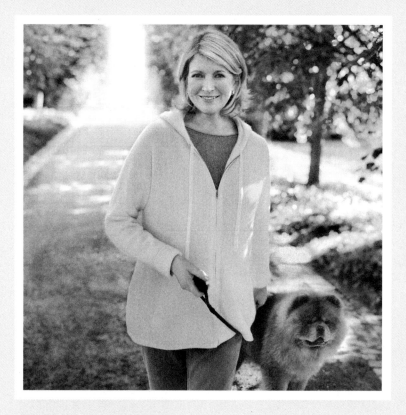

JUST MOVE ON

There are any number of incredibly challenging things that I have to deal with every day—I get mixed news on a financial report, or I have to make a speech in front of hundreds of people. So I long ago developed the ability to deal with stress: you just have to solve one problem immediately and, if you have to, let off some steam. A good way to do this is by going for a quick walk. And then, perhaps most important, you move on. You don't ruminate or worry, but keep moving forward. Life is a pile of problems that have to be solved one way or another, and the best way is to look at each one individually, figure it out, and move on.

IDENTIFY DEPRESSION

"Surprisingly, the rate of major depressive disorder (MDD) does not rise with age, it actually decreases," notes Dr. Marc Agronin, author of *How We Age*. "But that doesn't mean that it's still not a concern with age." Depression risk increases with the occurrence of other illnesses, as well as with loss of function. According to the National Institutes of Health, rates of major depression among older people range from 1 to 5 percent; that prevalence jumps to more than 13 percent among those who require home health care. Rates of depressive symptoms, or low mood (and subsequently lower quality of life), range from 15 to 30 percent in the elderly.

The problem with depression lies in detecting it. One of the biggest hindrances to addressing this problem is that doctors just aren't asking about it and patients aren't telling. "Doctors have to get better at detecting depression and anxiety because these increase an individual's risk for dementia and other medical problems," adds Dr. Agronin. "Assessing mental health should be done as routinely and regularly as any other vital signs, like pulse and blood pressure."

On the patient side, avoiding discussions of depression is a generational issue. "For many older people, mental illness still carries a real stigma," suggests Dr. Dennis Popeo. "As a result, very few people will volunteer that they're feeling depressed." Fortunately, "these patients do extremely well with talk therapy as well as antidepressants. It's never too late to start—I currently have ninety- and hundred-year-olds in therapy." Talk therapy is helpful in easing anxiety. Dr. Popeo advises, "Some therapies, like CBT (cognitive behavioral therapy) or PST (problem solving therapy), are more like 'skills training' rather than what most patients consider therapy (lying on a couch, talking about dreams and mothers) and might be more palatable to older folks."

Even relatively younger folks in their sixties and seventies are bound to be reticent on the topic. "It's important to understand that vague feelings of lethargy, fatigue, sleeplessness, and changes in appetite are all associated with depression," Dr. Popeo offers. "Getting help earlier rather than later can clear up symptoms and resolve depression so you can get back to the business of life." Your social support system can also help mitigate loneliness, which can play a contributing role.

Older people have a different pattern of symptoms than younger patients, according to Dr. Marc Agronin. Those over 70 experience more anxiety, physical symptoms (like weakness, shortness of breath, headaches, palpitations, abdominal or back pain), and noticeable mental deterioration (trouble focusing, forgetfulness).

DETECT ANXIETY

The older you get, the more time there is to ruminate. Normal worries can turn into pathology when someone is unable to function or limits their activities—refusing to take a trip or try something new—because of this anxiety.[12] A loss of identity or purpose can also trigger anxiety. And when you're experiencing anxiety, you become less resilient because it grows more difficult to face fears, force yourself out of your comfort zone, or share your concerns with friends.

"Older people may not want to admit or acknowledge their symptoms, mainly because they fear they will lose their independence," Dr. Popeo notes. "But if anxiety disrupts your normal functioning during the day and disturbs your sleep at night, you need help." Anxiety does respond to medication, such as antidepressants, anti-anxiety drugs (anxiolytics), and beta-blockers. Medications need to be carefully monitored, as there can be side effects or interactions with other drugs.

DEAL WITH GRIEF

While grief that comes from loss is an increasingly frequent occurrence with age, not everyone grieves in the same way. Most people know the stages of grief that were first set down by Elisabeth Kübler-Ross, but research has shown that people vary tremendously in their reactions to loss.[13]

Some people can suffer chronic, long-term grieving, while others have a shorter, more intense period of sorrow and then return to the business of living. Most people show a third pattern: an initial period of mourning and then a pattern in which they get back to life, interspersed with periods of sadness.[14] It's as if the brain is trying to find a middle ground between extreme sorrow and mirth, a new normal so that life can go on. But there is no one right way to grieve, nor one ideal duration of grief.

The good news is that an increased capacity for grief emerges with the passing years. "It may be because loss becomes a more frequent occurrence, or because a person develops better coping strategies," notes Dr. Marc Agronin. "There's also a sense of solidarity—you join the crowd of those who have lost someone."

If the effects of grief don't ease, check in with your doctor to see if you're depressed. The two states share many of the same symptoms, such as feeling hopeless, an inability to function or focus, and a sense of guilt. Grief can be roller-coaster-like, with good and bad days in spite of the pain, but with depression, feelings of despair and emptiness are pervasive and a sufferer should seek help.

BEGIN *a series of rituals*

Good rituals are essential because they help reconnect us to the sacred aspects of our lives. Try adopting any one of these mindful practices or develop your own.

WELCOME THE DAY

Many ancient cultures had some form of morning ritual, and even now most people have a pattern for starting their day, even if it's coffee from the same café. Savoring these few moments will put your mind into a positive frame and prepare your entire body for whatever stresses lie ahead.

Lie quietly for a few moments before getting out of bed and give thanks for this new day. Dab a few drops of an uplifting essential oil (grapefruit is nice for its freshness) on a cloth that you'll use solely for this ritual, and breathe in the aroma.

Get up and stand in front of a mirror. Smile at yourself and affirm that this will be a good day, full of blessings, opportunities, and wonder. Say aloud, "I look forward to a wonderful day," or any affirmation with personal significance. If there are difficult meetings or decisions ahead, affirm that you will tackle these with ease: "I will take the challenges of this day in stride."

Face east and perform the yoga exercise Sun Salutation. This sequence of twelve yoga poses is performed in one continuous flow in tandem with the breath. The series strengthens, tones, and promotes flexibility from head to toe, while helping the mind focus and relax.

SHARE THE FAMILY MEAL

Every culture around the globe has a tradition of blessing food, cooking and eating mindfully, and giving thanks for the gift of nourishment. Make time to create a setting for nurturing and togetherness with loved ones as often as you can, even if it's just once a week or once a month.

Set a specific day and time for a family meal. Every member of the family, even small children, should be in charge of contributing something—even if it's just stirring the pot or setting the table. Focus your intention as you chop, mix, and blend.

Before eating, light a candle, then hold hands and acknowledge the gifts in your life. Feel free to create a special family blessing. This could take the form of a favorite short poem or saying aloud, "We thank the earth, sun, and rain for producing this food, the farmers for growing, harvesting, and sharing it, and the cook for preparing it."

Eat your meal with mindfulness. Encourage silence as everyone savors the taste and texture of their food. Reflect on the long journey from farm to table, and how lucky you are to be eating such delicious, nourishing food. When the meal is finished, blow out the candle.

GIVE THANKS

For our ancestors, gratitude was ingrained, and as a result, every aspect of life presented an occasion for celebration. Offering gratitude is a way to open yourself up to giving and receiving more blessings. Sometimes it takes a simple ceremony to put us in touch with all we do have in our lives. Make this ritual a part of each day, each month, each year—or whenever you feel it's time to value and honor those you love, including yourself.

Pour a few drops of cinnamon oil into a diffuser or spray bottle, or crush two cinnamon sticks into a small bowl of warm water. Allow the aroma to permeate your space.

Make a list of all the family members, friends, and pets that matter the most to you. You could even include material things. By writing one or two reasons why each is important to you, you'll clarify your thoughts and honor the people and things in your life that shouldn't be taken for granted.

SLEEP WELL

Bedtime is when we drop our defenses and become vulnerable. This is why most religions have a tradition of bedtime prayers—and perhaps why most insomnia and disturbed nights are caused by overactive minds mulling over the day's problems. Mark the break from day to night and ease yourself into a state of physical and mental relaxation with this ritual.

Change (or bathe) with intention. As you take off your clothes, visualize all your daytime anxieties and concerns dropping away. As you wash, imagine that you are cleansing away all the negativity of the day.

Write down all the positive things that happened during your day.

Dab some essential oil on a handkerchief and place it near the bed. Lie down, breathe in the soothing scent of the oil, and cast your mind back over the day without judgment.

FIND *your perspective*

In any life, there are bound to be ups and downs. Taking the long-view perspective when considering your history can help you cope with loss. As anthropologist Mary Bateson notes, "Each new stage in the life cycle is related to what came before, ideally related in a way that is more than a sum of parts but, rather, an inclusive composition of grace and truth. It is often only in its final pages that a story reveals its meaning, so the choices made in later decades may reflect light back on earlier years."

Regularly visualizing your life as a whole, and its context within the universe, can minimize smaller disturbances and help you make sense of the bigger issues. "It helps if you look at your experiences to find opportunities for self-discovery," says Dr. Marc Agronin. "What did you learn about yourself in your struggle with grief? How have you changed and grown from the experience?"

You don't have to grasp everything; in fact, you may emerge with a sense that there is more to life than what you can see or fully comprehend. Some call this attitude spirituality or soulfulness, but that doesn't necessarily connote religiosity. Rather, it's a trust in the universe that you have a place in the order of things, that you matter. If you haven't thought about this life perspective, you may need to set aside some time devoted to finding it. As Plato noted, "The unexamined life is not worth living."

WRITE YOUR LIFE STORY

Put together a scrapbook of your life, depicting its different phases, your various roles. Invite family members and friends to contribute their memories or photos. Try to fit your life into the context of history—was it a time of prosperity? War? Peace? Who was president? What songs were popular? What did you wear? What were your hobbies? It can be immensely satisfying to trace the arc of your life through imagery. Future generations will appreciate that you've captured your personal history. And it will give you a sense of your life as a progressive, integrated narrative.

MAKE A SOUNDTRACK AUTOBIOGRAPHY

In *Musically Speaking,* noted sex therapist Dr. Ruth Westheimer recommends making a playlist of your life. "Search your memory banks for the pieces of music that were playing at various times of your life. Include songs from your childhood, as well as those that you associate with major events in your life," she advises. Burn them to a CD, record them, or just make a list of them. Sit and listen to them or hum them to yourself. Close your eyes and let the notes float into your brain and relive some of the most precious times of your life. "Music, like math, is processed on the left side of your brain. Using music to trigger recollection brings up a different view of those memories than looking at photos. You may even close your eyes so that you relive these experiences in a completely different, nonvisual way," says Dr. Westheimer.

RECORD YOUR STORIES

Take inspiration from StoryCorps, a national oral-history project, to tell the story of your life, so your loved ones have a permanent record in your own voice, and so that you can gain some perspective on your important contributions. Since 2003, people from all walks of life have been entering a mobile recording studio in cities around the country to record a 40-minute oral history. Participants take one copy home and the other goes to the American Folklife Center at the Library of Congress to become part of an oral history of America. Many of these recorded reminiscences also air on National Public Radio. The goal of this project is to capture and chronicle ordinary life in our times, an undertaking comparable to the body of work produced by the Works Progress Administration (WPA) two generations ago.

Why not make your own recording? Check out www.nationaldayoflistening.org or www.storycorps.org for basics on where to record and what to ask. Sit down with a relative or a small family group and talk through topics of common interest. Reminiscing is good for older people's brains because it cements connections between time, memory, and events. We are living in a unique era, when three, four, or five generations may be alive at the same time, so take advantage of it to capture multi-generational recorded recollections, if you can.

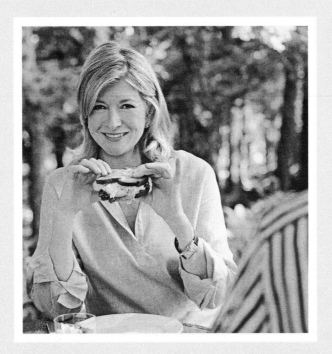

CHAPTER 5

Healthy Living Every Day

PRACTICE *prevention* 182

PAY ATTENTION *to aches and pains* 190

GET *the sleep you need* 194

KEEP UP *on maintenance* 200

MEDICATE *wisely* 223

Taking a preventive approach to health is vital to a good, long life. In 2007 I tore my labrum, the fibrous cartilage in the hip socket, while doing frog pose in yoga. After the injury I remember feeling horrible. I tried acupuncture, heat, a cortisone injection, and painkillers.

One doctor said, "Oh, it's just arthritis"; another said, "You'll need a hip replacement"; still another said, "It'll go away." But the pain didn't go away. In fact, it got worse. Finally, one doctor said, "Don't put this off—if you replace your hip now, you'll feel so much better and you'll heal 100 percent. If you wait a year, you'll heal 80 percent."

I had to make a decision, and I had to concede that I really was limping—I could see it in my television segments. So I interviewed doctors and had the operation. Within three days I was walking again and back at work. I did everything I could to recover, and worked through physical therapy every day.

The experience made me fearful of going through such an ordeal again, and letting my health get away from me. So I exercise and stretch (without straining) and eat right to protect the health of my bones and joints. But I will opt for another replacement if needed, because my new hip works very well. Plus, I now know that during recovery I can still lead an active life. That in itself is important prevention for so many other ailments, since the toll of being less mobile is far worse overall than the risks associated with certain surgeries.

PRACTICE *prevention*

Many of us are health procrastinators. Maybe you soldier through nagging pain in your hamstring or ignore the ache from that bunion or tennis elbow. Or maybe you put off getting a vision exam because everything seems to be okay. "An ache, a pain, or a symptom may seem trivial now, but few are truly without physical or psychological consequences in the long run," says Dr. Audrey Chun, director of geriatrics at Mount Sinai's Center for Living. Taking care of a minor annoyance now may prevent a permanent disability.

Here's a dramatization of a typical scenario: You ignore that corn on your toe, and don't mention it to your doctor because it seems so inconsequential. You're busy and have no time for a pedicure. Your foot hurts more and more, so you stop standing as much and drive or take the bus when you previously would have walked. Now your toe is permanently bent. Eventually, you forgo your regular exercise class and become increasingly chair-bound. Fast-forward several years or decades and your sedentary lifestyle takes its toll: you fall and break a hip. That fall was no accident; the seeds of disability were planted much earlier when that corn appeared. And that fall was probably preventable, if only you had taken care of that minor problem earlier.

Of course, no one wants to call a medical professional about each fleeting twinge. But there is a lot you can do daily to keep yourself healthier, now and in the future. This chapter begins with three general principles for living well today: practicing prevention, paying attention to aches and pains, and getting plenty of sleep—all of which are fundamental to healthy daily living and your overall wellness. Then it moves on to the specifics of preventing bigger health issues by maintaining your immune system, your eyes and mouth, your digestive system, your bladder, your sexual health, and your feet. If you're currently plagued by a health problem in one of these areas, you'll want to flip right to that section for tips on treatment. But these sections are worth a read even if you aren't currently experiencing a specific problem, because they'll give you a good idea of what to expect as you age and how you can best stave off serious health issues.

PUT A ROUTINE IN PLACE

Regular physical inventories can help keep you in tip-top shape and alert you to the start of a bigger problem. Make sure each of these checks is part of your routine.

DAILY CHECKLIST

☐ BALANCE

Rise up on your toes, then slowly lower down. Now lift your toes to stand on your heels, then lower toes back down. Finally, roll feet out to the sides of the foot and balance there for a moment, then roll inward to stand on the inner sides. Do this while you brush your teeth or wash dishes, or during any other routine standing activity; the "test" here is really just using your muscles, which are what stabilize your balance.

☐ FLEXIBILITY

Circle your shoulders, wrists, and ankles forward and backward. March in place, raising your knees up higher than your hips, then bend side to side, and forward and backward. Report any significant discomfort or changes in your range of motion to your doctor.

☐ URINE

Check that your urine is clear or straw colored every time you pee. This is a quick and clear indication that you're well hydrated (if not, drink more water!) and don't have any serious problems like a urinary tract infection or cancer. Let your doctor know if your urine has a strong odor, especially if you can't pinpoint it to a change in diet (like eating more asparagus than usual). And if there is blood in your urine, it is important to see your doctor immediately. "He or she will want to rule out bladder, urethral, or kidney cancer. In men, we would also want to rule out prostate cancer," says Dr. Michael A. Palese, associate professor of urology and director of minimally invasive surgery at Mount Sinai Medical Center.

For women: After you urinate, take a moment to practice Kegels (see About Kegel Exercises, page 214). Alternately tightening and relaxing the muscles of your pelvic can help prevent urinary incontinence. These pelvic floor muscles are what support your bladder and other pelvic organs.

For men: Observe any changes in your urinary habits. Are you noticing a slowing of the stream or incomplete emptying? Leakage just after urination? Do you have more frequency, intermittency, or urgency during the day? Is the urine stream becoming weaker? Are you straining to urinate or empty your bladder? How often do you get up during the night to urinate? If you note any of these symptoms, it's time to see your doctor. These can be early signs of benign prostatic hyperplasia (BPH), an enlargement of the prostate gland that occurs with age, as well as prostate cancer.

☐ BOWEL MOVEMENTS

Do a quick color check: if it's dark or tarry, or you see blood, contact your doctor. Blood in the stool can be a sign of many digestive-tract conditions, ranging from diverticulitis to polyps to hemorrhoids to colon cancer.

WEEKLY CHECKLIST

☐ **WEIGHT**

Getting on the scale once a week can prevent a 1- or 2-pound gain from becoming a 10-pound one. Small weight gains can easily be corrected by adjusting your diet or activity levels. You'll also be more likely to notice a sudden weight loss or gain, which can signal a more serious problem, such as fluid retention from congestive heart failure.

☐ **NAILS**

Think of them as ten little windows into your internal health. Heart valve infections can cause red streaks; liver disease leaves white lines; and brittle nails can be a sign of hypothyroidism. Stay alert to any dramatic changes in nail color and texture, and report them to your doctor.

☐ **FEET**

Injuries here heal slowly and can easily become infected. Check for sores, ingrown toenails, or blisters once a week as you're putting on your socks or shoes, as these can also affect balance and walking ability, which can in turn lead to joint and falling-related injuries. If you're diabetic, check your feet more often; damage to nerves may prevent you from actually feeling any soreness or discomfort and a sore may become infected. Use a small magnifying mirror for your checkup, if needed.

SET UP MEDICAL REMINDERS

If you tend to be forgetful when it comes to taking vitamins and medications—or even making it to doctor's appointments—consider setting up a system of reminders.

- If you're tech savvy, consider scheduling appointment reminders at reminderguru.com, a website that will send you e-mail, phone call, or text message reminders. A number of free or inexpensive phone apps are specifically designed for medical reminders. MedHelper (http://medhelperapp.com) tracks prescriptions, treatments, and schedules on Android phones. For iPhones, try RxmindMe Prescription Reminder (www.rxmind.me).

- If you prefer old-fashioned methods, a large wall calendar is the most obvious option; make sure it's big enough to write on and place it in a location that you walk by several times a day. For appointments, request that your doctor or dentist's office call you with reminders. If you need to take medication several times a day, set the kitchen timer to remind yourself. And don't forget to enlist the help of a trusted friend or family member—they'll bring a personal touch, no electricity required.

MONTHLY CHECKLIST

☐ MEASUREMENTS

Record your waist-to-hip ratio (WHR). This can help you keep your weight under control, and keeping a healthy weight can help prevent heart disease, diabetes, cancers, and other chronic conditions. In older adults, WHR may be a better predictor of who's at risk for a heart attack than body mass index (BMI), the classic estimate of an individual's body fat percentage based on weight and height.[1]

Simply measure your circumferences at these two points; divide your waist measurement by your hip measurement for your ratio. The ideal ratio for women is 0.8 or less; for men, 0.9. Check out www.bmi-calculator.net for an online WHR calculator.

☐ THYROID

Stand in front of a mirror and lift your chin. Now swallow (you may have to take a drink of water first). If there is a visible bulge along the side of your windpipe, just below your larynx, check in with your doctor. Swelling of the thyroid may indicate a tumor or thyroid disease.

☐ BREASTS

Lying in bed, place a pillow under your right shoulder; bend your elbow, and place your right hand behind your head. Using the middle three fingers of your left hand, trace small circles over the entire breast from your collarbone to your bra line and from your breastbone to where a dress seam would lie on your ribs. Move up and down in a series of parallel strips (imagine the lines a lawn mower would make), and use three levels of pressure on each area. Repeat on the other side. If you feel any thickening, lumpiness, tenderness, or puckering, or detect a bump, report it to your doctor immediately. (For a breast self-examination diagram, see page 332.)

☐ SKIN

Look for new moles and check existing ones for changes in size, shape, or color. Call your doctor if you notice any changes or if you have a sore that's taking a long time to heal in a sun-exposed part of the body, such as your outer ear, your chest, or the back of your hands. These may be early warning signs of skin cancer, the most common type of cancer. (For more on skin cancer, see page 235.)

☐ TEETH AND GUMS

Check for signs of gum disease: tenderness, puffiness, redness, bleeding after brushing, a change in the way partial dentures fit, recession (gums retracting so the roots of teeth are exposed), and any looseness or new gaps between teeth. These are all beginning signs of gum disease, the number-one cause of tooth loss, says Jeffrey Golub-Evans, DDS, of the New York Center for Cosmetic Dentistry. You should also tell your doctor if you spot open sores or pus in your mouth, changes in your bite or the way your dentures are fitting, or if you're experiencing bad breath that doesn't abate after cleansing. Changes in color should also be reported; teeth do darken slightly with the years, but color changes can also be a sign of large cavities, use of antibiotics (such as tetracycline), and high fevers.

☐ TESTICLES

Just after a shower, feel for any lumps or bumps by gently rolling each testicle between your fingers. A healthy testicle should feel and move like a peeled hard-boiled egg inside the scrotum.

GET YOUR SHOTS

Approximately 50,000 to 70,000 Americans die each year from vaccine-preventable diseases, including 40,000 flu-related deaths annually—95 percent of which occur in adults 60 and over, according to Dr. Gregory Poland, director of the Vaccine Research Group at the Mayo Clinic in Rochester, Minnesota.

The Centers for Disease Control and Prevention (CDC) recommends the following vaccines for adults aged 50 and older:

THE SHOT	WHO SHOULD HAVE IT	WHY	SPECIAL CONSIDERATIONS
INFLUENZA	Anyone 50 and older	The flu virus is constantly evolving from season to season, so an annual dose is recommended.	Speak to your doctor if you are allergic to eggs, or have had a bad reaction to a previous flu shot.
PNEUMONIA	Anyone 65 and older; adults over 50 with health conditions	Pneumococcal pneumonia can cause fever and respiratory problems.	If you have chronic lung or heart disease, diabetes, lymphoma, leukemia, or asthma, consider this shot if you're 50+ (these conditions make you more susceptible to pneumonia). If you smoke, get the shot.
TDAP (TETANUS, DIPTHERIA AND PERTUSSIS)	Adults 65 and older should get it if in contact with young children	A resurgence of pertussis ("whooping cough") has led to a CDC recommendation that adults 50 to 64 receive a booster immunization.	Get vaccinated, especially if you have young grandchildren or frequently spend time around infants.
ZOSTER (SHINGLES)	Adults 50 and older	Age is the primary risk factor for shingles.	If you have never had chickenpox or been immunized, get vaccinated to avoid catching shingles or infecting a child.

THE SHOT	WHO SHOULD HAVE IT	WHY	SPECIAL CONSIDERATIONS
MMR (MEASLES, MUMPS, RUBELLA)	Adults 50 and older who are unsure of their immunization status	Most adults 50 and older have either been exposed to these diseases or received a vaccination in childhood.	Getting a booster shot is cost-effective (about $35 per shot; likely to be covered by insurance) and isn't harmful, even if you're already immune.
HEPATITIS A	Adults age 50 and older	This virus causes liver disease.	Those who have chronic liver disease, close contact with someone with hepatitis A, or who travel to areas with a high incidence should get the shot.
HEPATITIS B	Adults 50 and older who are on dialysis, or who have renal disease or liver disease	This is another virus that can cause liver disease.	Talk to your doctor if you're unsure of your immunization status; getting a booster may be a good idea.
MENINGITIS	Adults 50 and older who were never vaccinated	Individual risk varies; consult your doctor.	Adults 55 and younger: meningococcal conjugate vaccine, which offers lifelong immunity.

Adults 56 and older: polysaccharide vaccine, which offers three to five years of immunity. |

SCREENING TESTS

We all need to monitor our health more closely as we age, and though screening tests can be a pain to schedule, they truly are some of the best weapons in your preventive health arsenal. If you're being screened for major health problems regularly, you'll have the peace of mind that comes from a clear result. And if problems arise, you'll know you're catching them as early as possible, giving you the best possible chance of a speedy recovery.

TEST TYPE	SCHEDULE
Dental cleaning and oral exam	Every 6 months
Eye exam	Every 2–4 years in 40s and 50s; annually starting at 65
Self breast exam/self testicle exam	Monthly
Mammogram & clinical breast exam	Annually, starting at 40; discuss with your doctor after age 80
Pap smear and pelvic exam	Every 1–3 years, more frequently after abnormal Pap; at 70, you may choose to stop having Paps if you've had no abnormal results in ten years prior
Full cholesterol panel	Annually
Blood pressure	Annually
Thyroid test (women only)	Every 5 years; after age 80, discuss with your doctor
Fecal occult blood test	Annually, starting at 50
Colonoscopy	Every 5–10 years, starting at 50; after age 80 discuss with doctor

TEST TYPE	SCHEDULE
Prostate Specific Antigen test	Annually, beginning at 45; after age 80, discuss with doctor
Bone density (DEXA) (women only)	Every 2 years, beginning at menopause; after age 80, discuss with doctor
Skin exam	Annually, starting at 40; every 6 months if you've had any suspicious moles removed
Hearing test	Every 10 years starting at 40; every 3 years starting at 80
Blood pressure screening	Annually; every 2 years starting at 80
Abdominal aortic aneurysm test	Once between 65 and 75 if you ever smoked; annually after 75

PAY ATTENTION *to aches and pains*

A twinge, some stiffness, an ache—these minor annoyances may become more frequent with age and take longer to heal. The following suggestions should take care of most problems, but if they don't, you'll need to get to the bottom of that pain with your doctor.

SOOTHE SORE MUSCLES

Exercise can decrease pain levels, boost your body's production of inflammation-fighting hormones, and moderate anxiety, but it can also exacerbate muscle soreness. Thankfully, there are a variety of ways to mitigate this discomfort.

REST YOUR MUSCLES

Pay attention to how you feel as you're moving, and don't try to push past muscle pain or fatigue. If your arms and legs feel depleted or your back is tight, these are signs you need to rest. A pulled muscle can sideline you for weeks.

USE ICE FIRST

If you do strain or sprain a muscle, ice can reduce swelling and inflammation as well as soothe pain. Wrap a cloth around an ice pack and apply it to your skin for 10 minutes, then remove for 10 minutes, then reapply for another 10. (The on-off approach will protect your skin from damage.) Keep a flexible gel pack in your freezer; in a pinch, a bag of frozen vegetables is a suitable stand-in.

TAKE A WARM BATH

A warm-water soak can help ease muscle soreness. Add 10 to 15 drops of lavender oil (traditionally used for joint and muscle pain) plus a half-cup of Epsom salts to a tubful of warm water. Warm water may also be a good place to stretch and strengthen your muscles. Water creates gentle resistance when you move, which helps build muscle strength, and its buoyancy makes exercise easier and more comfortable. Try swimming or water aerobics, and look for a facility with a heated pool.

TREAT CHRONIC PAIN

Some aches and pains can signal more serious problems, such as an injury to a tendon or ligament or even rheumatoid arthritis.[2] If you're experiencing symmetrical joint pain (on both sides of the body), joint pain with inflammation, or joint pain with fever, see your doctor.

KEEP JOINTS SUPPLE AND PAIN-FREE

It's common for your joints to become stiffer as you age, but there are ways to keep that from limiting mobility. Here are some things to try:

MOVE YOUR BODY

The very best prevention against annoying but inevitable aches and pains is to keep active. It may sound counterintuitive, but moving joints releases a lubricating, cushioning fluid that loosens up creakiness. Low-impact activities with smooth movements, such as swimming, kayaking, cycling, and spin classes, keep joints flexible. If joint pain is a problem, avoid activities that require quick changes in direction and stops or jumps, such as tennis or squash. And walk whenever you have the opportunity, because studies show walking helps preserve mobility in general. As you stroll along, focus on posture; correct alignment helps prevent pain and injury.

USE WET HEAT FIRST

A hot shower or even a warm, wet towel applied to an achy joint or stiff muscle can help loosen it up. Follow with some slow stretches to ease yourself into movement.

TRY MEDICATION

If you're still aching, take acetaminophen first. This over-the-counter pain reliever, found in brands such as Tylenol and Anacin-3, is safe and effective for ongoing pain, according to an FDA review of hundreds of pain relief studies. One caution: don't take it in combination with cold and flu remedies that already contain acetaminophen. An overdose (more than 4,000 mg a day) could severely damage your liver. But overall, acetaminophen is a better choice than aspirin, ibuprofen, naproxen, or other nonsteroidal anti-inflammatory drugs (NSAIDs), which may cause abdominal pain, diarrhea, or liver damage, and even lead to ulcers in about 15 percent of chronic NSAID users. NSAIDS can also interact negatively with blood thinners and other medications, so be sure to consult your doctor before using.

TAKE SUPPLEMENTS

Omega-3 fatty acids (the fats found in cold-water fish such as salmon) can ease arthritis pain, according to some research studies. The capsules may also ease neck and back pain; in one University of Pittsburgh study, 1,200 to 2,400 mg taken daily was as effective as a NSAID in reducing joint pain in 60 percent of test subjects.[3]

CONSIDER LOSING WEIGHT

If you're overweight, shedding extra pounds may help ease symptoms, as your hips and knees bear the brunt of your body's weight. For every pound you gain, your knees gain 3 to 4 pounds of added stress; for your hips, each additional pound translates into six times the pressure on these joints. Many years of carrying extra pounds can cause the cartilage that cushions your joints to break down, resulting in arthritis.

EASE AN ACHING BACK

Back pain is one of the leading causes of disability in the United States. If you're plagued by chronic pain, you should see an orthopedist. An MRI and other diagnostic tools can be used to assess your situation and help determine appropriate treatment if a concrete issue like a herniated disc, strained muscle, osteopenia, or arthritis is causing your distress.

In as many as 85 percent of cases, however, doctors are unable to pinpoint a cause of low back pain, says a 2010 *New England Journal of Medicine* report. Lifestyle and environmental factors like stress, poor posture, lack of exercise, and a job that requires you to hunch over a computer can all play a key role. If your back pain seems to be lifestyle related, doing your best to mitigate those circumstances (getting a better desk chair, taking frequent breaks from your computer, and so on) will help. But you might also want to pursue one of the following mind/body therapies, which can ease physical symptoms and improve how you process stress at the same time:

CHIROPRACTIC CARE

They've been around since the 1890s, but the medical community has long scorned chiropractors because their foundational theory—that a misaligned spine is the root of most medical problems—couldn't be scientifically proven. But according to the National Center for Complementary and Alternative Medicine, new research suggests that introducing a jolt of movement to the spine (the "manipulations" that a chiropractor performs) stimulates neurons in surrounding tissues, sending a message up the spinal cord to the brain to ease pain. In 2007 guidelines, the American Pain Society and American College of Physicians recommended spinal manipulation for low back pain that has persisted longer than a month. Find a practitioner at www.acatoday.org.

ALTERNATIVE THERAPIES

Consider acupressure, acupuncture, Reiki, and guided imagery to address your back pain issues. While studies on back pain and acupuncture have not definitively proven that inserting needles relieves pain, it may help. Researchers think the therapeutic intervention may stimulate the release of feel-good endorphin neurochemicals, which combat pain.

THE ALEXANDER TECHNIQUE

Somatic education therapies like Alexander teach you how to skillfully move your body through life while putting as little stress as possible on your muscles and joints. An Alexander teacher will start by investigating how you hold your head, because if the head isn't properly balanced, the cervical spine will compress, sending pain down to the lumbar spine and hips, and even all the way to your feet. A large randomized study published in the U.K. in 2008 vouched for the Alexander Technique's effectiveness in reducing back pain in almost six hundred sufferers.[4] Find a teacher at www.alexandertech.com.

SLEEP FOR A BETTER BACK

If you're sleeping in the wrong position, you may be forcing your spine out of alignment and compressing tight muscles or nerves for hours every night. No wonder your nightly slumber can contribute to pain in the neck and low back (along with a host of other ailments like numbness in your arms and fingers and chronic shallow breathing). The ideal sleeping position is on your back with no pillow, as this allows your spine to rest with its natural curves in place. But if you can't fall asleep in that position, try these suggestions:

IF YOU SLEEP ON YOUR SIDE

Look for a pillow that fills the space between your ear and the outer edge of your shoulder while you are lying on your side, while keeping both sides of your neck equally long. This promotes easier breathing and prevents you from overstretching one side of your neck. Place a second pillow (6 to 8 inches high) between your knees to keep you from hiking your leg up, which rotates the pelvis and contorts the lower spine.

IF YOU SLEEP ON YOUR STOMACH

Try to become a side sleeper, at the very least! Sleeping on your stomach is the worst position for your spine because it flattens the natural curve in the lower back and keeps your head turned to one side all night, which distorts the alignment of the spine in your neck. All of this can lead to chronic lower back pain, neck pain, and headaches. And because your body weight compresses your lungs, stomach sleeping also impedes your ability to breathe deeply. Instead, try lying on your side and placing a body pillow between your knees and hugging it with your arms to mimic the pressure offered by stomach sleeping without losing your spine alignment or compressing nerves and organs.

IF YOU SLEEP ON YOUR BACK AND LOVE THICK PILLOWS

Sleeping on a thick pillow pushes your head forward, exactly opposite the natural curve of the spine in the neck, which can lead to neck pain and headaches. Swap your big pillow for the thinnest pillow you can stand (soft down compresses the most). And if you wake up frequently with neck aches, try swapping that pillow for a neck roll (make one by tightly rolling a hand towel). Place the neck roll under the back of your neck for a few minutes to reset the spinal curve and ward off further pain, then go back to sleep using your usual pillow.

IF YOU SLEEP ON A MATTRESS THAT'S TOO SOFT OR HARD

There's no conclusive evidence that sleeping on a hard or soft mattress is better for the back, but many experts agree—not surprisingly—that you should sleep on what makes your back feel best. If you wake up with back pain after sleeping on a soft mattress, you may want to switch to a firmer bed or futon. Likewise, if sleeping on something rock hard leaves your back in knots, try adding a body-conforming foam pad to your bedding. If you share your bed with a partner, you may want to consider purchasing an adjustable-firmness mattress so each of you can customize your side of the bed.

GET *the sleep you need*

After age 55, sleep patterns change as your body clock resets itself and levels of hormones, such as growth hormones and melatonin, decline. You may find that you're tired earlier in the evening, that it takes you longer to drift off to sleep, and that you sleep less (and wake up more often) at night. The average person needs seven to eight hours of sleep. However, some people feel deprived if they get fewer than nine hours, while others are sluggish if they sleep more than five hours. Be sensitive to the fact that your needs change with the years. Physical conditions, medications, and depression can also sabotage sleep. Pain from surgery or joint inflammation also tends to worsen when you lie down because of the redistribution of blood flow in the prone position.

BE MINDFUL OF SLEEP CHANGES

As you age, it's not uncommon to experience shifts in your sleep patterns. Beyond the common sleep changes that come with age, you'll want to pay attention to more serious disorders that can affect your ability to get the deep, restorative sleep you need every night. See your doctor if you suspect you may suffer from any of the following:

SLEEP APNEA Sufferers of this disorder stop breathing—anywhere from 10 to 30 seconds—multiple times in the night. The condition generally causes you to snore very loudly, and wake up each time you gasp for a new breath, preventing you from achieving deep sleep. The disorder can lead to heart attack, high blood pressure, even death. Treatments include losing weight (if you're overweight), wearing a sleeping mask designed to keep airways open, and in some cases surgery. If you suffer from this condition, stop drinking alcohol or taking sleeping medications.

RESTLESS LEGS SYNDROME (RLS) This condition causes a creeping or aching sensation in the legs, particularly when you're lying or sitting down, and sufferers often feel the need to move their legs to stop the unpleasant sensation. This constant movement and pain often cause insomnia. RLS commonly occurs in people who also suffer from diabetes, chronic kidney disease, and Parkinson's disease, and in those with iron deficiency. Although there is no known cure, stretching, massage, and warm baths help some sufferers.

PERIODIC LIMB MOVEMENT DISORDER (PLMD) A movement disorder, PLMD causes legs or arms to move sporadically. Sufferers may not even realize they're kicking, but the movement can prevent you from falling into deep sleep. Those with RLS may also experience PLMD. Although there is no cure for the disorder, anti-Parkinson's disease medications can reduce or eliminate symptoms.

HOW SLEEP DEPRIVATION TAKES ITS TOLL

While it may seem like losing sleep isn't such a big deal, sleep deprivation has a wide range of negative consequences for your body and mind. Research suggests that only about a third of Americans get the seven to nine hours of shut-eye required to help keep their immune systems operating at full throttle. A study from Carnegie Mellon University found that those who averaged fewer than seven hours a night were three times more likely to catch a cold than those who clocked eight or more hours regularly. One potential explanation is that we produce the hormone melatonin during nighttime sleep, which prompts a key type of immune cell to destroy infected ones. Over time, less sleep leads to less melatonin secretion and a compromised immune system.

Perhaps more insidious are the effects that lack of sleep has on the mind. While you're snoozing, your brain generates new neurons, solidifies memories, and makes connections between old information and new. Princeton University researchers found that rats who were deprived of sleep for 72 hours formed significantly fewer new brain cells in the hippocampus than their well-rested counterparts, possibly because the tired rats produced more of the stress hormone cortisol, a chemical that's deadly to neurons. A number of studies conducted at Harvard from 2000 to 2005 reveal that students were better at remembering things they learned the day before if they had at least six hours of sleep—and far better if they logged a full eight hours.

You may be experiencing sleep deprivation if you suffer from any of the following symptoms.

- Fatigue, lethargy, and lack of motivation
- Moodiness and irritability
- Reduced creativity and skills involving problem-solving and decision-making
- Inability to cope with stress
- Reduced immunity; frequent colds and infections
- Concentration and memory problems
- Weight gain
- Impaired motor skills and increased risk of accidents
- Difficulty making decisions
- Increased inflammation
- Increased risk for cardiovascular disease, arthritis, and diabetes mellitus

PRACTICE GOOD SLEEP

The following schedule offers good guidelines for most people; adjust it to meet your individual sleep needs and to rise earlier or sleep in later.

6AM TO 12PM

WAKE UP AT THE SAME TIME If you're getting enough sleep, you should wake up naturally, without an alarm. If you need an alarm clock to wake up on time, you may need to set an earlier bedtime.

GET OUTSIDE Taking a walk or sitting outside to read the paper keeps your body's natural sleep/wake rhythm calibrated. Light enters the eye through the retina; this light-sensitive nerve tissue is directly wired to the master switch in the brain that controls your sleep/wake cycle. If you can't get outside, consider purchasing a desktop light box with a light output of at least 10,000 lux (a measure of light intensity).

12PM TO 6PM

SWITCH TO DECAF Drink herbal tea or water instead of coffee or tea after lunch. With age, you become more sensitive to caffeine, so even the small amount found in chocolate or colas can keep you up at night. Caffeine blocks a neurochemical called adenosine, which helps you feel drowsy.

HYDRATE Aim to drink most of your fluids during the day so you're less thirsty right before bed. This will make you less likely to wake up during the night because you need to urinate.

6PM TO 9PM

DEFY DROWSINESS If you find yourself getting sleepy hours before your bedtime, get off the couch and do something mildly occupying but not too stimulating, such as folding clothes or calling a friend. If you give in to drowsiness after dinner and let yourself conk out while reading or watching TV, you may wake up later in the night and have trouble getting back to sleep.

TAKE A BATH A warm soak two hours before you turn in is naturally soporific. Your blood vessels dilate to release excess heat—part of the natural cooling down of body temperature that precedes sleep. Just don't steep for too long (15 minutes is sufficient) or your skin can dry out.

9PM TO 12AM

RESERVE YOUR BED FOR SLEEPING Keep your bedroom free of work files, bills, and other clutter that will make it harder to wind down at night. Use your bed only for sleep and sex, so when you go to bed, your body gets a powerful cue: it's time to nod off.

SCENT YOUR SHEETS A single drop of lavender essential oil on your pillow or a spritz of lavender water on bedclothes can ease you off to dreamland. A study at the University of Leicester in England, as well as the Smell and Taste Treatment and Research Foundation in Chicago, found that this botanical can be as effective as medications used for easing insomnia.

SET A REGULAR TURN-IN TIME Go to bed at the same time every night. Stick to this schedule, even on weekends and vacations. Choose a time when you normally feel tired, so that you don't toss and turn.

KEEP YOUR BEDROOM DARK With the passing years, your brain experiences less delta-wave activity during sleep.[5] This leads to a greater sensitivity to light, from any source: moonlight, streetlight, early dawns, and late sunsets. Use heavy shades or curtains, charge electronics in another room, and turn the alarm clock to the wall. At the very least, use a sleep mask.

12AM TO 6AM

BLOCK OUT NOISE Even if you think you've learned to sleep through certain noises, such as sirens or airplanes passing overhead, studies show that these still disrupt your sleep. And the age-related decrease in delta-wave activity makes us even more sensitive to outside rumblings. If you can't avoid or eliminate such noise, try masking it with a fan, recordings of soothing sounds, or white noise, which can block out distracting sounds and aid sleep. White noise machines are widely available, or you can download sounds at www.freewhite noise.com or www.simplynoise.com.

KEEP A NOTEPAD BY YOUR BED The classic scenario for a night of lost sleep is to wake up during the wee hours and start worrying. Recognize there's little you can do at that time; calmly make a note of it, and tell yourself you'll

work to resolve the issue in the morning. Likewise, if you have a brilliant idea in the middle of the night, jot it down and fall back to sleep knowing you can be inspired by it tomorrow. Many cell phones and PDAs also have voice memo capacity that acts as a tape recorder.

TRAIN YOURSELF BACK TO SLEEP The key to getting back to sleep is continuing to cue your body for sleep, and for that you need to lie in bed in a relaxed position. It may be tough, but don't start stressing about the fact that you're awake and unable to fall back to sleep. Such thoughts only stimulate your brain, delaying sleep onset that much more. Instead, lie still and focus on your breathing. Note how your body feels. If your goal is relaxation and rest—not sleep—chances are, you'll drift off.

FIGHT FATIGUE

If you're practicing good sleep routines and still feeling weary and unrested more days than not, you may find the following strategies helpful.

BOOST YOUR INTAKE OF B VITAMINS

This family of vitamins—B_1 (thiamine), B_2 (riboflavin), B_3 (niacin), B_5 (pantothenic acid), biotin, B_{12} (cobalamin), and folate—is vital for the production of such neurotransmitters as dopamine and serotonin (responsible for modulating mood). Cover your B needs with a varied diet of lean meats, colorful vegetables, and whole grains.[6]

TAKE A WALK

Expending a little energy can actually give you energy. In research comparing more than seventy studies on exercise, researchers at the University of Georgia in Athens found that those who added an activity, such as a daily walk, experienced improved energy levels. Exercise even boosted energy in those suffering from serious medical conditions such as cancer, chronic fatigue syndrome, and depression.

BUILD SOME MUSCLE

Increasing your muscle mass and strength builds your body's energy reserves and stamina so you can meet the physical challenges of life. Never lifted weights? Check out the chair moves in Chapter 2 (page 118) to help you ease into a strengthening routine.

HYDRATE

With age, the body's thirst mechanism is less reliable, and dehydration may cause you to feel sleepy. Drink a glass of water when you wake up, drink at each meal, and sip throughout the day to stay hydrated. Water is the essential medium for all your body's chemical reactions.

RELAX

Stress can sap your energy. Try yoga, meditation, or even just sitting quietly in nature. Visiting your local church or synagogue during off-hours may also provide a soothing sanctuary.

SEE A PROFESSIONAL IF NECESSARY

Always report serious fatigue to your doctor. Depression, thyroid disease, cardiovascular problems, respiratory problems, blood loss, and blood dysfunction (like anemia) all are landmarked by fatigue. Also consult your doctor if you (or your partner) are troubled by snoring, frequent morning headaches, restless legs, or crawling sensations in your legs or arms. Your doctor can diagnose and treat any related health problems and may prescribe a sleep aid. If you suffer from chronic insomnia, ask your doctor to refer you for behavioral counseling. Patients who tried this counseling reported improvement in sleep after four weeks—and these benefits persisted at a six-month follow-up, according to a study published in the *Archives of Internal Medicine*.[7]

NATURAL SLEEP REMEDIES

For occasional insomnia, the following herbs and supplements (found at natural-food stores) may be especially effective. Be sure to discuss supplements you're interested in with your health-care practitioner before you take them.

VALERIAN

Probably the most well-known herb for sleep, valerian works by calming the nerves and relaxing the muscles. Since it's often described as smelling like dirty socks, take it "down the hatch" as a dropperful of tincture or in capsule form rather than sipping it as a tea. Keep in mind that for some people, valerian has a stimulating effect; try it on a weekend, just in case. You'll know quickly whether valerian works for you. If you're taking sedatives or medicine for depression or anxiety, use valerian only under the guidance of a health-care professional.

MELATONIN

This supplement is synthesized to match a hormone produced within the pineal gland, a pea-sized organ in our brain that regulates the body's internal clock. Melatonin supplements may help balance circadian rhythm. Because melatonin is a hormone, it should be used with caution; though 3 mg supplements are commonly sold in stores, some doctors advise patients to start with a dosage of 1 mg. As with valerian, you should notice the effects of melatonin quickly.

L-THEANINE

Found naturally in green tea, this amino acid raises levels of GABA (gamma-aminobutyric acid), a relaxation-inducing chemical in our brains, and can ease anxiety-induced insomnia without grogginess.

SLEEP-INDUCING TEA

For a relaxing bedtime beverage, you could try combining several herbs as follows: passionflower and skullcap soothe agitated nervous systems and can help with mental chatter; oat seed strengthens the nervous system and helps people who are too tired to sleep; and chamomile provides a gently relaxing base.

- 1 chamomile tea bag
- 30 to 60 drops passionflower tincture
- 15 to 30 drops skullcap tincture
- 15 to 30 drops milky oat seed (*Avena sativa*) tincture

Pour boiling water over tea bag, and let steep for 5 minutes. Remove tea bag, and add drops of tinctures to tea. Stir in a touch of honey if desired. Sip and enjoy.

KEEP UP *on maintenance*

To function at its best, the body requires regular upkeep. Maintaining different aspects of your health is much easier in the long run than recovering from an ailment resulting from neglect. Here's a blueprint for keeping everything going strong.

YOUR IMMUNE SYSTEM

With age, your immune system becomes more fallible, leaving you increasingly vulnerable to viral attack. The older you get, the more likely a seemingly benign cold or flu is a precursor to a more serious condition, such as pneumonia or bronchitis. That goes double for the flu—most flu fatalities occur in adults over 65. Here's how to stave off many illnesses:

WASH YOUR HANDS

Whenever you wash your hands, sing "Happy Birthday" to yourself twice to ensure that you've scrubbed for the recommended 30 seconds to dislodge germs. Any kind of soap will get the job done; it doesn't have to be antibacterial to clear germs from your skin. You should soap up after using the bathroom and before meals or food prep; wash more often during cold and flu season.

SNEEZE INTO YOUR SLEEVE

Stop sneezing into your hands; instead, aim for the crook of your elbow or your shoulder. That way you don't touch your nose, eyes, or mouth with your hand, so you'll be less likely to pass on germs.

AVOID EXCESSIVE GERMS

You can't avoid all pathogens, nor should you try; think of them as exercise for your immune system. Continuous exposure to germs keeps you strong and ensures that your immune system is continually stimulating new cell growth. You can avoid the most common accumulation points for germs: faucets, light switches, door handles, cutting boards, and sponges. If you need a stand-in for a sink, alcohol-based hand sanitizers will do the trick. You can also use disinfectant wipes to sanitize armrests and the folding table on airplanes, as well as phones, light switches, and TV remotes. But skip antibacterial products that contain triclosan; the chemical may be playing a role in our increasing antibiotic resistance problem.

IMMUNE BOOSTERS

As we age, our immune systems weaken, and our risk of contracting illness increases. Research suggests that raising nutrient intakes to adequate levels helps the immune system function normally. Talk to your doctor about whether you'd benefit from supplementation or taking a daily multivitamin, or from adding any of the following to your medical regimen.

VITAMIN D

Vitamin D is key to regulating the immune system, preventing it from overreacting and reducing inflammation oxidation (which produces cold and flu symptoms). This vitamin also stimulates the production of cells that line the respiratory tract and help prevent infection.[8] Twenty minutes of sun exposure on bare skin helps your body manufacture vitamin D, but the processing machinery in skin slows down with age. The Institute of Medicine (www.iom.edu) recommends that older adults take 600 IU of vitamin D daily. Over the age of 70, the dose jumps to 800 IU daily, to improve bone health.

VITAMIN E

This powerful antioxidant potentially fights off upper-respiratory infections. A study from Boston's Tufts University found that when elderly subjects increased their intake of vitamin E to 200 IU a day, they had significantly fewer colds than those who did not supplement.[9] Look for vitamin E in supplement form or in foods such as sunflower seeds, almonds, peanuts, and tomatoes, as well as in healthy polyunsaturated oils such as safflower and canola.

PROBIOTICS

These good bacteria ease digestion but also strengthen the immune system, helping prevent flu and other illnesses. Look for yogurt, kefir, kombucha, and other products with "live and active cultures" on the label. You could also look for probiotic supplements at a natural health food store.

FIBER

Soluble fiber promotes the formation and growth of probiotics (see above). Fiber-rich foods, such as bananas, almonds, artichokes, onions, and garlic, will help stimulate probiotic growth.

CATECHINS

Most commonly found in green tea, catechins are plant compounds that halt oxidative damage to cells. Steep tea for 3 to 5 minutes to get the full benefits and flavor it with fresh ginger (another anti-inflammatory) and pomegranate seeds (powerful antioxidants).

ELECTROLYTES

Staying well hydrated helps the body ward off illness. Coconut water contains the same balance of electrolytes as your body, so it may keep you better hydrated than regular tap water.

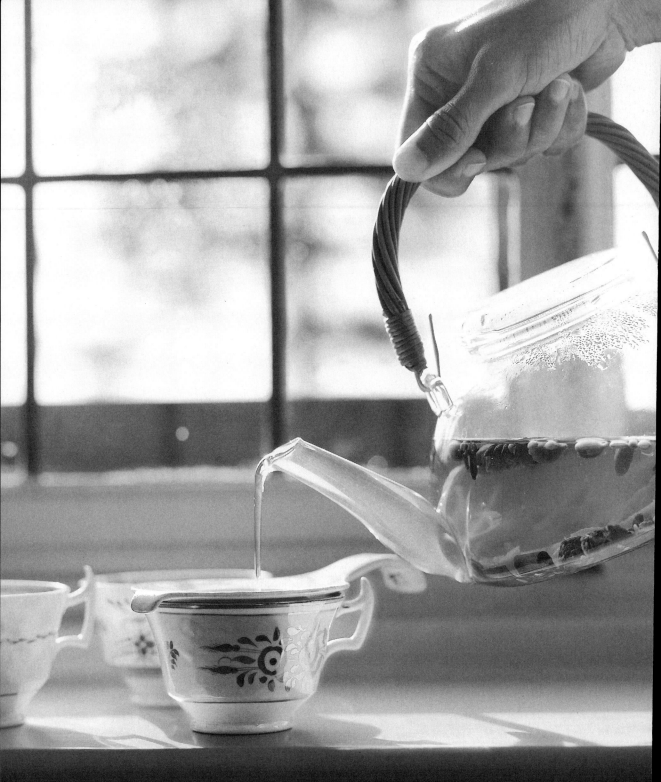

HOW I STAY HEALTHY THROUGH FLU SEASON

I can't let myself get sick—with my busy schedule, there's just no allowance for it. So I take a preventive approach to health, and always stay on top of early symptoms. As a result, I rarely miss a single day of work.

It's very important to keep my immune system in top shape, so in addition to essential preventive measures, like exercising every morning and eating healthfully, I have a few reliable strategies.

First, I get a flu shot every year—that is essential. I wash my hands thoroughly and often with natural soap (made with fats and oils, not synthetic detergents), which is important because I meet so many people. When I travel, I carry a natural hand sanitizer. I also get regular massages; though it sounds indulgent, it's an excellent way to manage stress, which can really compromise the immune system.

For sore throats, I prefer the old-fashioned remedy of gargling with salt water. I also rely on natural remedies, such as zinc lozenges, Flew Away, and InflamAway, to bolster my immune system during the germ-filled winter months.

But really, no remedy is as good as rest when you really need it. That's never been my strong suit, but I do take naps when I need to. Ten minutes is all I need to help maintain my energy during the day.

YOUR EYE HEALTH

You don't have to put on a pair of reading glasses to know that vision starts to shift after age 40. The structure of our eyes changes as we age, and conditions such as cataracts, macular degeneration, and glaucoma become more common. But lest you fear that severe vision problems are inevitable, research is proving that detecting these conditions early on can literally save your sight.

GET AN ANNUAL CHECKUP

Yearly screenings are optional until the age of 65; after that, an annual trip to the eye doctor is highly recommended. The earlier an eye disease is detected, the more of your vision that can be saved. Your ophthalmologist or optician should dilate your pupils, assess your eye pressure, test your eyesight and your eye muscles, and evaluate your eyeglasses or contacts.

WEAR SHADES OUTSIDE

Think of sunglasses as sunblock for the eyes. Wear them year-round to shade your eyes from the sun's damaging UVA and UVB rays. The most protective styles feature close-fitting lenses, such as wraparounds. Darker lenses aren't necessarily more protective; look for brands labeled 99 to 100 percent UV-protective. If you have a pair you like, but aren't sure how protective they are, have their UV-protection level checked at an optical shop; most have a machine called a photometer that gauges UV blocking levels. Consider photochromic lenses, which darken when hit by UV rays, eliminating the need for prescription sunglasses.

UPDATE YOUR PRESCRIPTION

You won't damage your eyes by wearing an incorrect or outdated prescription, but you will stress them and you do run the risk of injuring yourself due to not seeing clearly. Bring all your glasses and contacts to your annual appointment so they can be assessed. Feel as if you need "stronger" glasses? That means that you may need a prescription with more than one lens. For example, bifocals have a lens with a distance prescription on the top, and a reading lens (commonly in the shape of a half-moon) at the bottom.

If you work on the computer, you can have middle-distance lenses put into your prescription; often, these are called progressive lenses, because the lens type changes as your eye moves downward, from distance on top, intermediate distance in the middle, to reading at the bottom.

MOISTURIZE DRY EYES

Tears are your eyes' natural lubricant, but aging, stress, and even medications can reduce this organic protection, leaving eyes feeling gritty and scratchy. Long term, you may risk eye damage, pain, and vision loss. Talk to your doctor about your symptoms. One easy fix is to use over-the-counter artificial tears.

You can also station a humidifier in your home to boost the moisture content of the air during drier months. Schedule regular blink breaks if you spend time in front of the computer or the TV. Studies show that the average blink rate drops from twelve to six times a minute while you're glued to the screen. Look away regularly and blink to replenish tears. Finally, getting lots of omega-3 fatty acids (found in fish and flaxseed) may help eye symptoms, according to a Harvard Medical School study of more than 32,000 women.

EAT FOR VISION

A diet rich in leafy green vegetables and fatty fish may be one of your best defenses against eye-related diseases. A 2011 study published in the *Archives of Ophthalmology* showed that fewer older Americans are developing macular degeneration, and this is largely attributed to improved diet. Proper nutrition can also help ward off other disorders, such as glaucoma and cataracts.

USE SENSIBLE LIGHTING

With age, your pupils, which control the amount of light that reaches the retina, become smaller and less responsive to variations in light. A decrease in pupil diameter makes responding to abrupt changes in light level harder. You may require more time to adjust to changing levels of illumination, such as going from bright sunshine into a dimly lit room or restaurant, or the other way around, notes Julie Kardachi, of Fall Stop . . . Move Strong. Here are some smart ideas to cope (see also Illuminate Your Space on page 289):

- Increase the amount of ambient light throughout your home.
- Use individual lights—or task lighting—in specific areas for specific jobs, such as on your desk, over the kitchen countertops, or on bedside tables for reading.
- Use timed lighting that switches on and off at set times of the day to ensure consistent ambient lighting.

COMMON AGE-RELATED EYE CONDITIONS

It helps to understand if changes to the eyes are the result of a disease or the inevitable result of aging. Here's a primer on the three most common age-related ocular conditions:

CATARACTS

WHAT IT IS These growths cloud the clear lens of your eye, causing blurring of vision or worse. Your overall vision becomes foggy.

WHO'S AT RISK Age, family history, and having diabetes, myopia, or high blood pressure all elevate your risk for cataracts. In addition, chronic, unprotected exposure to sunlight or ionizing radiation (such as X-rays) increases the likelihood you'll develop them, as does taking corticosteroids for many years (often prescribed for multiple sclerosis, rheumatoid arthritis, and lupus).

HOW TO PROTECT YOUR VISION Maintaining a healthy weight and managing any complicating conditions (diabetes, hypertension) may lower your risk. A diet rich in vegetables and fruits may help, too. Antioxidants in pill form have yet to be proven effective against cataracts, however. Protecting your eyes by wearing sunglasses may also slow the development of cataracts. Surgery, in which the natural lens is replaced by a plastic lens that eventually becomes a part of the eye, generally restores vision.

GLAUCOMA

WHAT IT IS Glaucoma involves an increase in the pressure of the fluid inside the eyeball that damages the optic nerve, leading to loss of sight, starting in the periphery of your vision. Your risk of developing the condition increases each decade after age 40, from around 1 percent in your forties to up to 12 percent in your eighties.

WHO'S AT RISK African-Americans and Hispanics are more likely to develop glaucoma than Caucasians. Genetics may also play a role; if you have a family history, you're more likely to be diagnosed with it. Conditions such as diabetes and high blood pressure are also associated with higher rates of incidence. If you've taken corticosteroids (for multiple sclerosis, arthritis, or lupus), you may be more prone to glaucoma.

HOW TO PROTECT YOUR VISION Get your pressure tested by your eye doctor annually. As for lifestyle modifications, pace your fluid intake. Drinking large quantities in a short amount of time may increase the pressure inside your eye. Exercise may also reduce eye pressure for certain types of glaucoma; if you've been diagnosed, make sure your doctor tells you the exact type of glaucoma. Prescription eye drops (to reduce internal pressure) and oral medications may slow the progression of glaucoma. Laser or conventional surgery may also be a treatment option.

MACULAR DEGENERATION

WHAT IT IS Also called age-related macular degeneration, or AMD, this is a leading cause of vision loss among American seniors. At advanced stages, this condition can lead to vision loss in the center of your eyesight. There are two types: Wet AMD is caused when new blood vessels under the macula leak blood and fluid. Dry AMD is caused when light-sensititve cells in the macula break down, blurring vision. The dry form is more common.

WHO'S AT RISK The biggest risk factor is age. Other factors include gender (women are more likely to get AMD than men, but are equally likely to get the advanced form), race (Caucasians get AMD more often than African-Americans), and family history (if you have a first-degree relative with AMD, you're at greater risk). Smoking and obesity also increase your risk of developing AMD.

HOW TO PROTECT YOUR VISION If there's a family history, get your vision screened annually; AMD cannot be cured, but its progression can be slowed. Depending on the type you're diagnosed with, treatment may include phototherapy or injections or large doses of antioxidant supplements. Lifestyle plays a protective role: eat a diet high in leafy greens and fish, keep your weight and blood pressure at healthy levels, and if you smoke, quit.

BE MINDFUL OF CHANGES IN VISION

Beyond cataracts, glaucoma, and AMD, other age-related conditions can affect your vision. Check in with your ophthalmologist or optician if you notice any of the following:

- Extreme dry eyes that can't be soothed with do-it-yourself methods. This can be a sign of inflammation or disease.

- Blurred vision, especially if you've been diagnosed with diabetes. This can be an advanced symptom of diabetic retinopathy.

- Floaters (black or gray specks, strings, or cobwebs that drift about when you move your eyes) or flashers (sudden flashes of light in one or both eyes). Most are harmless, but these can also be the first signs of a detaching retina, so check in with your doctor to be safe.

YOUR ORAL HEALTH

Staying on top of your oral health helps to protect and preserve your teeth for life. Of course, a healthy smile is a social asset, but healthy teeth—that can bite into crisp fruits and vegetables and chew nutritious whole grains and nuts—make a vital difference in your quality of life. Keep the following guidelines in mind:

SCHEDULE REGULAR DENTAL APPOINTMENTS

The standard recommendation is to see your dentist twice a year for a cleaning and a checkup. Having trouble making regular appointments? Try scheduling your dental visits on your birthday and your half-birthday. It doesn't have to be your birthday, either—use your child's or spouse's date, if you'd rather. You know the classic preventive advice. Brush and floss twice daily. It's evergreen for a reason—it works. There are no excuses not to.

BRUSH UP ON YOUR TECHNIQUE

Whether you use a manual or an electric toothbrush, try not to grip the handle. If you do, you're more likely to apply excess pressure and end up damaging not only gum tissue but teeth as well, according to research conducted at the University of Newcastle upon Tyne in England. Instead, hold the handle with the same amount of pressure as you would a pencil. Researchers found that 2 minutes of brushing, with light to medium pressure, removed the most plaque. Sawing the brush back and forth against teeth may also be damaging. Instead, use short, vertical scoops to clean teeth from the gumline to the crown. Most electric toothbrushes are programmed to rotate in a specific motion; simply hold the toothbrush head to teeth, instead of trying to move the brush.

REMEMBER TO CLEAN YOUR TONGUE

Use your toothbrush or a special flexible plastic scraper to remove any filmy matter from your tongue. A study from the New York University College of Dentistry found that twice-daily tongue scraping reduced levels of the bacteria that cause cavities and periodontal disease. It also improved bad breath.

TRY A FLOSS HOLDER

If you're all thumbs using floss, or arthritis is making your fingers stiff, invest in a floss holder. There are two varieties widely available at drugstores: the disposable, single-use types that come prethreaded with floss, and the kind you thread with your preferred brand of floss. You can also try using an electric flosser.

SWAP SODA FOR GUM

The decline in the body's ability to mount an immune response makes some of us more vulnerable to cavities as we get older. This offers yet another good reason to stop drinking soda. Full-sugar varieties of soda are delivering sugar straight to the cavity-causing bacteria hiding in between teeth. Even sugar-free types of soda can harm your pearly whites: sodas contain strong acids that can erode tooth enamel.

Between meals, chew sugarless gum. Those that contain xylitol, a sugar alcohol derived from the fibers of fruits and vegetables, seem to help lower levels of cavity-producing acids made by oral bacteria, according to research from the Karolinska Institute in Sweden.

FIND OUT ABOUT FLUORIDE

Ask your dentist if you should be using a fluoride mouth rinse; you're a candidate if you live in a place that has unfluoridated water, have had cavities recently, or suffer from dry mouth. Ask your dentist, too, about whether you should have a fluoride gel treatment with your regular cleanings.

OPT FOR IMPLANTS OVER DENTURES

No matter how well a bridge or other "denture" device fits, it's no match for an implant. Implants are more expensive, but because they are fixed into the jawbone, they stimulate the bone and help prevent osteoporosis (weakening of the bone, which leads to more tooth loss) and bone loss.

TREAT DRY MOUTH

You've probably experienced situational dry mouth—say, when you're nervous—but persistent dry mouth is not normal. Technically known as xerostomia, dry mouth can result from conditions that impact the salivary glands. These conditions include the autoimmune disorder Sjörgren's syndrome, HIV/AIDS, and diabetes, as well as strokes and Alzheimer's disease. If you've undergone chemotherapy or radiation therapy for cancer, or are taking certain drugs (such as antidepressants), dry mouth may be a side effect.

The lack of saliva may make chewing, swallowing, tasting, or talking difficult. Since saliva also helps keep bacteria at bay, dry mouth may make you more susceptible to cavities and gum disease. To battle dry mouth, your dentist may prescribe a medication to stimulate the salivary glands or recommend that you use artificial saliva to moisten your mouth. For your part, sipping lots of water, chewing sugarless gum, sucking on sugar-free hard candies, or avoiding caffeinated beverages may stimulate saliva flow and ease discomfort.

BE AWARE OF THE EFFECTS OF OTHER CONDITIONS OR TREATMENTS

Chronic conditions, which seem to have nothing to do with your teeth, such as diabetes, cardiovascular disease, and arthritis, do impact oral care. Systemic drugs prescribed for chronic illnesses can cause dryness, allergies, and bleeding. And drugs administered after dental procedures, such as nonsteroidal anti-inflammatory drugs or antibiotics, may affect the proper function of beta-blockers, angiotensin-converting enzyme (ACE) inhibitors, or cardiac drugs, for example.

Your dentist may need to adjust treatment according to your condition: if you're diabetic, appointments should be carefully timed between eating a meal and receiving the appropriate insulin injection. If you have chronic obstructive pulmonary disease (COPD), you should not be treated in a lying (supine) position, but in a semiupright one for ease of breathing.

YOUR DIGESTIVE HEALTH

Unlike most other body systems, your digestive tract doesn't really experience much in the way of age-related changes. For most of us, changes brought about by age are minor enough that you don't really notice them. In fact, many of the changes in gut function are a side effect of another chronic condition such as heart disease or diabetes and the medications used to treat them.[10]

But a few things can go awry. Your stomach produces less acid, making it more difficult to absorb nutrients. You may produce less saliva, and experience declines in your senses of taste and smell (an integral part of taste) with the passing years. You may suffer from lactose intolerance or a sensitivity to gluten—even if you ate dairy and wheat when you were younger—owing to changes in the number or type of resident bacteria in your gut. You may get heartburn, especially if you've gained weight. And you may experience constipation or other alterations in your normal pattern of elimination, even if you've been regular all your life. Most of the changes that you do notice can be easily controlled by lifestyle changes.

CHECK THE TOILET BOWL

By middle age, your bowel habits have become pretty well established. They should not change substantially for any period of time unless there is a significant cause. So be on the lookout for any deviation. A visual check of your bowel movements can be revealing. If they are tan or white with a claylike texture, that could be a symptom of hepatitis or pancreatic cancer. Bowel movements that are creamy yellow (or if fat droplets appear in the water) could mean your body is having trouble absorbing dietary fat. And black stools could be a sign of bleeding of the gastrointestinal tract (unless you took Pepto-Bismol or ate beets recently, both of which are notorious for turning stool a reddish black).

Blood on or mixed in with the stool, a change in normal bowel habits, narrowing of the stool, abdominal pain, weight loss, or constant tiredness can all be signs of colon cancer, diverticulitis, or bleeding due to an ulcer. Any change that lasts three weeks or longer should be evaluated by your doctor.

CHECK YOUR MEDS

Nearly half of all medications have some gastrointestinal side effect, such as constipation or diarrhea. Antidepressants, anti-hypertensives, iron supplements, anti-Parkinson's drugs, prescription pain medications, aluminum- or calcium-based antacids, and antihistamines can cause constipation. And diarrhea can be a side effect of magnesium-based antacids, statins, beta-blockers, chemotherapy drugs, and medications used for rheumatoid arthritis and lowering triglycerides. Ask your doctor about changing your medication, but don't stop taking them.

CHECK FOR FECAL INCONTINENCE

If you find yourself unable to control your bowels, tell your doctor promptly. Some of the symptoms of colitis, or inflammation of the bowel, are diarrhea, rectal bleeding, and urgency (the frequent and immediate need to empty the bowels). This kind of incontinence can also arise from chronic constipation or nerve damage. Finding the cause should be a priority, because it impacts your quality of life.

HOME REMEDIES TO KEEP DIGESTION MOVING

Many digestive ailments can be alleviated through changes in diet. However, if dietary adjustments don't help, check in with your doctor instead of "doctoring" yourself.

IF YOU HAVE:	YOU'LL PROBABLY NOTICE . . .	TRY THIS FOOD FIX . . .
BLOATING	An uncomfortable sensation in your abdomen after eating; gas	Lightly toast fennel seeds or their cousin, caraway seeds, and chew a few after a meal. Or steep a teaspoon of seeds in boiling water for a tea.
CONSTIPATION	Hard stools, difficulty passing	Add more fiber to your diet—wheat bran and flaxseed meal are both good sources. Get plenty of fluids (at least 9 cups a day). Drink prune juice or eat prunes.
GLUTEN SENSITIVITY	Gas; bloating; stomach pain; diarrhea immediately after eating products that contain wheat or gluten	Avoid products containing wheat; look for substitutes with soy flour, brown-rice flour, potato-starch flour. Seek out products that are specifically labeled "gluten-free."
HEARTBURN	Burning sensation in the throat, near the breastbone; difficulty swallowing; nausea	Avoid spicy foods and large meals. Enjoy caffeine, alcohol, and chocolate during the day, not before bedtime. Drink fennel- or caraway-seed tea (see above). Or sprinkle seeds on vegetable or fruit salads. Keep an antacid, such as Tums, on hand.
INDIGESTION	Burning in upper stomach; a sensation of fullness or discomfort during or after a meal; gas; acidic taste	Avoid spicy or acidic foods, including oranges or tomatoes. Eat slowly, and drink fluids after, not during, meals. Drink ginger or peppermint tea after meals.
IRRITABLE BOWEL SYNDROME (IBS)	Crampy abdominal pain; excessive gas; a sense of bloating; a change in bowel habits	Try peppermint or spearmint lozenges, teas, or enteric-coated peppermint-oil capsules.
LACTOSE INTOLERANCE	Nausea; cramps; bloating; diarrhea	Try low-lactose dairy products and cheese, or stay away from dairy completely.

COMMON GUT WOES

Persistent digestive woes—such as bloating, burning, or gas pain—may indicate a larger problem. If you're experiencing chronic discomfort, you may suffer from one of the following conditions.

ULCER

WHAT YOU'LL FEEL Dull burning pain in the abdominal area when your stomach is empty. This pain may be mitigated by eating food or taking an antacid.

WHAT'S BEHIND THE PAIN Eating spicy food or being stressed do not cause ulcers; they're created by *Helicobacter pylori*, a bacterium that invades the mucosal wall of your stomach and first part of the small intestine (duodenum), causing infection and leaving sores.

SEE YOUR DOCTOR immediately if you notice bloody or black bowel movements or have had vomit that contained blood or material that looked like coffee grounds; these indicate a more serious, advanced ulcer. Get a checkup if you have ulcerlike pains for two weeks; you may have an *H. pylori* infection.

HOW IT'S TREATED Typically, a combination of antibiotics (to exterminate the bacteria) and an acid blocker is prescribed. Ask your doctor if you can add a probiotic to the mix. A study published in the *American Journal of Gastro-enterology* found that adding a probiotic produced fewer unwanted side effects (diarrhea, nausea, vomiting).

DIVERTICULAR DISEASE

WHAT YOU'LL FEEL Symptoms range from crampy discomfort to sudden pain and tenderness in the lower left side of the abdomen.

WHAT'S BEHIND THE PAIN Diverticular disease is actually two conditions: diverticulosis and diverticulitis. The first results from the outward bulging of small weakened areas in the walls of the large intestine. This condition increases with age; it's estimated that half of those over 60 have it. The condition is largely benign and symptomless. On the other hand, having diverticula increases your risk of diverticulitis, which occurs when the pouches become inflamed and infected. The pain arises suddenly and is typically confined to the sigmoid colon on the lower left side of the abdomen.

SEE YOUR DOCTOR if you experience sudden, severe left-sided pain (or pain that gets progressively worse over the course of a few days), or you notice blood after a bowel movement.

HOW IT'S TREATED Diverticulitis is treated by antibiotics. Since diverticulitis means you have diverticula, a high-fiber diet and regular exercise are typically recommended as a preventive measure. If untreated, diverticulitis can lead to abscesses and perforations of the intestinal wall. One British study found that vegetarians were 31 percent less likely to develop diverticular disease than meat-eaters.

GASTROESOPHAGEAL REFLUX DISEASE (GERD)

WHAT YOU'LL FEEL A burning pain (known as heartburn) in the back of the throat or behind the breastbone. In some cases, you may actually taste regurgitated stomach acid.

WHAT'S BEHIND THE PAIN Reflux occurs when the ringlike muscle that separates the stomach from the esophagus weakens or relaxes, allowing stomach acids to flow into the esophagus.

SEE YOUR DOCTOR if you start experiencing heartburn twice a week or you have been using antacids for two weeks. If untreated, the erosion of esophageal cells due to stomach acid may lead to esophageal cancer.

HOW IT'S TREATED Medications known as proton-pump inhibitors (PPI) are typically used to soothe GERD symptoms. Ironically, long-term use of PPIs predisposes you to weight gain, which is another root cause of GERD. If your doctor recommends a PPI, keep your eye on the scale. Acupuncture may improve the efficacy of your medication regime. Avoiding problematic foods such as citrus fruits, caffeine, alcohol, spicy foods, garlic, carbonated beverages, onions, and tomato sauces and salsas may ease symptoms. One small study showed that FenuLife, a fenugreek product, eased symptoms.[11] Also, avoid wearing clothing that fits tightly around the stomach. Finally, make sure another medication isn't causing GERD. Medicines such as calcium channel blockers and beta-blockers (used to treat high blood pressure), sedatives, nonsteroidal anti-inflammatories, anti-Parkinson's drugs, antidepressants, and certain osteoporosis drugs actually weaken the ringlike sphincter muscle in the esophagus.

IRRITABLE BOWEL SYNDROME (IBS)

WHAT YOU'LL FEEL A variety of stomach symptoms such as pain, bloating, and discomfort. Some people experience constipation; others, diarrhea; and still others, alternating bouts of the two.

WHAT'S BEHIND THE PAIN Research has yet to pinpoint the cause of irritable bowel syndrome, and because patients experience such a wide range of symptoms, there may be more than one factor at work. Current hypotheses include a malfunction of the gut lining, a bacterial infection, an immune system dysfunction, abnormal neurotransmitter receptors, and stress.

SEE YOUR DOCTOR if the discomfort or bowel changes affect your quality of life. IBS does not damage the intestines and does not lead to other serious conditions, but other conditions such as celiac disease can have similar symptoms.

HOW IT'S TREATED Leading a healthy lifestyle is the typical recommendation. Eat a wholesome diet and get regular exercise. Meditation and cognitive behavioral therapy may ease symptoms. Probiotics containing *Bifidobacterium infantis* 35624, as well as peppermint oil, were found to relieve IBS-related discomfort.

YOUR BLADDER HEALTH

Changes in your pattern of urination—leaks, spasms, frequency, and urgency—are distressing, not to mention uncomfortable, and can significantly impact your quality of life. Unfortunately, many people don't get the help they need because they are too embarrassed to talk about what they're experiencing, or they think nothing can be done.[12] Don't put off seeing a doctor, even if you feel you're managing your symptoms on your own. Without treatment, symptoms may get worse, and the underlying problem may become more difficult to treat. Make an appointment with your doctor to find the cause, and try the following strategies:

CHECK YOUR MEDICATIONS

Incontinence can be a side effect of diuretics, asthma drugs, narcotic pain relievers, calcium channel blockers, and angiotensin-converting enzyme (ACE) inhibitors. Ask your doctor if you can switch medications to see if symptoms improve.

SET A SCHEDULE

Sometimes self-conditioning works as well if not better than medications. If you have been diagnosed with urge incontinence, work out a schedule with your doctor for your urination. Typically, you go to the bathroom every hour or two whether or not you feel an urge, then gradually reduce the frequency to train your bladder to hold urine.

TRY ACUPUNCTURE

For short-term relief, acupuncture may be a safe and effective antidote to urge incontinence. The caveat: relief may last only four to six weeks, so you'll probably need follow-up sessions every few months.

EAT THE RIGHT FOODS

You may want to experiment with cutting the following foods from your diet, as they can irritate the bladder and make lower urinary tract symptoms worse: alcohol; caffeine; chocolate; dairy; carbonated beverages; spicy foods; and citrus, tomatoes, pineapples, and other acidic fruit.

And make sure you're getting plenty of fiber via leafy vegetables, fruit, and whole grains to keep yourself regular. If your colon is full of unexpelled waste, it puts pressure on the bladder and may lead to or worsen your incontinence symptoms. Your doctor may recommend a fiber supplement. Look for a brand that is labeled both soluble and non-fermentable. Whether it's natural or synthetic doesn't really matter; it's whatever agrees with your system, so experiment until you find a fiber supplement that works for you.

ABOUT KEGEL EXERCISES

Kegel exercises strengthen your pelvic floor muscles, which help prevent incontinence in women and can also make sex more pleasurable. To do a Kegel, contract the same muscles that you use to urinate. Simply squeeze, as if you were trying to stop the flow of urine. Hold for a count of three, then relax. Repeat ten times.

TYPES OF INCONTINENCE

CONDITION	WHAT IT IS	HOW IT AFFECTS YOU	MOST COMMONLY SEEN IN
OVERACTIVE BLADDER	Your bladder contracts more often than it should.	You need to go more frequently and/or urgently and may experience leakage.	People with nerve damage due to MS, stroke, injury, Parkinson's, or Alzheimer's disease. It is often associated with urinary tract infections and bladder irritants such as alcohol and caffeine, as well as BPH (benign prostatic hypertrophy).
STRESS INCONTINENCE	The bladder or surrounding muscles are weakened.	You leak when you laugh, cough, sneeze, or exercise.	Women who have had at least one pregnancy or vaginal delivery; men after prostate/pelvic surgery
URGE INCONTINENCE	Increased sensitivity of bladder muscles to the brain chemical that stimulates the bladder.	You get a sudden, powerful urge to go that often results in an accident.	People with nerve damage due to MS, stroke, injury, Parkinson's, or Alzheimer's disease. It is often associated with urinary tract infections, bladder irritants, and BPH (see above).
MIXED INCONTINENCE	Uncontrollable loss of urine	A combination of stress and urge incontinence	Often due to one or more of the conditions associated with stress or urge incontinence
OVERFLOW INCONTINENCE	Loss of urine due to weak muscles or a blockage of the urethra	You frequently leak small amounts of urine but are unable to fully empty your bladder.	Men or women with bladder damage, nerve damage from diabetes, a blocked urethra, or men with prostate problems
FUNCTIONAL INCONTINENCE	Urine control is normal.	You have accidents because you can't get to the bathroom in time due to a physical limitation or the inability to recognize the need to go.	People who have had a stroke, have severe arthritis, or have Parkinson's or Alzheimer's disease

YOUR SEXUAL HEALTH

The dual purpose of sex—procreation and recreation—means that sexual interest and sexual activity are a lifelong part of the human experience. As our longevity increases, we're enjoying sex well into our later years. And as it turns out, an active sex life also extends longevity. A twenty-five-year study of nearly three hundred men and women, ages 60 to 96, conducted at Duke University, found that the more sex men had, the longer they lived. Women who reported enjoying their sex lives lived up to eight years longer than women who were less enthusiastic. Here's how to get the most out of your sex life well into your golden years:

STAY FIT

Research shows that staying physically active and maintaining a healthy weight can increase the number of years of your sex life. Regular exercise can help improve libido and stamina, increase blood flow to erogenous zones, and reduce the instances of sexual dysfunction. Staying in shape can also work wonders for boosting self-esteem and confidence, both of which contribute to a healthier sex life.

TALK WITH YOUR DOCTOR

Social stigma prevents many aging baby boomers from talking about sex with their doctors. According to a 2007 study published in the New England Journal of Medicine, only 38 percent of men and 22 percent of women in the study reported that they'd discussed their sexual life with their doctor since turning 50. That's fifteen to thirty-five years of having sex without any necessary medical input. And aging does pose unique challenges to sexual expression and intimacy. Your doctor can recommend products and treatments for certain age-related sexual issues, as well as screen you for any sexually transmitted diseases, particularly if you're with a new partner. Don't be afraid to discuss sexual health concerns—be it lack of desire, discomfort, pain, or another physical issue—with your doctor. There are often simple and effective solutions that will enable you and your partner to reap all of the benefits of a healthy sexual connection for years to come.

USE PROTECTION

Pregnancy may no longer be a risk for you, but sexually transmitted diseases are a real danger. In fact, baby boomers are one of the highest risk groups for contracting STDs, such as chlamydia, gonorrhea, syphilis, and HIV. If you're having sex with a new partner, make sure to use condoms. You and your partner should be screened for any communicable diseases.

MIND YOUR CHANGING NEEDS

Clearly, levels of estrogen and testosterone can influence sexuality, but taking other factors into account can help you identify sexual issues that you might be able to address, rather than simply chalking them up to age and resigning yourself to living with them. For instance, decreased libido and sexual dysfunction may be side effects of pharmaceuticals. Drugs that lower blood pressure can reduce desire, cause vaginal dryness, and make it difficult for men to achieve and maintain an erection. Antihistamines, antidepressants, acid-blocking drugs, and medications for treating diabetes and lowering cholesterol are also notorious for impeding sex. So it's important to speak with your physician about possible side effects and alternatives.

HOW SEX IMPROVES HEALTH

It's no secret that sex is good for you. Some people even go as far as to swear that lovemaking is the secret to the fountain of youth. Although eternal youth may be wishful thinking, research has shown that there are measurable health benefits to having a healthy sex life. Further research is needed to prove or dispel some of the grander claims—such as sex preventing prostate and breast cancers—but there's strong evidence connecting sex with positive effects on the brain, heart, and immune and nervous systems. Here are a few of the proven benefits of getting busy.

REDUCES:	HOW:	ADDITIONAL BENEFITS:
STRESS	Replenishes stress-relieving hormones and potentially lowers blood pressure.	Lower blood pressure may help reduce strokes and heart attacks.
DEPRESSION	Like other physical activity, having sex can release chemicals in the brain that may make you happier and feel less stressed.	A good sex life can also help improve your body image and self-esteem.
COLDS AND FLUS	Enhances your body's production of IgA (immunoglobulin A), an antibody that protects you from coming down with colds and other respiratory infections.	Improved immunity, resulting in better overall resistance to illness.
HEART DISEASE	May reduce your risk for heart attack owing to the release of DHEA (dehydroepiandrosterone), which is known to improve circulation as well as dilation of arteries.	DHEA can also reduce depression.
SLEEP PROBLEMS	Helps you sleep better, thanks to the rush of the "bonding" hormone oxytocin that your body produces.	Getting more sleep, conversely, will likely improve your sex life.
PAIN	Oxytocin and endorphins released before and after orgasm may help relieve certain types of pain.	Oxytocin may also help wounds heal faster by regenerating cells.

ABOUT HORMONE REPLACEMENT THERAPY

If you're a woman and you're struggling with hot flashes, night sweats, or vaginal dryness, your doctor may suggest hormone replacement therapy (HRT). This type of therapy uses estrogen with or without progestin to treat these symptoms, along with a host of other menopause-related health issues, including mood swings, "brain fog," and insomnia.

HRT is often prescribed to address these problems—but you may be hesitant to start it because you remember panicky headlines about its link to an increased risk for heart disease. These were spurred by the long-running Women's Health Initiative (WHI), a large-scale study of women's health issues whose hormone therapy trial was stopped in midtrial because healthy women taking HRT had twice the risk of heart disease compared with women not on the hormones. However, the average age of subjects in the study was 63 (about a decade older than women entering menopause), while current recommendations call for considering HRT at the same age as you enter menopause.

Nevertheless, the decision to take hormones comes down to you and your doctor. Know that HRT does increase the risk for blood clots, strokes, and breast cancer, so if you have a predisposition or family history of these conditions or other risk factors for breast cancer, you may wish to forgo treatment. Ask your doctor about alternative therapies to ease menopausal symptoms and whether you should take bone-strengthening prescription drugs or simply rely on calcium and vitamin D supplements (bones are at risk once estrogen levels wane due to menopause).

For more information on the pros and cons of HRT, the North American Menopause Society's website has a very accessible position paper available at www.menopause.org.

AN ENLARGED PROSTATE

With age, the prostate, a walnut-size gland that surrounds the urethra (which is the tube that brings urine from the bladder to the penis), can become enlarged. The bigger the gland gets, the more it can put pressure on the urethra, causing urinary symptoms. This condition, known as benign prostatic hypertrophy (BPH), is typically diagnosed by a clinical digital exam and other tests to rule out prostate cancer or infection. Treatment ranges from lifestyle modifications to medications to surgery. Though BPH is not a sign of prostate cancer, you should mention any changes in urinary patterns to your doctor. If left untreated, BPH can lead to urinary tract infections, kidney infections, or even kidney failure. If you are experiencing urinary symptoms associated with BPH, try the following tips.

☐ **AVOID ALCOHOL OR CAFFEINE** Both are bladder stimulants, bladder irritants, and diuretics.

☐ **SPACE YOUR FLUID INTAKE THROUGHOUT THE DAY** Stop drinking any fluids two hours before you go to bed.

☐ **URINATE RIGHT WHEN YOU FEEL YOU HAVE TO GO** instead of putting it off until a more convenient time.

☐ **DOUBLE VOID** In this technique, you urinate, then wait for a moment and urinate again to more fully empty the bladder.

☐ **WORK OUT REGULARLY** The exact mechanism is unclear, but lack of physical activity tends to worsen symptoms.

☐ **LOSE EXCESS WEIGHT** Extra pounds press on your bladder and increase the incidence of incontinence, worsening BPH symptoms.

☐ **PRACTICE KEGELS** The same Kegel exercises that can help women prevent or minimize stress incontinence can also help men who are experiencing bladder control problems due to prostate surgery (removal of the prostate gland) or BPH. (See page 214 for directions.)

☐ **CONSIDER SAW PALMETTO EXTRACT** Although some studies have shown a benefit, remember to talk to your doctor before taking saw palmetto extract or any other herbal remedy. If you decide to try it, you should notice an effect after one to two months. However, symptoms associated with BPH do vary over time, and any improvement may be due to the changeable nature of symptoms and very possibly a placebo effect rather than due to the supplement.

WATCH FOR SIGNS OF PROSTATE CANCER

If you are a man, the older you get, the more likely it is that you'll be diagnosed with cancer of the prostate gland. Since this cancer shares many of the same urinary warning signs as BPH, it's critical to monitor symptoms, not to pass them off as "just" BPH, and to report any worsening of symptoms to your doctor.

The screening test for this cancer, the prostate-specific-antigen (PSA), is not a diagnostic tool; it merely identifies those at higher risk for developing prostate cancer. There is no absolute normal/abnormal value for a PSA test; your doctor must also take into consideration your age, your race, medications you are currently taking, the results of your last PSA, and other factors, such as prostate infection, to determine whether you need further tests or follow-up.

YOUR FOOT HEALTH

By age 50, you have walked more than 75,000 miles, and yet you probably tend to ignore the body part that made it all possible: your feet. Many of us still believe it's normal for feet to hurt—and to hurt increasingly with the passing years. Not true. Aging brings many changes to your feet, but pain shouldn't be one of them.

It's important to get to the bottom of your discomfort, because you'll need healthy, pain-free feet to help you keep your balance as you get older, to help prevent falls, and to keep you active. When your feet are too sore to walk, you lose strength and become increasingly sedentary, which is associated with a host of health conditions, from obesity to dementia. Finally, keeping an eye on your feet can even give you an early warning about serious health problems such as diabetes, arthritis, nerve damage, and poor blood circulation. Here's how to build a healthier foundation for your whole body:

KEEP FEET CLEAN

Wash your feet every day with warm water and soap. If you enjoy a foot soak, don't indulge for longer than 10 minutes, or your skin may become dry and start to crack. Dry feet well with a towel, especially between your toes to prevent fungal growth. Apply unscented moisturizer (fragrance is a potential allergen) on the tops and bottoms of your feet if the skin is dry or cracked, but not between the toes. Cut or file your toenails regularly, trim them straight across, and never shorter than the end of your toe. Make sure your feet are completely dry before slipping on your socks and shoes.

KEEP BLOOD MOVING

Avoid crossing your legs; it compresses the veins and arteries and reduces circulation to your feet. Whenever possible, put up your feet when you sit down, as a way to improve circulation and reduce swelling. (Keep a small footstool under your desk or in your living room so you can prop your feet up—higher than your hips, if you have the space.)

BUY THE RIGHT SHOES

The right shoes help you stay active and avoid falls, according to Julie Kardachi, a cofounder of Fall Stop . . . Move Strong. Keep these tips in mind:

SHOP LATER IN THE DAY Because feet tend to swell as the day progresses, you want to shop when your feet are their largest. Occasionally have a store clerk measure your shoe size; feet may grow larger as the arch flattens and swelling sets in.

CHECK THE WIDTH A shoe that is too narrow can cause calluses or force your toes to overlap.

TEST THE LENGTH The shoe should be long enough to allow a finger's width between the end of the big toe and the end of the shoe.

DETERMINE THE DEPTH The shoe should be high enough to accommodate the front of the foot, without excessive pressure.

CHOOSE SOLID SOLES Soles that are excessively slick or slippery, or, conversely, too "grippy," can cause trips and falls.

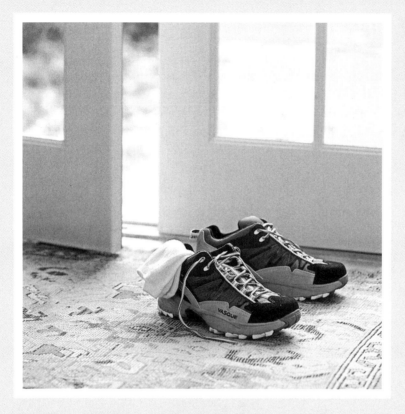

TREAT YOUR FEET WELL

I never wear the same shoes two days in a row. Rather, I rotate through high heels, medium heels, low heels, and flats. Also, I do not confine my feet. I never wear shoes at home, and when I'm riding in the car, my feet are bare so I can wiggle my toes and give my feet some air.

I also walk barefoot on gravel all the time. I like to walk on all different kinds of surfaces, particularly when I hike. Practicing walking on uneven surfaces (safely!) is good for foot health, because it strengthens the ankles and improves balance.

PREVENTIVE FOOT CARE

A variety of foot conditions can cause pain and throw off your gait, increasing risk of injury and falls. Even harmless-seeming calluses are a reason to see a podiatrist due to the imbalances they cause. That's especially true for diabetics. People who suffer from diabetes often have trouble with their feet. These problems are not only painful; they can be downright dangerous. Diabetes can cause nerve damage, compromising the ability to sense temperature or pain in feet. The Institute for Preventive Foothealth (www.ipfh.org) offers more information. Ask your doctor how often you need a foot check, and be attentive to the following foot conditions:

SORES AND CALLUSES

Particularly for diabetics, cuts, sores, calluses, and corns (the calluses that develop between toes) may develop into ulcers. This can be a very serious problem, especially because diabetes sometimes inhibits blood flow to the legs, causing sores to heal slowly. If ulcers become infected, or foot tissue starts to die because of poor or lack of blood flow (gangrene), a hospital visit may be required. To prevent calluses and corns, wear well-padded socks and properly fitting shoes with limited seams that might rub against the feet. Use a pumice stone to lightly sand calluses; never try to cut or remove them on your own.

BUNIONS

These bony protrusions often develop where the joints meet in the big toes. Ill-fitting shoes often are the culprits, but heredity can also play a part. If you suffer from arthritis, you're at particular risk; both inflammatory and degenerative arthritis can cause the protective cartilage that covers joints to deteriorate. Prevent bunions by wearing low-heeled shoes that don't cramp your feet. If you've already developed them, a doctor may prescribe anti-inflammatory drugs or suggest a surgical procedure to remove the swollen tissue.

HAMMERTOES

This condition causes the second, third, or fourth toes to bend at the first joint. The main causes of hammertoes include poorly fitting shoes, especially high heels that don't allow joints to lie flat; heredity; traumatic injuries; diabetic neuropathy; and nerve damage from stroke or arthritis. If left untreated, the condition can cause the tendons to contract and the toe to lose mobility. In extreme cases, a surgeon may have to remove bone or cut tendons to help straighten the toe.

WORK ON FOOT FITNESS

These moves increase circulation, prevent cramps, and keep your muscles in good shape:

- Try to crumple up a towel or pick up a marble with your toes while seated.
- Alternate flexing your feet and your toes, then pointing your toes downward; rotate your ankles in circles, first in one direction, then the other.
- Rise up on your tiptoes, then rock back to your heels, twenty times, while holding on to a sturdy table or chair back.

MEDICATE *wisely*

Part of the reason we're enjoying unprecedented longevity and quality of life is that there are so many effective medications available to control a broad range of chronic conditions and everyday aches and pains. That said, you should never be nonchalant about medications. Here are everyday ways to be smart about storing, using, and disposing of drugs.

MANAGE YOUR PRESCRIPTIONS

KEEP A MASTER LIST

Maintain a list of every medication you use, including OTC and prescription medicines, vitamins, herbals, and other supplements. Give this list to any health-care professional you see so he or she can update your records and help you use medicine safely. (See "Medicines in My Home" at www.fda .gov.) Keep a copy of this list, and let your loved ones know where it is. If you get sick, they will know exactly what you are taking. Another option: create a personal pill card, which provides a visual reminder of all of the medicines that you need to take on a regular basis. The Agency for Healthcare Research and Quality provides free software and graphics for safe pill-taking at www.ahrq.gov/ qual/pillcard/pillcard.html.

CONSOLIDATE YOUR CARE

Start by always filling prescriptions at the same pharmacy. You probably see several different doctors, and it's unlikely that any one of them keeps close tabs on every medication you take. Pharmacists keep digital records of the drugs dispensed to you, which makes it easier to consult them about medication contraindications or interactions.

BEWARE OF SIDE EFFECTS

The more medications you take, the greater your risk of drug interactions and side effects such as light-headedness, dizziness, or drowsiness. What's more, according to an ongoing study at the University of North Carolina School of Pharmacy, people age 65 and older who take four or more medications regularly are two to three times more likely to fall than someone who doesn't take as many.

Prescription drugs, such as antidepressants, antianxiety drugs, seizure medications, and pain relievers, along with over-the-counter drugs, such as allergy medications and cold and cough remedies, can work to subdue your central nervous system, reduce alertness, and slow reaction times, which can make you less alert, slower to react, and less steady on your feet. Talk to your doctor to assess your risk.

ADOPT A MED STRATEGY

If you take more than one medication, missing a dose or mistiming a dose becomes more likely. To avoid this, try taking medications at a set time every day, place bottles in obvious locations, or tie pill-taking to another behavior you won't forget (such as brushing your teeth). You could also try a medication reminder app or free e-mail reminder from a service like reQall (www.reqall.com/about/subscriptions).

KEEP A WELL-STOCKED MEDICINE CHEST

You'll find it easier to deal with minor injuries, aches, pains, and other ailments if you always have the right over-the-counter remedies on hand. All medicine should be stored in easy-to open containers with large-print labels. Ask your pharmacist for these no-cost extras. Most of these products will last longer if you keep them in a cool, dark place—think a corner of your pantry or kitchen door, not the humidity-prone bathroom.

- ☐ **Aspirin or a nonsteroidal anti-inflammatory (NSAID)** for everyday aches and pains, fevers, and stronger pains, such as strained muscles and sunburn

- ☐ **Nonaspirin pain reliever** If aspirin or NSAIDs cause stomach irritation, opt for acetaminophen.

- ☐ **Throat lozenges** to treat sore throat and cough

- ☐ **Antihistamine** to combat seasonal allergies or insect stings

- ☐ **Antacid** for occasional heartburn (but if you're using this remedy frequently, you may be suffering from gastroesophageal reflux disease [GERD]; see page 213)

- ☐ **Antidiarrheal medicine** such as Pepto-Bismol

- ☐ **Antibiotic ointment** for cuts and scrapes

- ☐ **Hydrocortisone cream** to calm itchy skin

- ☐ **Adhesive bandages** in a variety of sizes

- ☐ **Elastic (ACE) bandage** for sprains and strains

- ☐ **Tweezers and a pack of needles** to remove splinters

- ☐ **Rubbing alcohol** to disinfect cuts

- ☐ **Hydrogen peroxide** for disinfecting cuts

- ☐ **Cotton balls and swabs** for application of liquids and ointments

- ☐ **Tiger Balm or a capsaicin-based ointment** to treat sore muscles

- ☐ **Aloe vera gel** to ease mild burns

- ☐ **Digital thermometer**

- ☐ **Fingernail clippers**

ALTERNATIVE REMEDIES FOR YOUR MEDICINE CHEST

In addition to a stockpile of first-aid basics and over-the-counter (OTC) pharmaceuticals, it's worth keeping some of the more time-tested natural and non-drug-based treatments on hand. These homeopathic, herbal, and other naturally derived remedies can boost your body's own defenses and work as gentle alternatives to OTC drugs that would increase your risk of negative interactions and side effects. (That said, you should always tell your doctor when you are taking a natural remedy, as negative interactions can occur and many alternative medicines are not regulated for quality.) These solutions can generally be found in health-food stores and increasingly in mass drugstore chains.

FOR	TRY
CONGESTION AND ALLERGIES	Saline nose spray. These tend to be sodium chloride–based homeopathic sprays that flush out nasal passages.
COUGHS	Alcohol-free cough medicine. These safe, tasty syrups temporarily relieve coughs without causing drowsiness.
COLDS AND FLU	Echinacea blends, zinc lozenges, or Oscillococcinum. Echinacea can reduce the frequency and duration of colds, according to a 2007 evidence review by University of Connecticut researchers. Zinc has antioxidant effects and may decrease the ability of cold viruses to grow on the lining of the nose and throat. Oscillococcinum has been shown to reduce flu severity and duration when taken at the onset of symptoms.
MUSCLE OR JOINT PAIN	Arnica-based skin creams. The homeopathic preparation *Arnica montana* is a recognized anti-inflammatory that diminishes pain and swelling when applied at the site of pain.
MINOR CUTS AND BURNS	Calendula. Available in tinctures, creams, and oils, calendula acts as an antiseptic and anti-inflammatory.
SLEEP PROBLEMS	Chamomile extract capsules. In a first-of-its kind 2009 controlled trial, researchers at the University of Pennsylvania found that German chamomile–extract capsules provided significant calming benefits.
GASTROINTESTINAL TROUBLE	*Nux vomica.* Also known as poison nut, it addresses nausea and other digestive problems.

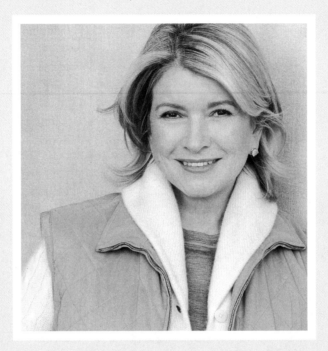

CHAPTER 6

Healthy Looks

TAKE CARE *of your skin* 228

MATCH *your makeup to your age* 246

CONSIDER *cosmetic enhancements* 250

ENCOURAGE *healthy hair* 254

I'm determined to succeed at aging gracefully. I always say, "It's never too early or too late to start." I know that age should not be an obstacle, but I don't always believe it when I look in the mirror. If I see a crow's foot, I put cream on it. If I look tired, I pat cucumber or witch hazel under my eyes. As we age, we have to keep at it on a regular basis; prevention, upkeep, and improvement are a vital part of an ongoing healthy lifestyle.

Today, we have a new understanding of how our genes and our environment affect appearance, particularly our complexion, face, skin, hair, and nails. We also know more than ever about how diet and lifestyle can prevent signs of aging. And there are wonderful and effective at-home products and professional procedures, all of which make it possible to look—and feel—younger for longer. I myself haven't had plastic surgery (yet!); perhaps I'll get to a point in my life where I decide I simply need it. But if you take preventive measures with your skin and are assiduous about maintenance, you will have so many more options later on.

That said, I believe that true beauty really is inherent, and comes from character and strength. The women I think are the most attractive are both confident and interesting, but they also take care of themselves.

TAKE CARE *of your skin*

We are all time travelers; our choices, our paths, our lifestyles leave their mark on the canvas of our bodies. The question remains—what are we going to do about the changes that the passing years etch upon our looks? If your immediate answer is "Everything!" or even "Nothing!" know that there is a considerable gray (!) area between looking as if the years have not touched you to being the proverbial "happy raisin." The goal for most of us is this middle ground we'll call aging positively. Acceptance of the changes that aging brings can be hard, but the key is to find a way (whether it's with doctors and the current antiaging arsenal of lasers, injectibles, and procedures, or simply letting the years roll on, or somewhere in between) to recognize, rather than deny, what's happening to us. It means having perspective about what can be maintained or changed and what must be accepted—and that there's no single solution that every one of us must look for. It's a valid point that we should be able to live our lives looking how we want to feel—whatever shape that takes. But more than anything, aging positively is about spirit. Being vital and attractive is about more than just looks.

For one thing, we know much more about the intrinsic process of aging. While we may not be able to stop aging (yet), we can avoid accelerating it and may even be able to slow it down. The basis for aging positively is being informed and being empowered with the information available, then acting on it. Having a preventive mind-set can really make a visible difference. Research has shown that while genetics account for up to 40 percent of the changes we associate with aging, the majority of those changes are due to lifestyle factors within our control. You have little to lose and everything to gain by making small alterations in your lifestyle (such as wearing sunscreen every day, adhering to a good skin-care regimen, and making healthier eating choices) that seem to slow the impact of the passing years. This chapter will show you the path to aging gracefully and looking your best in the process.

As we get older, it becomes all too easy to spend most of our time criticizing our skin—picking out every little wrinkle, sag, and imperfection, even those that are barely visible. We idealize that baby-soft skin of our youth (conveniently forgetting any blemishes or irritations that may have plagued us back then!), and we feel frustrated that the face in the mirror doesn't look the way it once did. But before you start thinking about how to improve your skin, why not take a moment to appreciate everything your skin does to improve you?

A CLOSER LOOK

On a purely structural level, our skin protects us from the elements while providing our bodies with support. According to Dr. Gerald Imber, a plastic surgeon in New York City and author of *The Youth Corridor*, human skin is only fifteen- to twenty-thousandths of an inch thick. That's thinner than most fabrics—and yet, you're wrapped in about 20 square feet of it. Our skin actually contains two layers: the dermis, or inner layer, and the epidermis, or outer layer; at the cellular level, skin is composed of connective tissue called collagen and the protein elastin, which allows tissues in the body to snap back into shape after stretching. It also performs other essential duties such as acting as a barrier against the loss of water from the body and the entry of bacteria into the body. Skin is also key in the regulation of body temperature; that's why you sweat and flush in the heat and shiver in the cold. Dr. Imber explains, "Even as it ages, the skin continues to perform these vital functions well. That's why the skin's health is just as important as its appearance."

THE IMPORTANCE OF SLEEP FOR YOUR SKIN

In addition to a healthy diet and skin-care routine, adequate sleep can prove your best ally in rejuvenating your skin. Just as with other body organs, the skin repairs itself during sleep. And lack of sleep will show up immediately on your face, with dark circles, bags under your eyes, and dull skin. Seven to eight uninterrupted hours are optimal, but if that's impossible, try taking naps. To get the best sleep possible, see the tips on pages 196–197.

FEED YOUR SKIN WELL

One of the most reliable routes to healthy skin is a balanced diet. Your skin needs a variety of vitamins and minerals to function optimally, and the best way to achieve that is by eating a diet rich in certain nutrients.

EAT MORE OF THESE

Antioxidant-rich foods such as brightly colored fruits and vegetables (red peppers, blueberries, strawberries, and purple grapes) help protect against damage from free radicals in the environment and shield your cells from premature aging.

Healthy fats found in salmon, nuts, olive oil, and flaxseed improve the quality of the skin barrier and increase the water-retaining capacity of skin, making it appear plumper (filling out wrinkles) and younger. These omega-3 and omega-6 fatty acids also decrease inflammation, which can damage skin over time.

Green tea is a great source of the powerful antioxidant group called catechins. Many studies show the benefits of catechins in boosting immune response and in possibly protecting against cancer. Green tea leaves are not baked during the production process, so they retain more active catechins than black tea. Decaffeinated tea has the same level of antioxidants as regular green tea (which is mildly caffeinated), so you can drink this skin tonic all day long.

Fiber promotes healthy skin cells and may protect skin from sun damage and reduce skin cancer risk. Soluble fiber—the kind found in citrus fruits, avocados, figs, and berries—has significant health benefits as well: it boosts the immune system and keeps inflammation at bay, which can keep skin looking and functioning at its best. It's easy to bump up your intake of soluble fiber. Stir in 2 tablespoons of ground flaxseed to your morning oatmeal (4 grams); eat a pear for a snack or dessert (3 grams); or enjoy an artichoke for dinner (4.7 grams).

EAT FEWER OF THESE

"White" foods such as white bread, pasta, rice, and sugar. These relatively empty carbohydrates increase insulin levels and cause inflammation, which can make skin appear older.

Food additives like MSG, found in many processed foods. By causing vascular dilation, these additives can contribute to a ruddy complexion.

Alcohol and spicy or salty foods can increase puffiness and inflammation. Persistent stretching and swelling over time will result in damage to the delicate skin of the eyelids, and permanent looseness may result.

HOW AGE AFFECTS SKIN

THE SKIN LAYER	WHAT HAPPENS OVER TIME	WHAT YOU'LL NOTICE
EPIDERMIS	The rate at which dead cells are sloughed off and replaced by newer ones begins to slow.	Skin can appear rougher and duller.
	New cells coming to this layer are irregular or uneven.	Skin is not so smooth; it develops small creases and wrinkles.
	Melanocytes (the cells in the skin that produce the pigment melanin) decrease. Those that remain increase in size and contrast with areas of the skin that no longer have any melanocytes.	Uneven or mottled appearance of skin.
	There's a generalized thinning of the skin layer.	More frequent scrapes or skin breakage.
DERMIS	Fibroblasts (which generate collagen) lose potency, so the process of skin repair slows down.	Skin loses some softness and elasticity, creating wrinkles. The destruction of collagen and elastin leads to wrinkling.
	Connections between the dermis and epidermis decrease, resulting in less sharing of nutrients and moisture-holding molecules between these two layers.	Dry, flaky, itchy skin.
	Attachment between the layers is less firm.	Even a minor injury can cause the two layers to separate and form blisters and bruising.
	Blood vessels thicken and dilate.	A spidery web of tiny red vessels on the face.

PROTECT YOUR SKIN

Just how—and how rapidly—you age is largely determined by genetics. However, this intrinsic aging plan is impacted by your individual response to age accelerators in your environment, such as sunlight, stress, and nutrition, as well as your general state of health. Many of these factors are under your control, so embrace the following preventive measures to keep skin looking as youthful as possible.

PRACTICE SAFE SUNCARE

Sun damage, in the form of wrinkles, laxity, and pigment changes, is cumulative over many years. Unfortunately, our skin is now paying the price for the bad habits of youth, before we were even aware that sun exposure could be so harmful. But any little change you can make today to counter the damage done is cumulative, too.

Follow these five simple rules of smart sun protection:

1. Cover up and wear sunscreen every day.

2. Reapply your sunscreen after about 90 minutes of sun exposure (more often if you're getting sweaty or wet at the beach or by the pool).

3. Avoid the sun at peak hours of intensity (11 a.m. to 3 p.m.). Try to schedule outdoor activities like tennis or golf for the morning or early evening.

4. When you apply sunscreen, squeeze it out on the back of one hand. Once you've finished applying it to face and neck, rub the back of your hands together. The hands are an often forgotten sunscreen spot and are among the first body parts to show damage from the sun.

5. When possible, cross over to walk on the shady side of the street—this small step can cut your UV exposure by 30 percent.

QUIT SMOKING

Even if you only smoke once in a while, you're still doing grave damage to your skin (not to mention your cardiovascular and pulmonary systems). Smoking constricts the small blood vessels and reduces blood flow to the skin, essentially starving and destroying your collagen, which causes sagging, drooping, and wrinkles.[1]

EXERCISE REGULARLY

Frequent exercise stimulates circulation, which supplies oxygen to skin cells while carrying away waste products and cellular debris. It also reduces stress hormones, helping to keep skin clear.

Work out without wearing makeup, so sweat can escape easily from your pores, and always wash off sweat and oil afterward. Drinking plenty of water after exercise will also help flush toxins and replenish the water you lost.

STOP YO-YOING

With age, the skin loses some of its elasticity and it won't snap back after excessive weight gain or loss. If you need to lose some weight to get to a healthier place, lose the pounds gradually (about a pound per week), which gives the skin a chance to shrink to fit your new frame. And beware of growing too thin: Your normal subcutaneous fat layer actually helps you look younger by plumping out hollows and wrinkles. It also makes skin look and feel healthy.

STAY HYDRATED

Up to two-thirds of older adults are chronically dehydrated because they simply don't drink enough water. In addition to leading to health problems like dizziness and heart palpitations, dehydration means parched skin. Water-dense foods can also supplement daily hydration; particularly in seasonally hot months, increase your intake of juicy fruits and vegetables such as cucumbers, watermelon, honeydew, cantaloupe, citrus fruits, pomegranates, grapes, eggplant, and tomatoes.

TAKE SUPPLEMENTS

For healthier skin (and a host of other health benefits), consider adding the following to your daily supplement routine:[2]

- ☐ 1,000 mg of vitamin C. This potent antioxidant is a necessary component of collagen production.

- ☐ 400 IUs of vitamin D (if you don't drink much milk or get outside often). You need vitamin D to keep bones strong, and without a solid framework, skin loses the integrity of its shape.

- ☐ A good multivitamin. Skin needs a range of vitamins and minerals to make collagen, and a multi can help fill in any gaps in your nutrition.

HUMIDIFY YOUR HOME

As you grow older, you may become more sensitive to temperatures, owing to diminished fat reserves, and you may keep your home heating turned up. To avoid skin dehydration, especially overnight, add moisture to the air with a humidifier or by placing bowls of water near heating sources.

SEE A PROFESSIONAL REGULARLY

You should see your dermatologist annually for a skin check—more often if you notice any unusual changes or growths. And a regular visit can also help you address certain signs of aging in a targeted way. Light peels that are done in a professional's office are easy, inexpensive, involve little downtime, and take only minutes. They can treat everything from tone and texture irregularities to pigmentation and wrinkles.

An in-office skin-maintenance treatment typically involves applying an acid over the facial skin—trichloroacetic and glycolic acids are common—which causes the bonds between surface cells to become unglued and flake off over the course of the following week. The treatment may sting or burn for a minute, and you may leave the doctor's office with slightly pink skin. Over the course of the following week, the treated area may look a little dry and flaky, but soon a healthy glow will emerge in the absence of so many dead cells—and effects last for months. Repeated peels are also effective for evening out skin discoloration and reducing whiteheads and blackheads.

A facial can also improve the appearance of wide and clogged pores. Women in their seventies and eighties are prone to developing "patulous," or gaping, pores, owing to the breakdown of surrounding collagen support due to sun damage. Older women with reduced vision also may not see both white- and blackheads, which can make the skin look dirty and uneven. A facial extracts those blockages and makes skin look fresher and more even in pigmentation.[3]

PREVENT SKIN-RELATED HEALTH PROBLEMS

While we tend to focus on the look and health of our facial skin, it's important not to neglect the skin that's less exposed to the public eye—or yours. First and foremost, be vigilant about monitoring any changes to skin texture and color and bring them to the attention of your doctor. What's going on at the surface of the skin is often a bellwether for what's happening in the rest of your body.

DON'T IGNORE THE ITCH

Dry skin is not just red or rough to the touch—it can also itch. While the causes of dry, itchy skin range from dehydration to stress, sometimes itching is associated with graver diseases, such as diabetes or kidney disease. If moisturizing can't cure the problem, consult your doctor.

CHECK FOR BRUISES

The older you are, the more easily you bruise and the longer it can take for a bruise to vanish because skin is thinner and slower to heal. But bruising can be a sign of nutritional deficiencies, blood-clotting disorders, and even cancer. If you notice that you bruise easily and often and can't recall how you got a bruise, see your doctor.

KEEP TABS ON SWELLING AND DISCOLORATION

Many age-related skin problems reflect underlying systemic disease. For instance, the heart condition known as vascular insufficiency or chronic venous insufficiency, can lead to blood collecting in the legs, causing discoloration and swelling. If you begin to notice any changes, see your doctor for a checkup.[4]

TRACK CHANGES IN YOUR SKIN

Check moles, birthmarks, or other parts of the skin, using the following ABCDE system. Don't wait for the area to hurt—skin cancer isn't usually painful. See your doctor right away if you notice any of these signs.

- [ ] **A**symmetry (one half of the growth looks different from the other half)

- [ ] **B**orders that are irregular

- [ ] **C**olor changes or more than one color

- [ ] **D**iameter greater than the size of a pencil eraser

- [ ] **E**volving, meaning changes in size, shape, symptoms (itching, tenderness), surface (especially bleeding), or shades of color

KNOW THE SIGNS OF SKIN CANCER

With more than 2 million people diagnosed annually with skin cancer, it is the most common type of cancer in the United States. The disease's main cause is exposure to ultraviolet radiation from the sun. This adds up over time, so even if you haven't sunbathed in years, your childhood exposure still impacts your current skin status. Use of sunlamps and tanning booths also increases your risk. People with fair skin that freckles easily—and contains less protective melanin—are generally most prone.

Skin cancer falls into two categories: nonmelanoma—which includes basal-cell carcinoma and squamous-cell carcinoma—and the more dangerous melanoma. The latter is more rare than the other types—affecting an estimated 76,250 people in the United States in 2012, according to the National Cancer Institute—but it can spread to other organs and can be fatal.

It's extremely important to book yearly appointments with a dermatologist to give your skin a complete once-over, but you should also check monthly for cancerous spots. Pay particular attention to changes such as a new growth, a sore that doesn't heal, or a bleeding mole. Here are other symptoms to look for:

TYPE OF CANCER . . .	FOUND ON . . .	LOOK FOR . . .
BASAL-CELL CARCINOMA	Head, face, neck, hands, arms, and other body parts exposed to the sun.	Pearly bump that bleeds or won't heal. Growth could be white, light pink, flesh colored, or brown.
SQUAMOUS-CELL CARCINOMA	Head, face, neck, hands, arms, and other body parts exposed to the sun; may occur on areas that have been injured or inflamed	Rough, scaly area with flat, reddish patches
MELANOMA	Anywhere on the body, including in the mouth and eyes	Brown, black, or blue growth. Pay particular attention to any that are asymmetrical, have uneven borders or color, are larger than 6 mm wide, or continue to change appearance.

DEVELOP A MORNING SKIN-CARE ROUTINE

If you have a skin-care routine of any sort, you're one step ahead—consistency is key. But if you've been using the same products for years (or the bar of soap in the shower to wash your face), a few tweaks may prove helpful. While some targeted ingredients are proven to help temporarily improve the look of your skin, the biggest changes you'll likely see are from sticking to a consistent routine with simple products. Here is a basic routine that is effective starting at any age.

STEP 1

CLEANSER

This step is important because it primes the canvas for the rest of your healthy skin-care regimen. Your skin type will dictate whether or not you need to wash your face once or twice a day. If you cleansed thoroughly the previous evening and have normal to dry skin, a splash of water in the morning should be sufficient. If you have oily skin, wash again with a gentle cleanser to remove overnight oil buildup.

To cleanse effectively, gently massage face in circular motions, avoiding the eye area. And don't miss the areas around your forehead and ears, which are where excess dirt and grime can accumulate. Rinse with tepid (never hot) water and follow with a cold-water splash to constrict blood vessels and firm the skin.

STEP 2

TONER

A companion to a cleanser, toner helps remove residue and restore proper pH balance to the skin. Depending on your skin type, you'll want to choose a toner that soothes, disinfects, or exfoliates.

STEP 3

MASK

Facial masks treat a range of issues, including enlarged, congested pores, dryness, and irritation, while helping to tighten and firm the skin. Look for masks formulated for mature skin that include ingredients such as collagen, coenzyme Q10, and vitamin C. Many of these masks also include natural exfoliators, such as oatmeal or seaweed. Some masks can be used daily, while others are designed to be used several times a week.

STEP 4

ANTIOXIDANT SERUM

Many skin-care products contain some sort of antioxidant ingredient—popular ones include green tea or the vitamins A, C, or E. Antioxidants help to block free radicals from damaging healthy skin cells. Free radicals are produced in the living cells of the dermis, so you want to drive the active antioxidants into the skin, where they're needed. While antioxidant ingredients are common in moisturizers, consider applying a serum—which is lightweight and typically more concentrated than a cream—after cleansing and before your daily moisturizer.

STEP 5

DAILY MOISTURIZER

A good daily moisturizer plumps the skin almost immediately by retaining moisture in the superficial layers of skin. Look for hydrating ingredients like squalene, glycerin, or hyaluronic acid, which help the skin absorb moisture and are suitable for oily or combination skin. Dry skin may benefit from a cream that features petroleum and silicone, which create a moisture-locking barrier on top of the skin. Although most basic moisturizing creams can be applied close to the eyes, eye creams often contain ingredients that help treat specific issues. Puffiness, for example, is often treated with cucumber or caffeine extract, and dark circles with vitamin K, so it's worth investing in a separate eye product if you have those or other eye issues.

STEP 6

SUNSCREEN

Apply a daily sunscreen about 15 minutes before you go outside, because it takes a little time for the active chemicals to be absorbed and become effective. You can use an SPF-enhanced moisturizing face cream, but you'll want to use a different moisturizer at night so you don't sleep with SPF on.

Sunscreens are labeled with an SPF (sun protection factor), which refers to the time it takes for skin to burn under laboratory conditions with the sunscreen versus without. Always aim to wear a minimum of SPF 30, which blocks 97 percent of the sun's damaging UVB rays. Higher SPF lotions protect more, but only minimally—SPF 100 protects only 2 percent more than SPF 30.

When choosing a sunscreen, look for ones that cover for both UVA (the aging rays) and UVB (the burning rays). There are several types of sun-blocking ingredients, but all are either chemical blocks (like Parsol 1789, Helioplex, or Mexoryl) or physical blocks (zinc oxide or titanium dioxide); many sunscreens contain a combination of both. Chemical sunscreens absorb the sun's UV rays. Physical blocks stay on the surface and work by reflecting rays—though formulas have improved, they may take a little longer to blend. No matter what you choose, sunscreen only lasts two to four hours, so be sure to reapply frequently.

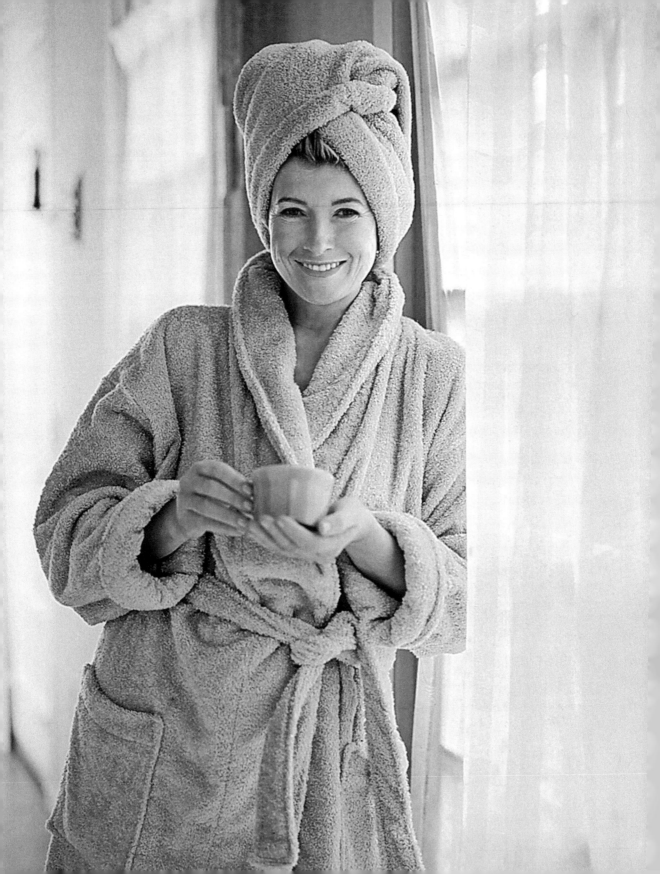

MY SKIN-CARE ROUTINE

I take excellent care to cleanse and pamper my skin because I have to wear makeup very frequently for public appearances and interviews, and it is subjected to so much wear and tear. Clean skin is so important to maintaining one's healthy appearance.

1. I get up around four o'clock to start my work for the day and put on a facial mask of collagen or ginkgo; there are so many good ones now. I don't rinse it off until I shower, an hour or so later, and it leaves my skin very silky.

2. In the shower, I wash my entire body with an exfoliant or silicone soap, and then slather moisturizer all over (if I'm feeling lavish, sometimes I'll use rich facial products on my body).

3. I also drink the juice of a lemon with hot water, which I find very cleansing and detoxifying.

4. If I'm planning to be outside, I always use a moisturizer with sunscreen. Alexis reminds me to be diligent about it—she absolutely will not spend time in the sun, but because I love the outdoors, I need that daily sun protection.

At the end of each day, I remove the makeup using a reliable, traditional technique: baby oil and a cleanser with a hot washcloth. If it's everyday makeup I'm removing, I use a silicone soap—it's the cleanest soap I've ever found. You absolutely must go to sleep with a clean face, to prevent irritation and clogged pores—if there's any color coming off on your pillow, you haven't done a thorough job.

AVOID THESE BEAUTY-PRODUCT INGREDIENTS

Certain ingredients in our cosmetics can irritate sensitive skin. Others are potential endocrine disruptors and possible carcinogens. Carefully read labels on all cosmetics and avoid any that contain the following chemicals:

- **Diethanolamine:** This ingredient appears on shampoo labels as "DEA." While it's typically added to increase lather, DEA has been shown to increase liver tumors in lab animals.

- **Formaldehyde:** A skin and respiratory system irritant and considered a human carcinogen by health agencies, it's still found in some nail polish and hair-straightening salon treatments. Look for nail polishes that state they're formaldehyde-free.

- **Hydroquinone:** This skin-lightening agent is found in skin creams and under-eye-circle treatments; some evidence links it to cancer in lab animals.

- **Parabens:** Found in toothpaste, shampoo, makeup, and moisturizer, these are identified by "methyl-," "ethyl-," "propyl-," "butyl-," and "isobutylparaben" on labels. Animal studies reveal that these have estrogenic effects.

- **Phenylenediamine:** Hair dyes may contain so-called PPD; this component can cause irritation to the lungs and nervous system.

- **Petroleum distillates:** These often appear on product labels as "petroleum" or "liquid paraffin." The European Union has restricted or banned these ingredients because of their association with cancer.

- **Phthalates:** Hiding in some nail polishes, shampoos, and fragrances, these plasticizing chemicals are suspected endocrine disrupters. Look for nail polishes that are free of dibutyl phthalates (called "DBP" on many labels), and opt for natural fragrances or fragrance-free products.

- **Sodium lauryl sulfate:** An ingredient commonly found in face and body cleansers and shampoos, the strong cleansing agent can be too harsh for dry or sensitive skin.

- **Synthetic fragrances:** Listed broadly as "fragrance" on labels, some synthetic fragrances can irritate sensitive skin or cause headaches. Look instead for fragrance-free products or those that list only essential oils, not fragrance.

- **Talc:** In many body powders and some makeup, talc is a suspected carcinogen, so be sure to shop for cornstarch-based or talc-free formulas.

INDULGE IN A FACIAL MASSAGE

There is nothing quite as effective as a well-performed facial massage to stimulate circulation and the lymphatic system; the latter regulates the amount of fluid (affecting swelling) in tissues. If you can't have a facial massage regularly, give yourself a mini massage when applying your night creams, with some gentle sweeping and tapping movements.

1. Using your fingertips, begin with small, sweeping strokes on the forehead, going from brow to hairline.

2. Moving to the midface, use light, consistent strokes and rub from the sides of the nose to the temples.

3. Stroke from the middle of the chin to the end of the jaw line below the ear.

4. Starting at the forehead, locate the eight pressure-point areas (O), and massage each spot.

5. Gently tap the entire face to finish.

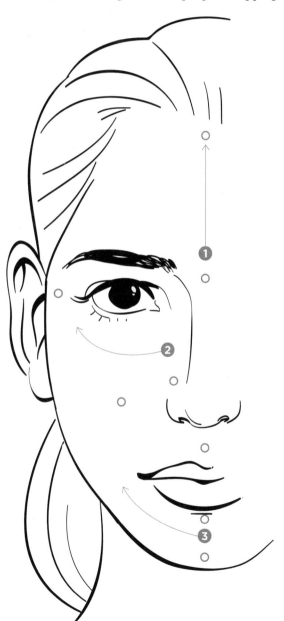

DEVELOP AN EVENING SKIN-CARE ROUTINE

Nighttime is when the skin rejuvenates and repairs, so the products you use before you sleep are the ones that will have a transformative effect on skin. Removing accumulated makeup, oil, and dirt from the day will help keep your complexion blemish-free, while applying other products can target specific issues, such as brown spots and wrinkles. The following basic routine will go a long way to keeping your skin looking its best.

STEP 1

CLEANSER

Everyone needs to wash his or her face before bed, to remove makeup or just the daily build-up of environmental dirt, grime, and surface-skin oils. Choose a formula that's suited to your skin type; you'll know you're using the right one when your skin feels clean but not tight after cleansing. Oily skin tends to fare well with gel or foam cleansers, while cream- or oil-based formulas are ideal for drier skin types. Using a mirror with magnification and a light can help ensure that you remove makeup completely.

STEP 2

EXFOLIANT

This is the product you'll need more and more as you age. When you're young, the top layer of skin turns over to reveal a new, plumper layer roughly every twenty-four to forty-two days. By age 30, that rate begins to slow so that as you reach 80, skin takes 50 percent longer to renew itself. That's why older skin can look so dull and blotchy.

Products containing beta and alpha hydroxy acids are effective at promoting cell turnover. In so doing, they help remove surface irregularities, brown spots from sun damage (or hyperpigmentation), and fine wrinkles. Opt for combination products (for instance, AHA plus cleanser or moisturizer) or a stand-alone formula. For the latter, Dr. Gerald Imber, a plastic surgeon in New York City, recommends acid concentrations as high as 10 percent. "These may be irritating at first," he cautions, "so use them at bedtime, followed by a soothing moisturizer." Some products are gentle enough to use daily, but if you have sensitive skin, you may want to start using them only every other day or three times a week until you see how your skin responds.

And don't neglect your body! Chronically dry skin can lead to a greater susceptibility to irritation and infection, as well as contact dermatitis and allergies. Keep your skin supple from head to toe with physical exfoliation once or twice a week. An exfoliating sponge, loofah, or washcloth are all effective for stimulating cell turnover for most body parts (except the face, where the skin is too delicate). You could also try brushing dry skin with a soft-bristled brush before showering, or dry yourself post-shower with a towel that hasn't been washed with fabric softener. Always follow exfoliation with a moisturizer.

STEP 3

ANTIOXIDANT SERUM

An accumulation of free radicals, caused by sun and environmental exposure, can exacerbate wrinkles and age spots. Fighting these free radicals with antioxidants will help the skin repair itself. While many nighttime moisturizers contain antioxidants, a serum is usually more concentrated. As directed in the morning routine, on pages 236–237, apply your serum after cleansing and before you moisturize.

STEP 4

NIGHT CREAM

When choosing a night cream, consider your primary concerns. Whether it's a bleaching cream for under-eye circles and discoloration or a prescription-only formula for wrinkles, a dermatologist can prescribe a product for particular needs. Some proven topical skin-care ingredients include these:

- **Retinol:** It is a mild form of prescription Retin-A, one of the most effective treatments for diminishing fine wrinkling. Both ingredients help normalize erratic skin cells, which can help improve skin texture and reduce pigment irregularity.

- **Peptides:** Best for fine lines around the mouth and eyes; ample science demonstrates that peptides can reverse early lines.

- **Glycolic acid:** One of the oldest and best ingredients used for skin care, glycolic acid is great to get the skin to turn over, smooth the surface, and erase blackheads.

- **Hyaluronic acid:** By delivering hydration deep into the skin, it temporarily plumps out wrinkles.

- **Squalene:** Derived from olives and shark livers, this oil softens the skin surface by absorbing water from the environment.

STEP 5

EYE CREAM

Eye cream can help firm skin and smooth fine lines, although it isn't a necessity. Often other moisturizers work just as well. Whatever you use, just be careful not to daub it any higher than the bone under your eye, or it might migrate upward and leave your eyes red and irritated.

TREAT TROUBLESOME SKIN CONDITIONS

When basic skin care isn't improving a skin condition, or troublesome spots suddenly crop up, it may be the result of a larger problem. You can improve many skin conditions with an at-home treatment, but it's important to see a dermatologist to get a proper diagnosis before you do so.

ADULT ACNE

RECOGNIZE IT Just like the pesky breakouts you may have had as a teen, adult acne can be caused by fluctuating hormones, stress, cosmetics, and bacteria. Acne can range from small white bumps to larger red sores. While it often shows up on the face, especially the chin, nose, and forehead, it can appear anywhere on the body.

CAUSE When sebum (the oily substance that keeps skin moisturized) clogs pores, bacteria can grow and become inflamed, creating a breakout. Hormones and stress are sometimes the reason for the overproduction of sebum; hands as well as objects such as telephones and clothing can introduce bacteria, which cause inflammation.

TREAT IT Over-the-counter washes and creams often contain benzoyl peroxide or salicylic acids, which help to kill the bacteria that cause acne. Since many acne products are designed for teenage skin, which is very oily, it's important to use products that are designed for adult skin, or to incorporate them one at a time, so you don't overdry the skin. If over-the-counter solutions aren't working, a dermatologist can prescribe topical or oral antibiotics. Laser treatments can also help address bacteria and regulate oil production, as well as minimize acne scars.

ECZEMA

RECOGNIZE IT An itchy condition that shows up mostly as red patches and small raised bumps, eczema is an inflammation of the skin that tends to flare and subside. It shows up most commonly on the arms and behind the knees.

CAUSE While it's not clear what causes eczema, hot baths, stress, changes in temperature, and irritants such as soaps, dust, and cigarette smoke often exacerbate it. There also may be a connection to dry skin and the body's immune system malfunctioning.

TREAT IT Avoid drying soaps and other irritants and limit bathing. Applying moisturizers or cool, wet compresses can help relieve itching; using a humidifier and wearing cotton clothing further calms irritation. A doctor may recommend prescription steroid creams, oral antibiotics, or antihistamines.

PSORIASIS

RECOGNIZE IT Thick, red painful patches covered with silvery scales define this skin disease, which causes skin to grow rapidly. There are many different types of psoriasis (including scalp and nail), which can appear as small spots of scales or larger red patches, or even dry, cracked skin that bleeds. It's most commonly seen on the scalp, knees, elbows, and lower back. A chronic condition, there are times when psoriasis may get better or worse, but it never goes away entirely.

CAUSE It isn't known what causes psoriasis, but it's thought to be a combination of the body's immune system getting weakened and a genetic susceptibility. Possible triggers include infections, stress, cold, or skin injury.

TREAT IT Simple measures like bathing in water with Epsom salts to remove scales and soothe itching, using an over-the-counter cortisone cream, and getting moderate amounts of natural sunlight can help improve symptoms. There are ways to treat psoriasis topically: prescription steroid drugs and tar shampoo are the most common. By suppressing the immune system, they slow cell turnover, which reduces inflammation.

Over-the-counter options include salicylic acid, which helps to slough skin cells, and moisturizers, which can help with itchiness and dryness. Light therapy (controlled doses from a light source, administered by a doctor) can help by exposing your skin to UV rays, slowing cell turnover.

ROSACEA

RECOGNIZE IT The hallmark of this inflammatory skin condition is redness (flushing) and small, red bumps. It is seen most often on the cheeks and nose, though it may also appear around the mouth, and sometimes it affects the eyes.

CAUSE The triggers for rosacea are different for everyone, but common causes of flare-ups include hot food or beverages, spicy foods, alcohol, sunlight, high or low temperatures, stress, and hot baths.

TREAT IT Rosacea doesn't have a cure, but treatments can help control the condition. At home, try to identify and avoid your triggers and use a gentle cleanser and moisturizer. If that's not working, a combination of prescription oral and topical antibiotics are often used. Laser treatment is effective for redness caused by blood vessels. These anti-inflammatory compounds are thought to help by decreasing some of the bacteria that inhabit the skin. Symptoms can return if medication is stopped, so long-term treatment is often recommended.

SKIN TAGS

RECOGNIZE IT These flesh-colored noncancerous growths can appear anywhere on the body, although they're most often seen in areas where skin folds or rubs, like the eyelids, neck, underarms, or under the breasts.

CAUSE Genetics and obesity may play a role in who is prone to getting skin tags, but reduc-

ing friction in some of these areas may help prevent them.

TREAT IT There's not much you can do to treat skin tags at home, but as long as they're not getting irritated and red, they usually pose no threat. If they're bothersome, a dermatologist can remove them.

MATCH *your makeup to your age*

It's easy to get stuck in a makeup rut, relying on favorite products and colors you've used for many years. Yet it's very important that your cosmetics evolve as you age, to account for your changing skin's needs.

Every couple of years, assess whether your go-to look is still working for you. "Women will change their clothes, but when it comes to hair and makeup, they go with what they've always done," says veteran makeup artist Charlie Green. "Makeup can make you feel confident, put-together, professional, and it can put a spring in your step. Wearing it and keeping it fresh is a nice touch—even if you're just doing it for yourself." Look hard at your reflection in the mirror—are your eyelids a little heavier than before? Is the skin duller, paler, or drier? Are your lips the same shape? All of these details inform the best strategy for updating your look.

Now consider your tried-and-true makeup routine in light of some of the changes you've observed in the mirror. Perhaps it's time to highlight your eyes more, or to bring more color to your cheeks, or some prominence to your thinning lips. You are the artist, and you can decide how to paint the prettiest picture.

Keep in mind, however, that your makeup style doesn't have to recede just because you're older. If red lipstick or bright eyeliner is your signature look, don't stop wearing what you love. Just make sure that when you choose one feature that you want to stand out, you keep the rest of your look subtle and understated.

It's important to get a good makeup lesson every few years. Find a professional who can show you how to adjust your makeup. Or try a makeup artist at your favorite department store makeup counter—often these stylists are very skilled and the lesson is free, though you'll need to be smart about the fact that they're trying to sell you products. If they put a new color on you, see if they have a good reason for doing so. If you ask questions and listen, you can pick up some good tips.

Finally, invest in high-quality makeup brushes. Putting these and other well-made tools to work can change the way your makeup works. Big, fluffy brushes distribute powder evenly, foundation brushes can help liquid makeup look flawless, and targeted brushes for eye makeup let you apply it in just one swipe. To care for your brushes, wash them weekly with a mild shampoo and lay them flat to dry (standing them on their end sends water into the barrel of the brush, loosening bristles).

BE AWARE OF EXPIRATION DATES

Like most toiletries, makeup has a shelf life. As a product ages, it can irritate your skin, and some of its ingredients eventually break down into carcinogens. Many products now use a Period After Opening (PAO) icon, which indicates how many months the item should last after you crack the seal. If your makeup doesn't have this icon, use a fine-tip permanent marker to note the discard date on the product itself. Here's a general guideline of when to toss old cosmetics:

PRODUCT . . .	SHOULD LAST . . .	TOSS SOONER IF . . .
MASCARA AND LIQUID EYELINER	Three to four months	You get an infection, such as pinkeye, or it dries out
POWDERS: EYE SHADOW, BLUSH, FACE POWDER	Up to two years	It gets suspiciously crumbly or shiny
LIP GLOSS, LIPSTICK, BALM	A year with a wand, two years with direct or brush application	You get a cold sore or other lip infection
PENCILS	Up to three years, with sharpening	It becomes either unusually dry or melts
LIQUID FOUNDATIONS	Up to two years	The color changes or separation occurs

ESTABLISH A MAKEUP ROUTINE

For a polished look that suits the needs of your face now and keeps you looking your best, use this easy guide to a basic makeup application.

STEP 1

PRIMER

The key to flawless makeup is proper skin care—good moisturizing creams create a beautiful canvas for your personal palette. Age-related skin changes mean that foundation can settle into fine lines or rapidly soak into dry skin. To prevent this from happening and to prepare a smooth surface for foundation that will last all day, try a clear gel primer with a silicone base over your daily moisturizer. Apply it in the areas where skin collects oil—forehead, nose, chin, and the top of the cheeks—and feather it out across the face.

STEP 2

FOUNDATION

Foundation is the building block of all your other makeup, so choose one that blends in well with your skin. If skin tends to be dry, a liquid foundation can make it look dewy. If skin is prone to oiliness, a powder (pressed or loose) will help absorb excess oil. A lot of new foundations have a "cream-to-powder" finish (you'll see that phrase stated on the packaging), meaning that they go on like a cream but look matte and powdery when they dry, and work for most skin types.

To find a foundation that matches your skin perfectly, test a few shades—but not on the back of your hand, which tends to be darker than your face. Instead, swipe swatches on your cheeks. If you're using a liquid, allow the product to dry, as the color may change. If you can, sample the product by a window or step outside to see what it looks like in natural light. Don't get wedded to one shade: you may need to change the hue with the seasons, or climate (if you've moved to the Southwest, for example, or taken an extended vacation).

STEP 3

BLUSH AND BRONZER

Blush, either liquid or powder, should be applied to the apples of the cheeks, which you can find by smiling and locating the fatty round part just under the cheekbones. Bronzer is a lovely way to attain a warm glow without venturing into the sun. Look for a powder that could be the color of your skin when you're tan, and avoid products that are orange or sparkly, as these don't look natural on anyone. After blush, apply bronzer anywhere the sun would hit (forehead, the bridge of the nose, the top of the cheekbones, and chin) using a big, fluffy brush and blending in a swirling motion. A little goes a long way, so go easy on the amount you use.

If you don't want to add color, but are looking for a way to brighten skin, try illuminators, which reflect light. Try them along cheekbones, on brow bones, and down the bridge of the nose. Just be sure to pick creams, not powders, which have larger particles that can look overly glittery.

STEP 4

EYES

Eye shadow rubs off easily and typically starts to crease as the day goes on. To prevent this, use an eye shadow primer. Much like skin primer, this cream creates a base, giving eye shadow something to hold on to. Apply it to lids with a flat brush before your shadow.

When applying shadow, consider the changing shape of your eyes. If you bring shadow all the way to the outer corner of the eye, it can cause them to appear droopy. Instead, apply color in the inner corner and then sweep it outward, letting it diffuse as it hits the outer edge. When shopping for shadows, look for cream shadows, which are easier to blend than powders.

An aging eye will tend to develop a "hooded" look, meaning that the delicate skin of the lids begins to droop. Use eyeliner to frame the eyes. Then curl your lashes from base to tip before applying mascara. This will make the eyes appear bigger.

STEP 5

BROWS

Shaping your eyebrows can define your face, even if you don't wear makeup. If you've never shaped your brows, try seeing a professional first to determine the best shape for your face—then maintain it at home by tweezing. To prevent a sparse brow, pull just a few hairs each day until you achieve the look you like. You can always do more the next day, but they grow about twice as slowly as the rest of your hair, so pluck with caution.

STEP 6

LIPS

If your lips become dry and cracked seasonally, apply a daily lip balm. A swipe before bed will help lock in moisture and repair lips while you sleep. Look for a moisturizing lipstick that does double duty by conditioning lips (vitamin E, aloe, and shea butter are common ingredients) while adding color. Those who intend to be out in the sun should choose a lipstick or balm with SPF; lips actually have less melanin than other parts of the skin and are more prone to sun damage.

To prevent lip color from bleeding into the fine lines around your lips, powder lightly around the edges of the lips or pat gently with a concealer. If your lipstick tends to wear off quickly, stay away from greasy formulas and try a "long-wearing" lipstick. If you'd rather not worry about how long your color lasts, stick to neutral, sheer colors. It's less noticeable when they wear off, so you won't need to reapply as frequently. To enhance your pout, try a dab of gloss atop your lipstick in the middle of both lips, which will reflect light and make lips appear fuller.

CONSIDER *cosmetic enhancements*

To get a glimpse at where you're headed physically, New York City plastic surgeon Dr. Gerald Imber suggests breaking out the family photo album. "If your grandparents or parents had under-eye bags or jowls, chances are you will, too. Decide whether you're okay with the family physical traits or not." If you want to follow a different path, you have choices.

When topical treatments aren't enough, more invasive procedures can be discussed with a plastic surgeon. However, healthy lifestyle habits and good skin care have a huge effect on the well-being of your skin, and treatments from dermatologists can restore a glow. Given the new technologies available today, it's possible to get great results without ever going "under the knife."

FREEZE FACIAL LINES

You've no doubt heard of Botox, and perhaps its European competitor, Dysport—injectibles for achieving smoother, more youthful complexions. These products, made from a safe and purified form of botulinum toxin (derived from bacteria), are incredibly effective at smoothing frown lines and wrinkles caused by routine facial expressions or smoking; however, they cannot address sagging or deeper wrinkles.

Botox and Dysport work by blocking the neurotransmitter that tells the nerve to tense the targeted muscle at the injection points, and they have been approved by the FDA to treat the vertical frown lines, or "elevens," between the brows; they are also commonly used to relax smile or squint lines and the striated horizontal grooves across the brow. "Occasionally, too, I use an injectible to soften the dimpling of the chin that some patients develop with age, as well as the vertical bands of the neck," Dr. Imber notes.

Botox and Dysport are most effective when used before the skin has a great deal of lines and laxity. You'll see results within twenty-four hours to a week, but these usually wane within three to four months. These injections—although available at many spas, hair salons, and medi spas—should be administered by a licensed dermatologist or plastic surgeon. This should help to ensure that the products are full strength (some discount places will dilute products to provide a "deal") and that the person administering the treatment has the skill to tackle any problems that, while rare, may occur.

TREAT LINES WITH FILLERS

The class of FDA-approved cosmetic fillers, which include collagen, hyaluronic acids, and one's own body fat, work at filling in many of the telltale lines of age, such as na-solabial folds (between the nose and the corners of the mouth), marionette lines (running from the corners of the mouth to the chin), thin lips, sunken cheeks, depressed under-eye troughs, and concave forehead temporal areas. As the face loses fat over time, causing concavities and hollowness, these fillers allow a cosmetic surgeon or dermatologist to sculpt more youthful facial contours.

A good filler should not produce hypersensitivity or inflammation, nor should it clump or cause pain beyond just a pinch at the injection site. A topical anesthetic can be applied to the skin before injection to further prevent discomfort. Each filler performs optimally when injected at a certain depth, and a skillful practitioner may use more than one kind at once to achieve a desired look.

Be sure you're receiving treatment from a licensed cosmetician or plastic surgeon—expertise on the part of the doctor is crucial—and note that not all lines can be filled. "To change the surface texture of your skin, you'll need a resurfacing treatment," says New York City dermatologist Catherine Orentreich. Below and on the next page is a list of current options.

FILLER: HYALURONIC ACID

Found naturally in the connective tissues of the body, hyaluronic acid decreases with age and the body's exposure to UV light. This light filler, made synthetically, is best for fine lines, where the wrinkles aren't too deep, and some deep folds.

BRAND NAME	BEST FOR	PROS	CONS
RESTYLANE	Under-eye area, nasolabial folds, medium-deep wrinkles, lips	Lasts up to 8 months, but the more frequently you're treated, the longer it lasts	Though rare, bruising can occur (lasts up to a week).
JUVÉDERM	Hollow cheeks, fine or deep wrinkles, large areas	Lasts up to a year	Bruising occurs rarely; lasts up to a week.
HYDRELLE	Deep wrinkles, nasolabial folds, thicker-skinned areas of the face	Lasts up to a year; minimal swelling or bruising	Rarely, severe redness and tenderness occur.
PERLANE	Deep wrinkles, re-contouring jaw line, lips	Six months to well over a year	Touch-ups may be needed.

FILLER: COLLAGENS AND COLLAGEN STIMULATORS

These calcium-based (Radiesse) or synthetic (Sculptra) fillers gradually increase skin thickness, adding volume to the face. Sculptra is a collagen stimulator and the only product approved for this purpose. It not only fills the skin but also helps the body produce its own collagen, so results last a little longer.

BRAND NAME	BEST FOR	PROS	CONS
RADIESSE	Cheekbones, jaw line, hands, nose reshaping	Lasts one to two years	Unintended bumps may arise when used on lips.
SCULPTRA	Replacing volume over large areas (called "the liquid facelift")	Lasts up to two years	Must be injected in several sessions spaced over months; must massage area for 5 minutes, five times a day for a week; results not immediate.

FILLER: SEMIPERMANENT AND PERMANENT FILLERS

While permanent options for lines and wrinkles are worth considering for nasolabial folds or scars such as deep acne scars, some doctors caution against using them because if they wind up moving or if your face changes as you age, they may not look natural and will then have to be removed.

IN THE SYRINGE	BEST FOR	PROS	CONS
BODY FAT (your own—removed by liposuction procedure, typically from belly, thigh, or rear)	Cheekbones, nasolabial folds, under-eye area	Lasts from six months to forever; no worry about allergic reactions because it comes from you	Time intensive—involves lipo-suction plus procedure.
SILICONE	Lips, deep wrinkles, scars, cheek volume	Permanent	May migrate and form granulomas, or a small clump of cells.

IMPROVE SKIN TONE AND REPAIR WRINKLED SKIN

To reverse sun damage, redness, fine wrinkles, or brown spots, consider laser treatment. Lasers (an acronym for Light Amplification by Stimulated Emission of Radiation) come in different wavelengths and strengths—the lights are strong enough to vaporize the top layer of skin and cause new skin to grow. A good laser may tighten the skin temporarily and help get rid of wrinkles. They help the skin look youthful by making the surface smoother and more even. Unlike fillers, though, which require very little downtime, lasers can put people out of commission for five to seven days, so you need to be able to take some recovery time. If you have dark or olive skin, you'll want to talk to your doctor because there's a risk of pigment damage.

MACHINE	BEST FOR	PROS	CONS
NON-ABLATIVE LASERS (E.G., FRACTIONAL)	Facial redness, thready veins around nose and on cheeks	Decreases redness; minimum downtime; noninvasive; may help superficial wrinkles	Photosensitivity, slight bruising, may require several treatments; doesn't tighten skin.
PHOTO DYNAMIC THERAPY/ INTENSE PULSED LIGHT (IPL)	Sun damage (e.g., AKs, or actinic keratoses) and acne; oil-gland expansions (aka sebaceous hyperplasia)	Treats brown and red spots at the same time, improves skin texture, may help fine lines and wrinkles, stimulates collagen production; especially good for those over 60 because they have the most sun damage. Covered by most insurance and Medicare.	You must avoid sun for 48 hours posttreatment; sun sensitivity can last approximately 3 months.
ABLATIVE LASER RESURFACING	Improving sun damage, brown discoloration, and redness— known as the "photofacial"	Results evident after one treatment; often last up to a year	Skin is raw then pink for a month or two; painful (can require sedation).

ENCOURAGE *healthy hair*

A healthy head of hair is a signifier of youth. As we age and hormone levels change, hair color, texture, and thickness are invariably transformed. Through the years, too, pigment-producing cells shut down, turning hair gray or white, and there is a conversion of terminal (the longer, thicker strands) hair to vellus hair (thin, fine, and short). Many people fight these changes by overtreating their hair to retain their old look and style, or just the opposite—giving in to changes in shade and texture without making any effort to tailor their grooming. But our hair-care routine needs to adapt, too, so we can look our best and maintain the healthiest hair and scalp into our later decades.

CLEANSE AND CONDITION PROPERLY

Hair care begins at the scalp, which is where the oil is produced that both protects hair and makes it limp and greasy. To select a type of shampoo and decide how often you need to wash, you must determine how oily or dry your scalp is. (Note that this may have changed over the years, so the grease-busting shampoo you've relied on for years may be undermining your hair health now.)

If you have oily hair that gets limp by the end of the day, a daily shampoo is probably best. If your scalp doesn't easily become greasy, your hair may do better by washing just a couple of times a week. On days when you don't shampoo, you can still wet your hair in the shower—the water alone will help eliminate some oil and debris without stripping it of essential oils.

Whenever you shampoo, saturate your hair completely with water before applying the product to avoid buildup, and massage the scalp to loosen debris. Wash the suds out thoroughly to avoid dandruff or itchy scalp. As hair grows finer over the years, conditioner is important to help prevent breakage. It also helps the cuticles on the hair shaft to lay flat to prevent frizz—the hair appears shiny and healthy. While your shampoo selection depends on your scalp type, choose a conditioner based on your hair texture. If it's dry and frizzy, look for a heavy-duty conditioner. If it's healthy and balanced, try something lighter. Always apply conditioner at least an inch away from the scalp—oils and waxes from the product can stay on the scalp, leading to fungal overgrowth.

STYLE GENTLY

Styling products help to shape hair and give it volume, but when overused, they can dry out strands, weigh them down, and lead to flaking and dullness. Limit the number of products you use and apply them an inch or two away from the scalp so they don't cause buildup. Foams and mousses are ideal for adding more volume, since they don't tend to weigh hair down. Gels, waxes, and pomades help tame texture, but can also be heavier and goopier. Hair spray often contains alcohol, which in large amounts can damage hair, but as long as it's applied in a light coat, it shouldn't be drying—the alcohol evaporates so quickly that it doesn't have time to penetrate the shaft.

Heat styling is very hard on hair, drying out strands and weakening the bonds. When you use a dryer, hold it several inches away from your head. If you use curling or flat irons, apply a heat-protective spray to the hair first to help minimize damage. Foam rollers are a nice alternative for styling, as the heat isn't as intense. Brushes and combs that pull on the hair can weaken the hair over time, so if you often find yourself trying to untangle hard knots, consider a softer brush.

COLOR CAREFULLY

Gray and white hair is the result of the gradual shutting down of pigment-producing cells in the hair follicle. Because of the contrasting colors, gray hair seems to occur earlier in people with dark hair, but gray strands emerge simultaneously in those with lighter colored hair; they just aren't as visible.

If you decide to color your hair, consult with an expert about the best shade for you, or try pulling out old photos from childhood—the shade of your hair when you were much younger can be a good gauge of what natural colors would look good with your skin tone. When hair is colored, the cuticles on the hair shaft (which normally lie flat like shingles on a roof) are lifted in order to deposit color, so afterwards, the hair is dry and slightly damaged. Choose moisturizing shampoos made for color-treated hair and deep-conditioning treatments to keep hair soft and make color last.

TAKE CONTROL OF HAIR LOSS

Balding in men is usually a condition called androgenetic alopecia, related to fluctuating hormone levels. The pattern of hair loss is very predictable, beginning above the temples and moving to the crown of the head.

While baldness does men no favors, it's especially hard on women. Hair loss can occur in women as early as 40. If you notice early hair loss, immediately see a dermatologist— some even specialize in hair loss. The time to address the problem is when you first notice some loss, not when you've lost a whole patch of hair. The younger you are when starting a medication like Minoxidil (the active ingredient in Rogaine), the better the result, as regrowth is increasingly more difficult as you age.

Often, mild cases of hair loss can be addressed or camouflaged by a different hairstyle, a perm, or strategic coloring. But be sure your styling habits, such as heat styling or aggressive brushing, aren't contributing to the hair loss first. You can also treat fading or thinning eyelashes and eyebrows cosmetically. Besides having them dyed, which lends definition to the face, try lash curlers and lengthening mascara formulas.

For more serious cases of hair loss, you may want to consider surgical techniques. "Hair transplantation for women is simply not prescribed often enough," according to Dr. Catherine Orentreich. "A transplant can be helpful in solving a cosmetic problem, such as filling in a thinning front, or replacing hair lost as a result of a facelift." Note that transplants redistribute hair, but do not address the problem of thinning hair.

Beyond age, there are several other reasons for premature hair loss that require early intervention. If you find your tresses dwindling, have your doctor test you for the following conditions:

Nutrient deficiency: Make sure you're getting enough iron and protein. Supplements can help, so get tested to see if your levels are low.

Medication side effects: Some drugs that treat disorders, including hypertension, high cholesterol, depression, and cancer can lead to hair loss. If you take one of these medications, check with your doctor to see if the two are connected. Switching medications may help stem further loss.

An autoimmune disorder: Some hair loss is normal for women, due to hormonal changes. But if you have outright bald patches, you may be suffering from the autoimmune disorder alopecia areata, in which the body's immune cells attack its own hair follicles, inhibiting hair growth. A dermatologist can treat this with steroid injections, which force the immune cells to back off.

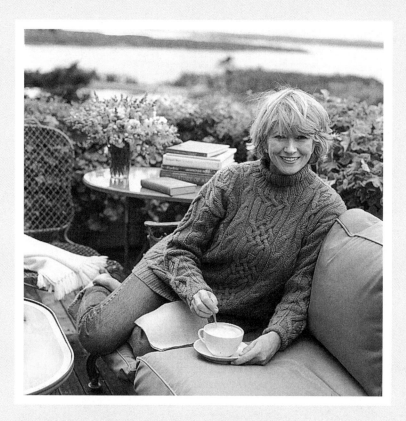

GIVE YOUR HAIR A BREAK

Women subject their hair to so much daily abuse. I have
my hair blow-dried almost every weekday, which can be extremely drying and damaging, so I need to take really good
care of it. I wash and condition it almost every day, but don't
use any products after that, especially hair spray—I hate it! I'm
also convinced that the green juice I drink every day, rich in
nutrients and fresh enzymes (see page 52 for recipe), keeps my
hair strong and shiny. On the weekends, I like to give my hair
a break and don't wash or even comb it at all, unless I have to
go out. I think it helps restore balance to my hair and scalp,
and it's so nice to just relax about it.

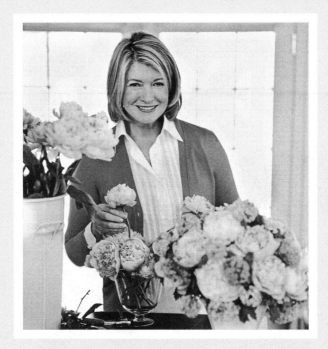

CHAPTER 7

Healthy Home

DISCOVER *smart design* 260

SAFETY-PROOF *your home* 262

EDIT *your home, room by room* 268

ARRANGE *furniture well* 280

CULTIVATE *an indoor garden* 284

CONSIDER *color* 288

ILLUMINATE *your space* 289

MAINTAIN *a healthy home* 290

Your home should be a reflection of how you want to live—right now, and for the next phase of your life. It needs to have a good layout for your changing physical needs, and offer you a sense of security and calm. It's a place to think, do, make, and enjoy. When you get down to it, we need only a few of our creature comforts to live well—for me, that means having plenty of room to entertain, good light so I can read in bed, and sufficient space for all my animals.

Although I'm fortunate to have more than one home, the truth is that my ideal home will someday probably be one large room with a kitchen attached. Day to day I live, write, and create in my kitchen and crafts room, because these are the areas of a home that are most inviting to me. Think about how you can focus on the essential spaces in your own house and make them the best they can be. Happiness doesn't come from wanting to be somewhere else. Happiness comes from finding beauty and stimulation in your every-day surroundings.

DISCOVER *smart design*

Whether you live in an old farmhouse, a suburban family home, or a city loft, you've surely worked hard over the years to make your home beautiful and livable. And like most of us, you hope to stay in your home for as long as possible. Aging in place is important because it lets us retain our freedom and our dignity—and research shows that rates of depression and memory loss are lower when elderly adults can maintain their continuity, surrounded by personal possessions that trigger memories and bring happiness.[1] However, if your home isn't suited for your changing needs, aging in place may become difficult, or even impossible. This is why a smartly designed or remodeled home can serve you well now and in the future.

Even if you don't currently need easier access to your bathroom, kitchen, or living areas, now may be the time to improve your home's long-term efficiency. One way to do so is by implementing universal design, a concept used to create objects, environments, and systems that are accessible and usable by nearly anyone—regardless of age or ability. Remodeling according to universal design standards involves eliminating barriers that could make it harder to navigate, such as poor lighting, stairs, or hard-to-reach appliances. Modifications could be as simple as changing lighting fixtures to installing a ramp or lift for easy wheelchair or walker access. If you live in a multi-level home, you may want to consider arranging it so that you can eventually live on just one floor.

If downsizing, consider whether the layout of a potential living space is appropriate for the long term. Look for a home with universal design elements, such as walk-in bathtubs and showers, easy-to-grasp cabinet and faucet handles, and adjustable kitchen countertops to reduce bending. Many newly constructed homes already have these standards in place, particularly in planned communities designed for people over 50.

Whether you remodel or relocate, taking steps now to improve your home's functionality will help empower you well before the time comes to make a stay-or-go decision.

PUT UNIVERSAL DESIGN INTO PRACTICE

To help create an attractive, safe space that anyone—regardless of age, ability, or size—can enjoy, integrate these universal design features from the National Association of Homebuilders. A Certified Aging-in-Place Specialist (see below) can also advise you on how to modify your home. For more safety-proofing tips, see pages 266–267.

FOR THE	INSTALL
KITCHEN	A raised dishwasher to avoid back strain; a side-by-side refrigerator with slide-out shelves for easier access; larger cabinet and drawer pulls; a cooktop with controls on front; a pull-out cutting board; a lower, side-opening oven.
BATHROOM	Two to three shower grab bars; lever-handled faucets; curbless shower, featuring no or low threshold so users can easily walk or wheel in; tub and shower controls closer to entry point; higher toilet with no-slam seats and lids.
COMMON AREAS, INCLUDING HALLWAYS	Improved lighting with recessed fixtures; lever handles on doors and windows; lower light switches and thermostats; raised outlets; wider doors to accommodate wheelchairs and walkers.
ENTRYWAY	Zero-step entrance; shelf or table by front door for packages and other items; handrails at existing steps and porches; plentiful outdoor lighting.
STAIRWAYS	Handrails on both sides of stairway, 1¼-inch diameter; contrast strips on top and bottom stairs; adequate lighting.

ENLIST THE HELP OF A CERTIFIED AGING-IN-PLACE SPECIALIST

If you'd like to modify your home according to universal design standards, consider hiring a Certified Aging-in-Place Specialist (CAPS). This expert will take your current and future design needs into account to help you come up with a plan for remodeling an existing home, or designing a new one. CAPS design principles focus on creating aesthetically pleasing, barrier-free environments. Both construction and design professionals can be certified under the CAPS program. To find a CAPS professional, visit the website of the National Association of Homebuilders (www.nahb.org).

SAFETY-PROOF *your home*

Beyond staying physically fit, creating a safe environment at home is one of the best ways to ensure that you'll be able to age in place for as long as you want. Of course, the risk of falling or other age-related issues may be years off, as we're living longer and stronger than ever before. But a little advance planning now can bring peace of mind and a higher quality of life later. There are many straightforward precautionary measures you can take to improve the livability and safety of your home, which should allow you to stay in the home you love for many years to come.

FALL-PROOF YOUR HOME

It might seem surprising, but the greatest danger in your home may lurk right below your feet. Falls account for an average of 5.1 million injuries and nearly 6,000 deaths annually.[2] According to the Home Safety Council, falls are by far the leading cause of unintentional home-injury death among adults 73 and older, and the second leading cause of death of adults 60 to 72. "Walk around every room in your home with an eye to spotting risk factors for falls," recommends Julie Kardashi, cofounder of Fall Stop . . . Move Strong, in New York City (www.fallstop.net). "Falls don't just happen to 'old' people, they happen to those who don't believe they're at risk."

Thankfully, most falls can be prevented through home modification and changes in attitudes. Celeste Carlucci, also cofounder of Fall Stop . . . Move Strong, says, "Along with the environmental fixes, we recommend strategies and behaviors that keep people safe, such as pausing if the phone or doorbell rings. Jumping up the second it sounds is one of the top causes of falling at home." She warns, "Avoid multitasking. Stay aware of and conscious of whatever task you're doing. That keeps your attention where it should be: right in front of you." It's also crucial to make an honest assessment of your fitness level. If your mobility has decreased, don't ignore the problem. "So many people 'furniture crawl' or 'wall crawl' around the house; that's a recipe for falling," says Carlucci. Instead of holding on to furniture or walls for stability, use a cane or other walking device.

In addition, never stand on a chair, table, or other surface on wheels, and avoid sitting on furniture that is too low and difficult to stand from. Similarly, invest in a bed that is easy to get in and out of.

SAFE-HOUSE CHECKLIST

Follow these tips from the Home Safety Council, a national nonprofit organization solely dedicated to preventing home injuries, to make your home a true safe haven.

- Use nonskid pads under all rugs.
- Make sure stairs are well lit, with light switches at top and bottom.
- All railings should go from the top to the bottom of the staircase and be easy to grab, at 36 to 39 inches from floor.
- Doors should have easy-to-grip lever-action handles instead of round knobs.
- Furniture arrangements need wide paths for traffic, clear of cords and other trip hazards. (See page 281 for more on this.)
- Keep a lamp or flashlight within easy reach of your bed.
- Install smoke detectors on every level and near sleeping areas so you'll hear them anywhere in the house; change batteries twice a year. (Battery-operated alarms can now be connected by wireless technology so you don't have to worry about batteries going dead.)

- Keep electrical and telephone cords out of walkways.
- Arrange items so they are easy to reach in closets and cupboards.
- Install night-lights for better visibility in the dark.
- Place a slip-proof rug next to the bathtub and a rubber mat or nonskid texture strips inside the tub or shower.
- Replace glass shower doors with nonshattering material.

FAST FIXES FOR FALLS

Falls are often caused by hazards that are easy to overlook but simple to fix. Here's a checklist to help you uncover and remedy risky areas in the home.

THE PROBLEM	POSSIBLE CULPRITS	FAST FIXES
THE SLIP	☐ Loose carpeting on stairways	☐ Tack or tape down all carpeting securely.
	☐ Area rugs without nonskid backing	☐ Replace or install nonskid backing; tape edges of rugs to floor.
	☐ Slippery bathroom and shower floors	☐ Install nonskid strips (consider contrasting strips to aid depth perception). Remove soap scum on a regular basis. Wipe up spills and damp bathroom floors immediately.
	☐ Slippers, backless sandals, or bare feet	☐ Wear sturdy, low, wide-heeled shoes with nonslip soles indoors.
THE WOBBLE	☐ Stacks of papers, books, magazines on the floor, tables, desk, or bookshelves	☐ Rearrange so items aren't stacked, or, better yet, toss outdated periodicals in the recycling bin.
	☐ Anything stored on the stairs	☐ Stick to the rule: nothing stashed on the stairs (even temporarily).
	☐ Frequently used objects stored on high shelves	☐ Organize items you need on a daily basis so they are within reach.
	☐ Deep bathtubs/low toilets	☐ Install grab bars and nonskid tub mats; consider a shower/tub bench to make getting in and out easier; install a toilet riser.
	☐ Rickety chairs	☐ Replace with sturdy chairs with arms, which are easier to get into and out of and better for posture.
	☐ Steep stairs	☐ Install sturdy handrails that extend from the top to the bottom of stairs.

THE PROBLEM	POSSIBLE CULPRITS	FAST FIXES
THE TRIP	☐ Upturned edges of carpets or floor coverings, or loose threads on carpet	☐ Tack or tape edges to the floor (or replace the carpet).
	☐ Pets, pet toys, and pet beds	☐ Train pets to snooze out of high-traffic areas.
	☐ Electric cords or computer cords that cross traffic areas	☐ Tack or tape cords along walls.
	☐ Uneven floorboards; door saddles/doorsills	☐ Repair loose or uneven floors; paint door sills a contrasting color; remove elevated shoulders.
	☐ Furniture crowding	☐ Create space between furniture in high-traffic areas.
THE BLINDSIDE	☐ Dim lighting	☐ Install bright lighting (at least 60 watts); don't let burned-out bulbs languish; consider motion-detection night-lights.
	☐ High-glare floors	☐ Do not polish floors.
	☐ Carrying loads that block your vision, especially on stairs	☐ Move smaller loads; always be sure you can see where you're going.
	☐ Lack of lighting	☐ Buy night-lights for bedroom, bathroom, and any high-traffic area; install light switches at top and bottom of all stairways.

SAFETY-PROOFING, INDOORS AND OUT

Any number of factors can cause safety hazards in and around your home. To help you avoid trouble down the line, here's a simple guide to potential hazards, with easy solutions compiled from the Home Safety Council, Electrical Safety Foundation International, and the National Safety Council.

Many of these precautions may sound excessive now, when you're healthy and fit. But they're well worth the peace of mind they'll give you. And elderly family members (and young children!) will appreciate how accessible these changes make your home. For more tips on preventing indoor falls, see pages 264–265.

BEDROOMS

PREPARE FOR EMERGENCIES	☐ Install a smoke alarm and carbon monoxide detector in or near every bedroom.
	☐ Keep a lamp and flashlight (with extra batteries) by your bed in case of power outages.

BATHROOMS

PREVENT POISONINGS	☐ Keep all medicines in the bottle or box they came in. Make sure you save the label. It may have information your doctor or pharmacist needs to help you in an emergency.
	☐ Use a pill holder to remind you how much of your medications you've taken and when you took them.
	☐ Do not keep medicines or hypodermic needles inside purses, nightstand drawers, or other places children and pets can find them. Instead, store them in a cabinet out of reach.
	☐ Throw out anything that has passed its expiration date, or that has changed color, odor, or taste.
PREVENT SCALDS	☐ Set your water heater at 120°F or just below the medium setting to minimize your risk of burns and scalds.
	☐ Install special tub spouts and showerheads that prevent hot water burns. These fixtures sense if the water gets hot enough to cause a burn and shut off the flow of water.
PREVENT FALLS	☐ Install grab bars by the bathtub, shower, and toilet.
	☐ Put nonslip strips in your tub or shower and use a bath mat with a nonskid bottom next to the tub and shower.
	☐ Keep the bathroom floor clean and dry. Mop up spills as they occur and run the fan when you shower to minimize the humidity that can create damp spots.

KITCHEN

PREVENT FIRES

☐ Always stay in the kitchen when the stove or oven is on. Cooking is the number one cause of home fires—usually because someone forgot a pot on the stove.

☐ Keep your cooking area clean. Don't let grease build up on the range top, in the toaster oven, or in the oven.

☐ Before cooking, roll up sleeves and use oven mitts. Loose-fitting clothes can touch a hot burner and catch on fire.

LIVING ROOMS

PREVENT ELECTRICAL FIRES

☐ Make sure entertainment centers and computer equipment have plenty of space around them for ventilation.

☐ Examine extension cords before each use for cracking or damage. Avoid extension cords in high-traffic areas, under carpets, or across walkways, where they pose a potential tripping hazard.

OUTDOORS

PREVENT FALLS

☐ Put bright lights over all porches, walkways, and at the top and bottom of all staircases.

☐ If you have steps outside your home, keep them free of ice and snow and install handrails on both sides. To prevent a tripping hazard, periodically check steps, walkways, and paths for broken or loose bricks, cement, or stone.

☐ Fix broken or chipped steps and walkways as soon as possible.

☐ Before you mow your lawn, check the area for broken sticks, stones, toys, and anything else that could shoot out from under the mower or damage the blade.

☐ Paint the bottom basement step white to make it more visible. Mistaking the lowest step for floor level can cause you to lose your balance and fall.

☐ Carry smaller loads up and down stairs. Always hold on to a handrail.

PREPARE FOR EMERGENCIES

☐ Pick a spot outdoors where everyone in the household should meet in case of a fire. Practice evacuations to that spot.

EDIT *your home, room by room*

Take a good, hard look around your house. Does it reflect your life as you live it now—or is it a shrine to the past? Children grow up and life changes so quickly, it's easy to find yourself living in a house filled with old relics and memories but bearing little resemblance to the life you currently lead. Try to view each transition as an opportunity to look at who you are now and how you want to live. And while it's important to honor your family's history, that doesn't mean you need to live in a museum or provide a lifetime of free storage for your son's baseball-card collection.

In fact, living with that kind of cumbersome, dust-gathering clutter may take a serious toll on your health. Forty percent of adults experience considerable anxiety and embarrassment over the amount of stuff in their homes.[3] According to a 2008 study by the Australia Institute, a whopping 88 percent of houses contain at least one cluttered room.[4] Clutter saps our energy. If you can't remember when you last cleared out a closet, a room, or your whole house, now is the time to reclaim that space. Living well requires a focus on the present, especially as you approach a new stage of life. The good news is, the older we become, the better we are at living a well-edited life. We know now that less is more and we value quality over quantity in all things.

STRATEGIES FOR DECLUTTERING

If the prospect of ridding your home of clutter seems daunting, take it step by step. Set small, achievable goals for yourself, such as reorganizing one drawer, or cleaning out a small closet. At the change of every season, sort your wardrobe into "Keep," "Donate," and "Repair" piles—and get the latter two off to a charity drop-off site or your tailor by the end of the week. Reexamine your closets every six months and rearrange the shelves, rods, and bins according to your new storage needs. For the rest of your home, take advantage of occasional spare moments for small tasks, and set aside longer periods of time for bigger projects, such as clearing out a bedroom or garage. Finally, take a consistent, daily approach to decluttering.

KEEP IT OR TOSS IT?

Start by making a list of everything you most want and need from your living space. A cozy reading nook? Space for your yoga practice? A hearty table for gathering with family and friends? Then take stock of your possessions, noting which meet those needs and which feel extraneous. Keep only those things that are useful, beautiful, or both. If you get stuck over an item, evaluate it by asking the following key questions. But remember, if you really have to mull it over, you probably don't need it.

- **Have I used/worn it in the past year?**
  If not, you probably won't use or wear it next year, either. Toss.

- **Is it in good condition?**
  And if not, will I spend the time or money to get it repaired?

- **Is this worth the space it's taking up?**
  If you love classical music, then by all means keep your grand piano. But if it only gets played by the piano tuner, ask whether you could use that space for something else. And donate the piano to a worthy recipient.

- **If I threw this away, could it be easily replaced if I needed it later?**
  If the answer is yes, by all means, toss it.

- **Am I keeping this because it belonged to someone I love?**
  This is especially difficult when sorting through the belongings of a loved one who has passed away. Remember that these are mementos of that person's life, not yours—and that parting with someone else's possessions is not an indication of how much (or how little) you loved them.

- **Does it carry negative energy?**
  Don't keep gifts from people you dislike, photos from unhappy times or failed relationships, clothes that are too small, or medicines from an old ailment.

MAKE THE MOST OF YOUR ENTRYWAY

Whether it's a front-hall closet or a series of hooks on the wall, implementing a few organizing and design strategies will help create a welcoming entryway where you can begin to unwind the second you step in the door.

❶ SEATING AREA

A long bench or a group of chairs provides an easy place to take shoes on and off, particularly in cooler months when you or your visitors may be wearing a lot of outerwear. A bench has the added benefit of providing a convenient storage space underneath. This simple wall-mounted half bench saves space by only using front legs.

❷ COAT HOOKS

Large coat hooks keep essentials off the floor, providing a convenient place to hang outer-wear, baskets, dog leashes, and scarves. The hooks pictured here are mounted into the shelving unit, so there's no need to put extra holes in the walls.

❸ SHELVES

A shelf installed above the row of hooks provides additional storage space, perfect for stashing separate bins for scarves, gloves, hats, and other accessories. In this entryway, the shelf is cut to the same length as the bench, which helps define the space.

❹ BINS

A row of identical storage bins gives this entryway a pleasing, uniform look. Sunglasses, purses, and scarves can be corralled in the bins, neatly tucked under a bench or on a shelf. Choose from metal, wicker, canvas, or even wooden bins (such as old wine boxes). Sort through the boxes weekly to prevent them from becoming cluttered. Add casters to the bottom of the bins for easy access.

❺ KEY HOOKS

Designate a row of small hooks or a bowl as the place you drop your keys as soon as you come in the door. You can also store a spare set of keys here.

❻ MAIL SORTERS

Use baskets, letter trays, or standing racks to sort incoming and outgoing mail. Dedicate one basket to junk mail so it can be immediately recycled. File bills and other correspondence in separate in-boxes.

❼ NONSLIP RUG

An absorbent, nonslip rug will help prevent falls and keep your entryway tidy.

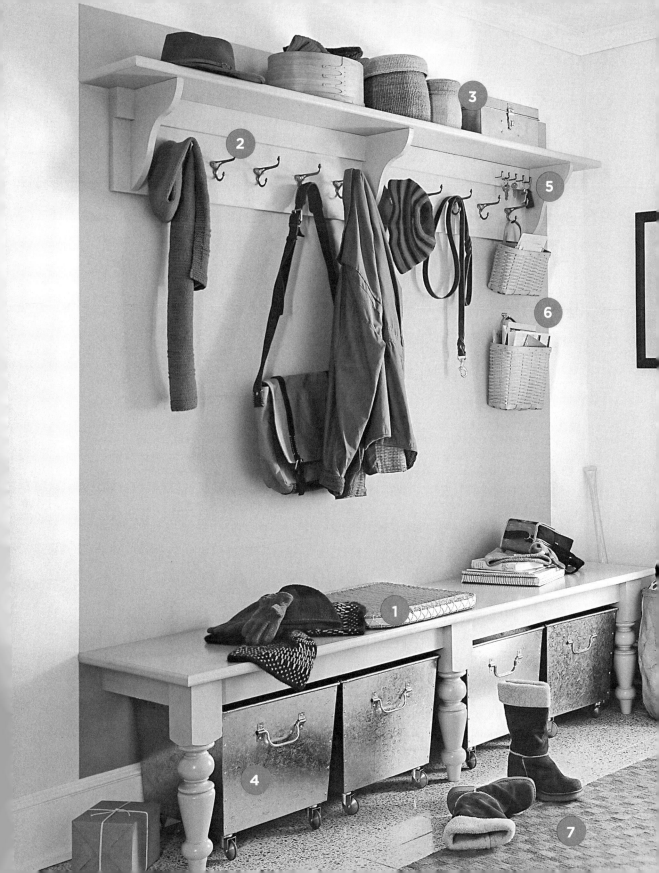

MAKE YOUR KITCHEN WORK FOR YOU

In any kitchen—spacious or compact—thoughtful organization will help maximize cupboards, countertops, and drawers. Implementing just a few changes can help make cooking and cleanup easier and more enjoyable.

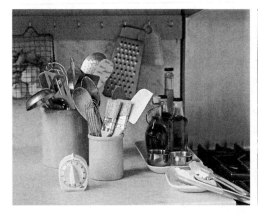

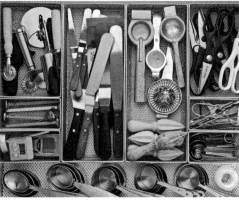

Store items where you use them. Cooking tools are best kept near the stovetop; house mixing bowls near the countertop you use for food preparation; plates, glasses, and flatware are best near the dishwasher. Keep things you use most often at eye level.

Keep like with like. Store all bakeware in the same cupboard, all wooden spoons in the same ceramic crock, all spices in the same drawer. Group glassware and dinnerware by function so everyday plates, bowls, cups, and glasses all reside in one area.

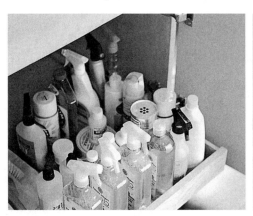

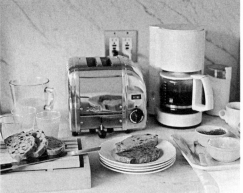

Create accessible storage. Sliding drawers under the sink grant easy access to cleaning supplies. Similar drawers also work perfectly for organizing garbage and recycling bins.

Arrange appliances. Keep small appliances you use daily, such as a toaster and coffee-maker, on the counter. Install a drawer on a deep lower shelf for appliances used occasionally, such as a rice cooker and blender.

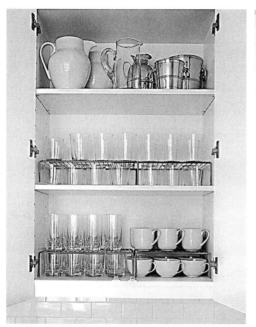

Add shelf dividers. Instead of wasting space on a single layer of teacups or juice glasses, try adding expandable—and inexpensive—wire risers: Slide one onto a cabinet shelf and you've instantly doubled the storage capabilities.

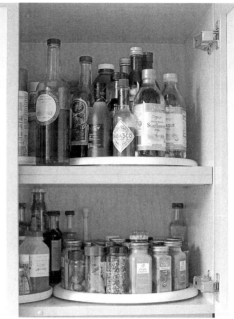

Improve access. To avoid awkward reaching in tight spots, use lazy Susans (revolving trays) to organize condiments, spices, or vitamins in corner cabinets. Put wire baskets on gliders (sold at home centers) on shelves in bottom cabinets for easier reach.

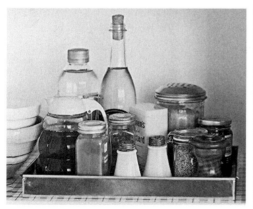

Declutter shelves. Gather the small items you store on a shelf into a spare baking tray, then treat it like a drawer, carefully sliding it in and out for easy access. The pan will also catch drips, minimizing cleanup.

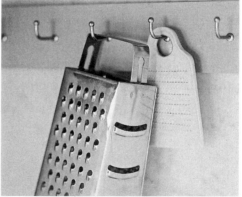

Hang tools. A row of small hooks offers quick access to items that would otherwise be lost in a jumbled drawer. The hooks can also be used to support wire baskets to store pantry staples like onions and garlic.

BEAUTIFY THE BATHROOM

The same principles that work in the kitchen apply to bathrooms. Group like items together and maximize storage where you can. Cosmetics, skin-care products, and medications all have finite shelf lives. Once a year, toss out those items that are expired, no longer used, or damaged.

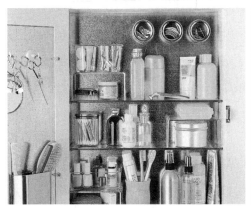

Magnetize the medicine cabinet. Insert cut-to-fit galvanized metal inside the cabinet door; adhere the metal with caulk. Use magnetized hooks, notepad holders, and spice canisters to store small items. Double shelves' storage space with acrylic risers.

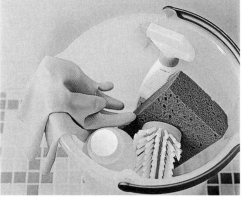

Designate a tote bucket for supplies. Store all of your essentials—gloves, brushes, sponges, all-purpose cleanser—in a bucket so you can carry them from room to room. Keep the bucket under the bathroom sink or in a closet.

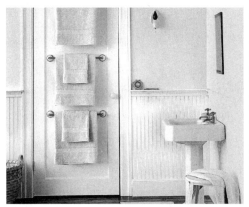

Add three bars instead of one. Stacking towel bars on the door provides extra hanging space. A flat or single-paneled door should fit three bars. Hang the hardware according to package instructions, evenly spacing the bars.

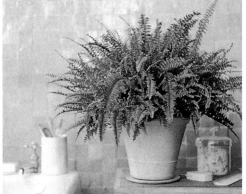

Purify the air. Ferns are masters at clearing indoor air—the Boston fern, above, tops the list of air-purifying species. Place one fern (or many!) in a bathroom with a window or diffused natural light, and let warm steam from the shower act as a virtual greenhouse.

SET UP AN EFFICIENT LAUNDRY AREA

Whether your laundry room is a tiny closet or a roomy basement, organization is key. As we age, toting heavy laundry baskets can become more cumbersome; installing a washer and dryer near your bedroom will make the job easier, though the cost or installation may be prohibitive. Rolling carts are a lower-cost solution.

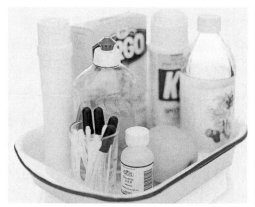

Make a stain-treatment kit. No single product takes care of every spot or spill. Keep a variety of your favorite cleaners organized on a shallow tray or in a dish, so they're on hand whenever you need to tackle tough stains.

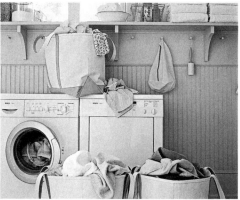

Separate clothes into more efficient loads. In addition to sorting laundry by color, try mixing large pieces with small ones in each load to help clothes get cleaner. Also, dry items of a similar weight together.

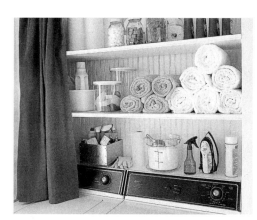

Hide supplies. Keep laundry supplies tidy and out of sight with built-in shelves and a curtain that can be pulled across them when the laundry is done. Organize smaller items in separate receptacles, such as clear glass jars and airtight plastic containers.

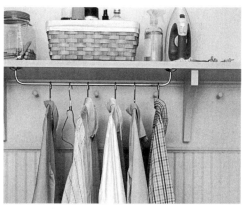

Maximize shelving. Bare walls in a laundry room are a lost opportunity. A smartly installed laundry shelf stores supplies on top and—with the addition of a bar—serves as a drying rack below. Use a hand-towel bar, or even a pot rack for this purpose.

ESTABLISH A HOME OFFICE

Housing your office supplies and paperwork together, in clever ways, will not only help you stay clutter-free. It may inspire you to tackle your tasks more frequently.

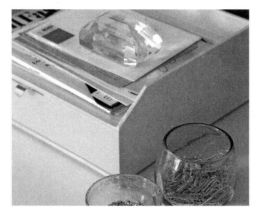

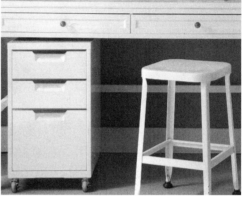

Designate a daily action drawer or box. Use this to contain projects and files that you refer to daily. Keep the file at your fingertips, and edit weekly or monthly as projects finish.

Use a filing cabinet. Store important paperwork, like medical records and insurance policies, in an easily accessible cabinet. Choose one with one drawer that locks, for storage of especially valuable or irreplaceable documents.

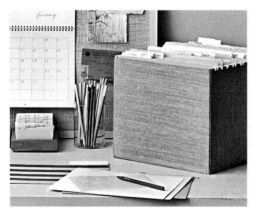

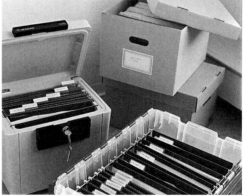

Keep "operational" documents in an accordion file. This includes licenses, renewal forms, and deeds, all of which can move to the file cabinet when necessary.

Move "archival" paperwork to storage. Keep hard copies of your past seven years of tax returns in a safe, fireproof box in an upstairs closet or attic.

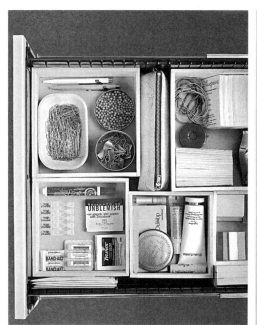

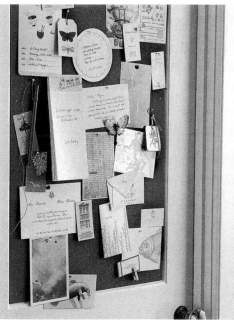

Organize desk drawers. Instead of allowing paper clips, breath mints, bandages, and such to accumulate with abandon, arrange them in a variety of small boxes and tuck them inside desk drawers. You'll be delighted to look inside and more likely to find exactly what you need in no time.

Install a back-of-door bulletin board. Make the most of every inch by cutting a corkboard to fit inside your office or closet door or within a cabinet panel. Trim a piece of sheet cork (available online or at home-supply stores) to the dimensions you want to cover and hang with tiny nails.

FILE REGULARLY AND EDIT ANNUALLY

After the bills are paid, the easiest way to keep track of them is to arrange them, by month, in a thirteen-pocket accordion file (use the last pocket for tax documents, such as W-2s). Each year, replace the file and use the previous year's file to do your taxes. Then go through month by month to determine what to scan or keep.

Once a year, go through all your files (even the sentimental correspondence file!) and shred unnecessary papers. Give your computer the once-over, sorting folders, deleting out-dated files, and backing up important data onto an external drive. This is also a good time to cull your book collection and donate unwanted titles to libraries, prisons, shelters, churches, or schools. If you work in an office or live in an apartment building, set up a communal book-shelf. Minimize additional book clutter by making use of your library card and consider an electronic book reader: OverDrive Media Console lets you borrow eBooks from their catalog of 400,000 titles for free (www.overdrive.com).

DECLUTTER YOUR CLOSETS

Clean, orderly, well-kept clothes and coat closets will simplify getting dressed and out the door. They also offer the chance to make the most of your storage.

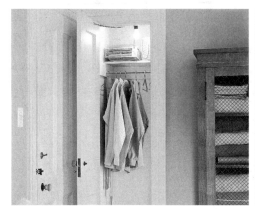

Illuminate the interior. Consider battery-operated lighting if your closet has no power source. Better yet, have an electrician install recessed ceiling lights that turn on automatically when the door is opened. An incandescent light can also help prevent mildew.

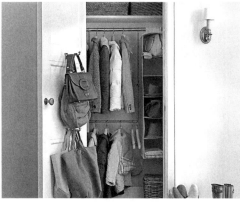

Add an extra rod. Two or even three short rods installed one above the other, rather than one high one, will maximize hanging space for short items like shirts, skirts, and folded trousers. Reserve another area for longer items such as coats and dresses.

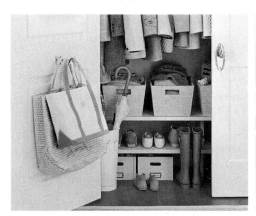

"Increase" your floor space. Installing shelves or cubbies at the base of a closet gives you more room for additional bins and boxes. Adjustable shelves will allow you to change the arrangement of your closet as your storage needs evolve.

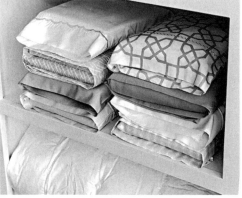

Keep linens together in sets. In the linen closet, store sheet sets together in one pillowcase to make it easier to find what you need when making a bed.

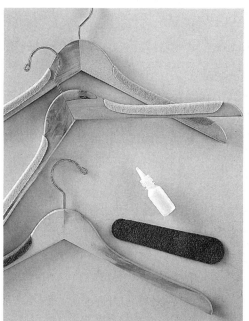

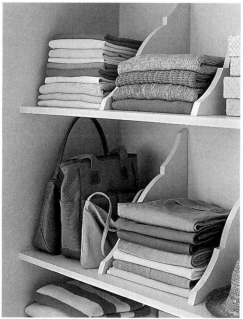

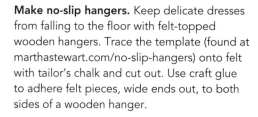

Make no-slip hangers. Keep delicate dresses from falling to the floor with felt-topped wooden hangers. Trace the template (found at marthastewart.com/no-slip-hangers) onto felt with tailor's chalk and cut out. Use craft glue to adhere felt pieces, wide ends out, to both sides of a wooden hanger.

Divide shelves with brackets. Stacks of shirts, sweaters, and linens need support to keep from toppling. Wooden shelf brackets, available at hardware and home stores, divide the stacks quite nicely. Arrange the closet's contents to determine where to place the brackets. Paint brackets to match shelves; let dry. Position brackets, securing each by drilling in two screws from the underside of the shelf.

LONG-TERM CLOTHES STORAGE TIPS

- Before packing away anything, wash or dry-clean items and remove any stains.
- Lay each garment out on a piece of acid-free tissue paper, and fold the garment and the tissue together; this helps prevent creasing.
- Pack whites and colors into separate containers, if possible, and store clothes in buffered acid-free cardboard or a cedar chest, clean trunk, or hanging fabric bag.
- Natural fibers need ventilation, so airtight plastic boxes aren't the best container choice for long-term clothes storage. Regular cardboard boxes should not be used either, as the acids in the cardboard can cause clothes to yellow.
- Date and label the boxes with their contents, then find a stable environment for them. Damp basements and hot attics are the worst places for clothes. A guest-room closet, on the other hand, is a good place.

ARRANGE *furniture well*

Have you ever cocooned yourself in a rustic cabin, or basked in the serenity of a spa, and thought, *I could live here forever*? Your home should feel just as happy, welcoming, and comfortable—because your everyday environs have a huge impact on your daily sense of well-being. Cluttered, badly arranged rooms can make you feel stressed and tense as soon as you walk in the door. If your house has started to drain your energy, the first step is to pinpoint the problem. The solution might be as simple as moving a piece of furniture. Call it an "energy makeover" for your home—and for yourself.

PROBLEM #1: TOO MUCH CLUTTER IN LIVING SPACES

HOW THE ROOM LOOKS Messy (with papers and other items accumulating on floors and flat surfaces) and cluttered, with no space for new things.

HOW YOU FEEL Overwhelmed, creatively blocked, embarrassed (which can limit social gatherings), depressed, or financially disorganized, as you lose track of bills, bank statements, and other paperwork.

HOW TO FIX IT Everything needs a place to "live." Boxes and baskets work well; use several that match to create a sense of organization, intention, and harmony. Minimize clutter by the front entrance, in hallways, and crammed behind doors, which can keep energy from flowing into the room. Limit yourself to just a few purely sentimental objects in each room. (For more on editing your belongings, see pages 268–269.)

PROBLEM #2: COUCHES AND CHAIRS BLOCKING DOORWAYS OR POSITIONED WITH THEIR BACKS TO THE ROOM'S ENTRANCE

HOW THE ROOM LOOKS Empty and uninviting, since we tend to feel uncomfortable sitting with our backs to others on ill-placed furniture. Blocked doors and pathways are a major trip hazard.

HOW YOU FEEL Unwelcome, uncomfortable, restless, or nervous.

HOW TO FIX IT Arrange furniture so that it faces the entrance of the room. Move seats and sofas away from doors and hallways so they don't prevent energy from flowing or obstruct natural paths of movement. If you have two sofas in a room, put them facing each other so that you see their sides as you enter the room; neither sofa should have its back to the entrance. Additionally, you can place a chair perpendicular to the couches to "greet" you as you enter. Chairs placed diagonally in corners also help open the space. Minimize the number of occasional tables and other small furniture items and keep them out of the flow of traffic. You will gain a safer living space with a welcome feeling that invites connection, conversation, and comfortable gatherings.

FURNITURE PLACEMENT MATTERS

In older houses, the fireplace is often the focal point around which furniture in the living area is arranged. In many homes today, the fireplace has been supplanted by the entertainment center, especially in living areas devoted to casual family gatherings rather than formal entertaining. Here are some suggestions for optimal furniture placement.

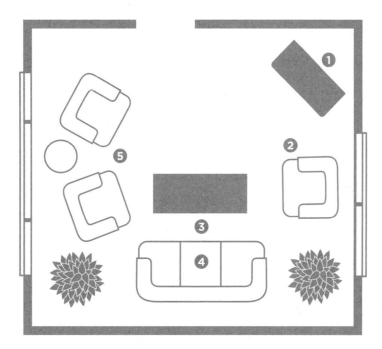

1. Place your television so that it is within 45 degrees of the straight-on view from the seat you will sit in most to watch. For comfortable viewing, place it a distance that is between three and six times the width of the screen from that seat.

2. Allow 36 inches of space around furniture for walking.

3. Leave enough room between the sofa and coffee table (about 14 to 18 inches) to allow easy access and to ensure your knees don't bump the table once you're seated but also to be close enough for you and guests to comfortably reach it.

4. Consider the depth of the seat cushion in relation to your own height: if it's too deep, your feet won't touch the floor; if it's too shallow, you won't be able to settle in.

5. Strategically group furniture. Pull pieces away from the walls to create conversation areas and more intimacy.

MAKE THE MOST OF A SMALL SPACE

Downsizing to a smaller living space doesn't mean you have to sacrifice comfort. Integrate any of the following design elements, along with innovative storage, to make a small apartment—or even just a room—feel more spacious and homey.

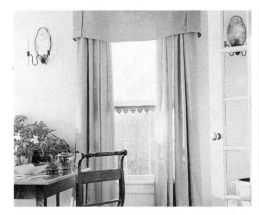

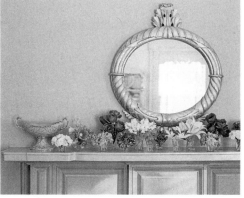

Hang drapes from floor to ceiling. This helps anchor a room and provides a cocooning effect. A simple valance disguises the workings of the window treatment, while implying a sense of architecture.

Add a mirror. A strategically placed mirror makes a small space feel larger. Place one over a mantel or couch or in an entryway and notice how the reflection seems to expand and brighten the room.

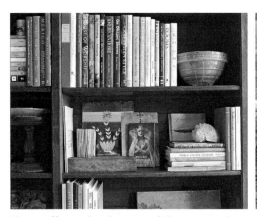

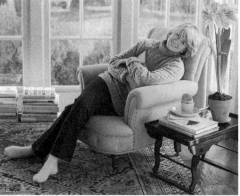

Show off your books. An artfully organized shelf of books can help divide a room into separate living spaces, while also holding sentimental belongings. Prominently display the books that are most meaningful to you.

Create a nook. Designate one chair your "quiet area" and pull it into a corner, preferably near a window. Keep books, magazines, and handicrafts easily accessible by placing them on a side table or in a nearby basket.

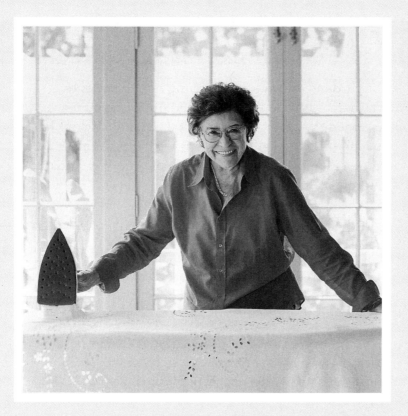

FOLLOWING MY MOTHER'S EXAMPLE

I've certainly kept many of my mother's methods and habits. I learned from her that life is better if the home is prepared, that nature is more easily observed through sparkling-clean windows, and that less time is wasted if closets and storage areas are orderly and organized. And, most important, that housework is a task that, once done, allows for flexibility and enjoyment in other parts of our daily existence.

CULTIVATE *an indoor garden*

Nurturing an indoor garden can have far-reaching health benefits. Research has shown that houseplants lower blood pressure, increase creativity, and even speed the recovery of hospital patients. If your home lacks greenery, you may find yourself low on energy, stressed out, and agitated—and for good reason. A home without plants can feel cold and lifeless, with stuffy or musty air.

Beyond their ability to brighten a room, houseplants serve as powerful air purifiers. A NASA study in the early 1980s was the first to scientifically prove that plants could actually remove volatile organic compounds (VOCs) from the air in sealed test chambers. Additionally, researchers at Pennsylvania State University found that chambers containing ordinary houseplants removed higher amounts of ozone—the main component in smog—at a higher rate than chambers without any plant life.[5]

According to the principles of feng shui, plants are a restorative addition to any room. The more healthy plants you have in your house, the better. Not only are they thought to provide healing energy, they can bring new opportunities into your life. Additionally, research has shown that blooming plants give off fragrance that can increase happiness, encourage deep breathing, and reduce stress.

Regardless of whether you're a green thumb or have struggled to keep a cactus alive, growing plants indoors is well worth the minimal effort involved. Even keeping just a few houseplants can greatly improve your health and the feel of your home.

PLANTS THAT FIGHT AIR POLLUTION

In addition to the toxin-fighting powerhouses on the following pages, the plants below are thought to have air-cleaning properties.[6] Place them throughout your home, and you're sure to breath easier.

- Areca palm
- Australian sword fern
- Boston fern
- Dwarf date palm
- English ivy
- Golden pothos
- Dracaena 'Janet Craig'
- Lady palm
- Peace lily
- Reed palm
- Rubber plant
- Snake plant
- Spider plant
- Weeping fig
- *Zamioculcas zamifolia*

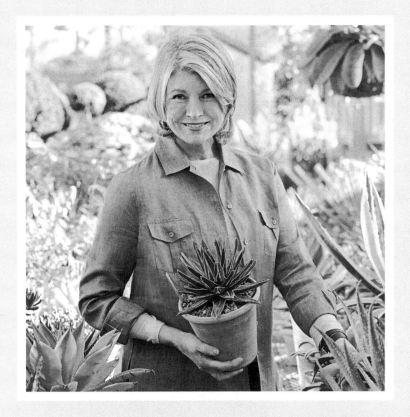

MAKE ROOM FOR HOUSEPLANTS

We grew many things in our yard in Nutley, New Jersey, where I was raised, but we rarely, if ever, had plants in the house. Cut flowers, yes, but not what I like to call "house-plants." My maternal grandmother's sunroom was filled with begonias, ferns, and other luscious plants, and I longed for the day when I would have my own collection. Houseplants scrub the air of impurities and lend beauty to every room.

BRING THE GARDEN INDOORS

The eight houseplants shown here can improve your mood with fragrance, boost the flow of positive energy in a room, and wipe out airborne toxins.

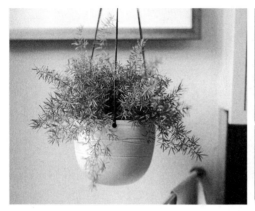

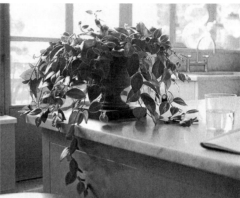

ASPARAGUS FERN This fern's feathery vines help circulate energy, particularly in gloomy or stagnant rooms. It flourishes in humidity and low light. Replant or separate the root ball and plant in two pots.

HOYA Also called waxplant, waxvine, or waxflower, the Hoya's luxuriant leaves, coupled with the fragrance of its white-and-pink flowers, make it a popular houseplant. It blooms best in bright, indirect sun.

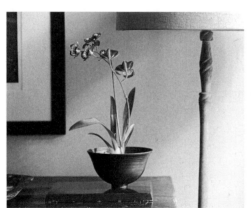

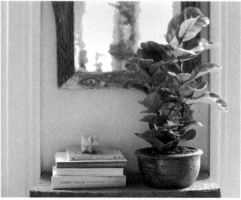

MILTONIA ORCHID Its subtly fragrant and colorful flowers help improve mood. Pot this orchid in a general bark or orchid mix and keep evenly moist. Expose it to bright, diffuse light up to two hours daily, and treat with monthly high-nitrogen fertilizer.

FICUS LYRATA Its broad, arcing leaves make this species (also known as the fiddle-leaf fig) a powerful health-improving plant by feng shui standards. Keep soil barely moist and place the plant where it can receive medium to bright, indirect light.

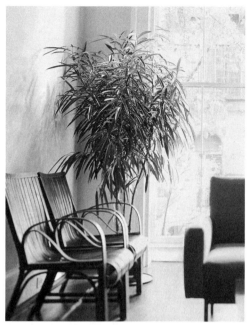

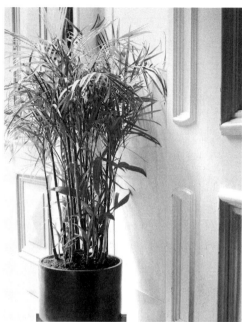

FICUS ALII This tree's ability to remove chemical vapors increases with size (some can reach 10 feet). Give it lukewarm water (to prevent leaf loss) once the top inch of soil dries out. Keep it in bright to medium light and a pot just big enough to contain the roots.

BAMBOO PALM This tree effectively removes benzene, trichloroethylene, and formaldehyde from indoor air. Keep it moist but not wet (leaf tips turn yellow when overwatered). It thrives in medium light. For symmetrical growth, rotate the pot once a week.

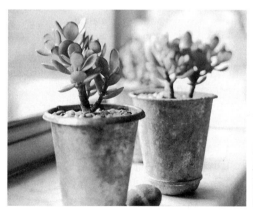

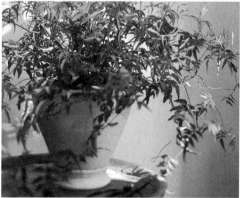

JADE Said to promote abundance, prosperity, and good luck, jade plants require very little water—about once every two weeks. Avoid too much direct sun. If the plant becomes too top-heavy for the trunk, cut back the stems to the lateral branch.

JASMINE With its sultry-sweet fragrance, jasmine is a powerful stress buster. It flowers best in cool areas (ideally 55°F to 65°F) with diffused light. Keep it away from radiators and other dry-heat sources. Water when the top half-inch of potting mix is dry to the touch.

CONSIDER *color*

If your house feels at all drab or uninspiring even after you've edited and solved space issues, it might be time for a color makeover. After all, the hues we use to decorate our homes have a significant impact on our mood. Color can trigger depression or dampen cognitive performance, according to new studies. Choosing the right colors can help you feel uplifted, inspired, or relaxed, depending on the shades you choose.

Sticking to one cohesive color palette throughout your house will enable you to easily move things from room to room. Notice the colors you're personally attracted to. Are there particular hues you like to wear? Do you feel most comfortable in a particular setting? Perhaps you gravitate toward the steel and chrome of the city? Or maybe you prefer the neutral browns and greens of a temperate forest? You'll likely find that color scheme you've always been attracted to will begin to emerge. Use it confidently for a whole room. To create more intense moods, choose items with deeper, more saturated shades. Use favorite photos, works of art, or beloved objects to guide your color choices. Above all, don't worry about trends; surround yourself with the colors you love.

COLOR CHOICES, ROOM BY ROOM

Color is a personal choice, of course, but there are some combinations that are classic, and with good reason. Consider the following suggestions from color experts:

- In the kitchen go for warm and nurturing colors like mustard yellow. For an updated look, balance it with cooler blues and grays. If you're worried about making a mistake, choose mellow colors with a similar value.

- In the living room opt for comfortable and bright. Reds and yellows can be challenging to work with. Grounding them with oatmeal gray results in an inviting palette that's perfect for a laid-back gathering space.

- Refined and relaxing colors work well in bathrooms; try pale gray, green, and blue accents against white walls.

- The bedroom should be soothing and sophisticated. Purple can seem young and playful, but when paired with graceful grays, subdued browns, and chalky whites, the result is a grown-up palette that brings a sense of comfort and elegance to a bedroom.

ILLUMINATE *your space*

You can create warmth, serenity, and coziness by using lamps or installing dimmer switches on overhead lights throughout your living space. During the day, let in as much natural light as you can; one study showed that 30 to 60 minutes of direct sun exposure per day improved sleep patterns in nursing home residents.[7] Be sure to get the right amount of light where you need it as well—consider task lighting above kitchen counters and desks, for example, and bedside lamps for late-night reading.

OPTIMIZE YOUR LIGHTING

Where you put your lights depends on their style and intensity. A variety of lamp styles should be used, depending on your needs. Keep the following in mind:

☐ The bottom of a table lampshade should be at eye level, to prevent glare.

☐ Arrange task lamps so the bulb is about 15 inches above the work surface.

☐ Hang a pendant so the bottom of the shade is between 5½ and 6½ feet from the floor (depending whether you need to walk under it easily). If you're hanging one over a table, arrange it about 30 inches from the surface.

☐ If a floor lamp is more than 3 feet above your head when you're sitting, the harsh light of the bulb will be visible. Adjust the height or place the lamp farther from your sitting area.

☐ For maximum brightness and energy efficiency, look for Energy Star–qualified bulbs—including incandescents, CFLs, and LEDs—that use less electricity (measured in watts) for the amount of light they produce (measured in lumens). For example, older, inefficient 100-watt incandescents, which give off about 1,600 lumens, have been replaced with 72-watt bulbs that produce the same amount of light. These bulbs will save you money on your electric bill in the long run.

☐ In rooms where you spend a lot of time, use full-spectrum lightbulbs that mimic daylight. They're better for your mood and brain, and they require less strain if you're using them to read by.

THREE WAYS TO GET MORE NATURAL LIGHT IN YOUR HOME
- Lighten your curtains. Trade heavy drapes for sheer shades.
- Decorate with mirrors. They can brighten a room's shadier corners.
- Maintain clean floors, which will reflect light better than drab walls and carpets.

MAINTAIN *a healthy home*

One key benefit of a well-edited home is that it's much easier to clean than one overflowing with dust-catchers and clutter. This is important because a clean home is a healthy home. "Clean" doesn't mean scrubbed, scoured, and bleached within an inch of its life. Rather, pure—a home that has fresh air flowing into it and as little dirt and as few toxins as possible.

Maintaining a healthy home is vital as we age and become more vulnerable to the effects of toxic exposures. Yet staying on top of your cleaning can also become more challenging as dust and dirt become trickier to see! Here are simple strategies to sustain and even improve the health of your home—now and in the future.

HEALTHY FLOORS

Not only do your home's floors take a beating from your daily traffic patterns but they also accumulate more dirt than almost any other surface in the house. The materials your floors are made from will dictate how easy they are to clean and how well they wear over the years. Your floors can also be a major source of toxic chemical exposure, depending on the material they are made from. Some of these chemicals can irritate airways and affect breathing, particularly in older people and children.

If you're looking for new flooring or are considering refinishing your old parquet, it's important to choose nontoxic, durable materials. Though popular and inexpensive, petroleum-based polyvinyl chloride (PVC) flooring, bought rolled or in tiles, and laminates (which may contain wood pulp or wood chips) can pose health and environmental problems. Even "green" options aren't always so healthful. Bamboo flooring, for example, is made from fast-growing, sustainable bamboo, but like laminates it's also frequently produced with adhesives containing formaldehyde. Hardwood such as oak is routinely sealed with oil-based polyurethane, a respiratory irritant. Recycled-rubber flooring sounds great, but can be made from old tires, and often has a strong odor. It pays to know what's underfoot. On the following pages, you'll find important considerations to keep in mind when choosing floors and floor coverings.

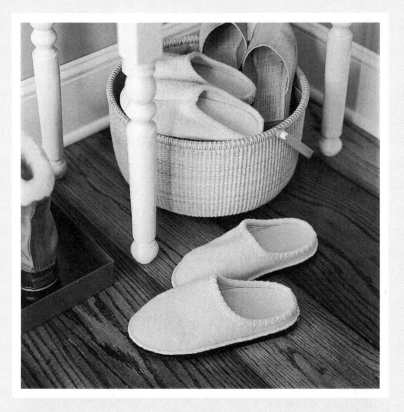

LEAVE YOUR SHOES AT THE DOOR

I rarely allow outdoor shoes in my home, because they track in dirt, heavy metals, and even pesticides from visitors' lawns. Going shoeless indoors makes maintaining floors and rugs effortless. Moreover, walking in socks or thin house shoes is so wonderful for foot health. It works all the muscles in the foot, enhancing range of motion, and it improves balance. I keep a boot tray filled with stones (from garden centers) next to each entrance for outdoor shoes. Ice and snow melt and drain through the rocks so boots don't stand in a puddle. I also maintain a basket with a ready supply of slippers for visitors and one-size-fits-all booties to slip over workboots.

ABOUT CARPET

Carpets and rugs retain heat, muffle sound, and offer a soft landing for tired feet. But, as anyone who vacuums knows, they also harbor a lot of dirt and dust, which can aggravate lungs and trigger allergies. More concerning, many carpets are treated with stain protectors, fire retardants, and moth-proofing insecticides, while synthetic carpets contain volatile organic compounds (VOCs). These chemicals can cause serious side effects. Avoid some of these health threats by choosing your next carpet wisely.

CARE FOR EXISTING CARPET

Invest in a vacuum cleaner with a HEPA (High-Efficiency Particulate Air) filter. The average carpet has nearly 70 grams of dust per square meter. The HEPA filter helps ensure that the dust doesn't blow around in the air, where you can inhale it.

Make sure your home is well ventilated. Good ventilation will minimize the effect of chemical components or additives.

Dispose of any wet carpet. If you've had flooding, get rid of the carpet right away; the chances of keeping it mold-free are slim.

SHOP SMART FOR NEW RUGS

Consider area rugs. These can be less toxic than wall-to-wall carpeting, since the latter is usually glued to the floor with adhesives that can also off-gas chemical fumes. But bear in mind that throw rugs can pose a trip hazard. Choose heavyweight, larger area rugs and secure them with a nonskid pad.

Choose carpets and rugs made of sustainable materials. Materials such as sisal, coir, wool, or organic cotton are good choices.

Look for rugs with jute, latex, or other natural backings that are sewn on, rather than glued with toxic adhesives, and ask for a wool underpad, too. Many eco-friendly alternatives are available, including low-VOC nylon and wool modular floor tiles, with backing made of some recycled materials.

Choose untreated floor coverings. Check that they have not been treated with fire retardants, stain protectors, or other chemicals.

INSTALL WALL-TO-WALL SAFELY

Ask your installer to air out a new carpet. Request that this be done in a clean, well-ventilated area. Have the carpet tacked down instead of glued.

After installation, leave the house for several hours. Synthetic carpets (often nylon and olefin) can emit noxious gases, including VOCs. According to the Consumer Product Safety Commission (CPSC), the government

agency that monitors products that may pose a health risk, you should also open doors and windows, and keep the air circulating throughout your home with window fans and air conditioners. If you have an air-ventilation system, keep it running for at least forty-eight hours after the carpet is installed.

ABOUT HARDWOOD FLOORING

Valued for their beauty and longevity, wood floors last for generations if properly cared for. Though extremely durable, these floors will inevitably need to be repaired, refinished, or even replaced. There are multiple finishes and materials to choose from that will help keep your floors attractive and your home free from toxins.

CARE FOR EXISTING WOOD FLOORS

SCREENING For floors that are merely dull but not badly damaged, screening will remedy minor scratches that have penetrated the wood itself. The existing finish is abraded with a mesh screen that's attached to a rotary buffing machine, which prepares the surface for a new coat of finish. To adhere properly, the new finish must be compatible with the old one.

REFINISHING Floors with stains, gouges, or deep scratches should be refinished. This involves sanding down the surface to bare wood with a drum or belt sander, staining (to enhance or change the color of the wood), and then coating with several layers of polyurethane. This is a messy, strenuous job best left to a wood-flooring professional. Oil-based polyurethane can also be toxic. Better to choose a low-VOC sealant.

REPLACING If you're looking to have new hardwood floors installed, an eco-friendly option is reclaimed wood, which may have had a former life, and in some cases can be of an even higher quality than the new wood flooring you'll find in stores. If you decide to replace flooring that's in decent shape, ask your contractor if he or she knows a vendor who might be interested in purchasing the wood (or just taking it off your hands), so it can be put to use again. The Forest Stewardship Council (FSC) certifies hardwood flooring that comes from managed forests (look for the FSC seal). It's best to have wood prefinished at the factory, so that you don't have to seal it at home.

ALTERNATIVES TO HARDWOOD FLOORS

LAMINATES Look for those with low-VOC emissions. Borrow a couple of boards from a retailer and keep them in your living room. Does the smell bother you? If so, check out other brands. You may find some natural-wood flooring at a comparative price. Make sure any sealants on your floors are water-based and contain no or few VOCs.

STONE AND TILE Although they aren't renewable, stone and tile are good choices for floors exposed to a lot of sunlight because they will slowly release the heat they absorb into your home.

OTHER NATURAL FLOORING If you're interested in rubber flooring, look for natural—not synthetic—rubber, and make sure it's free of contaminants and chlorine. Cork, palm, and bamboo floors are made from renewable resources. Buy only brands that use no- or low-VOC adhesives. You can also purchase true linoleum that is made with cork and linseed oil.

COMBAT DUST—ESPECIALLY IN BEDROOMS

If you're waking up with a stuffy nose; itchy, watery eyes; or you are having difficulty breathing, odds are good that the dust situation in your house isn't under control. Your bedroom is likely the cause, as more than 2 million microscopic dust mites live in the average bed. Dust will also gather on blinds, carpets, and around collectibles, filling shelves and nooks. Here are a few ways to combat the problem:

HAVE YOUR LEAST-ALLERGIC FAMILY MEMBER DO THE DUSTING.

Allergy sufferers should wear a paper face-mask if they're planning to do any cleaning themselves. Better yet, wait 30 minutes before entering a just-cleaned room so airborne pollutants have a chance to escape or settle back down.

PROTECT YOUR BEDDING.

To avoid dust-mite saturation, encase your mattress and pillows in standard protective allergy-proof covers, and wash all linens weekly in hot water. Wash pillows and duvet inserts every two weeks if any symptoms persist. (If your symptoms aren't severe, once a season will do.) Synthetic bedding can go in the washer and dryer; load pillows in pairs to keep machines balanced, and add two tennis balls (slipped into a white sock to prevent dye transference) to the dryer to help fluff them back up. Down or feather bedding and bulky items will do better being frozen or hung outside on cold, windy days for three to five hours per week.

CONSIDER INSTALLING FORCED-AIR FILTERS.

Look for filters with a minimum efficiency reporting value (MERV) of 8 or higher on all central air vents (ratings range from 1 to 20). These will pull dust and other particles out of the air as they circulate through your heat or air conditioning. No central air? A freestanding HEPA filter in your bedroom or other main living spaces can do the same job. Be sure to clean all filters on vents and your furnace before turning them on for the first time each season.

OPEN WINDOWS.

Keep fresh air circulating through the house as often as possible. Dust mites can survive into early winter, so even on cold days, it's worth it to turn off the heat and open the windows whenever you can (try it for a few hours while you're out running errands).

BEWARE OF COMMON CHEMICAL HAZARDS

Even the most scrupulous homekeepers can have a dirty house if one of these dangerous—but invisible and often scentless—chemical hazards is present. Fortunately most are easy to prevent once you know how to spot them.

CARBON MONOXIDE

Unintentional carbon monoxide (CO) poisonings account for about 500 deaths and 15,000 visits to the emergency room each year.[8] While everyone is susceptible to this odorless, colorless gas, older adults are more vulnerable to CO poisoning because they are more likely to have a health condition that lowers their tolerance to it.

WHERE IT LURKS In enclosed or semi-enclosed spaces around your stove and heating system.

HOW TO AVOID IT Install carbon monoxide detectors near kitchen and sleeping areas. Have heating systems and stoves checked annually. Avoid the use of nonvented combustion appliances, and never burn fuels indoors except in stoves or furnaces designed for that purpose. Be attentive to possible CO symptoms; they are easily confused with flu, but if you feel better when away from home and notice family members or pets feeling the same way at the same time, your symptoms could be the result of CO poisoning.

MOLD

Molds require only moisture and oxygen to flourish. One of the worst allergy offenders, mold can cause itchy eyes, runny noses, asthma, and other respiratory disorders.

WHERE IT LURKS Refrigerators, washing machines, shower walls, dank basements, under sinks—anywhere there's water.

HOW TO AVOID IT It's impossible to clear your air of all mold spores, but if you keep moisture under control, you can prevent the spores from landing and growing on surfaces. Measure indoor moisture levels with an inexpensive humidity meter available at hardware stores; 30 to 50 percent humidity is optimal. And don't forget to check your attic and basement—standing water or humidity over 50 percent in these areas can contribute to mold growth throughout your house. Run a dehumidifier to fix the problem. Empty the drip trays beneath your dehumidifier and refrigerator regularly. Use exhaust fans in bathrooms and kitchens; the best fans vent to the outside and include a HEPA filter to eliminate moisture buildup. To prevent mold from invading your washing machine, run a cycle once a week with 1 cup of hydrogen peroxide and no clothes, and keep the room dry.

HOW TO COMBAT IT If mold growth covers an area larger than 10 square feet or has spread inside the ducts of your central air system, the Environmental Protection Agency recommends hiring a professional to clean it up. You can tackle smaller jobs yourself by scrubbing the mold off of hard surfaces with a mixture of detergent and hot water, then fixing the source of the water damage, whether that means tightening leaky plumbing or sealing up cracks in walls and roofs. (Throw out infested porous materials like carpets or ceiling tiles.) Visit www.epa.gov for more information on handling mold in your home.

COMBUSTION GASES

Most of us forget that our gas stoves actually produce open flames, and wherever there's an open flame, nitrogen dioxide and carbon dioxide can build up.

WHERE IT LURKS Kitchen, living room (if you have a gas-powered fireplace), furnace room, or basement.

HOW TO AVOID IT Make sure your gas appliances are properly adjusted—a blue flame is best. If the flame has a lot of yellow or orange, a sign of higher pollutant levels, ask the gas company to tweak the setting. If you are buying new, opt for a model with a pilotless ignition, which doesn't have a continuously burning pilot light.

ASBESTOS

A mineral fiber (similar to fiberglass), asbestos is easily inhaled or swallowed. Once inhaled, asbestos particles, which are too small to see, accumulate in lungs and can cause chest and abdominal cancers and other fatal lung diseases. Symptoms do not appear until many years after exposure.

WHERE IT LURKS In insulation, fireproofing, some types of paint, and acoustical materials as well as ceiling and floor tiles.

HOW TO AVOID IT As long as asbestos-containing materials are in good condition, with no threat of being disturbed, it is fine to leave them alone. But as soon as any project begins that could disturb it, or if asbestos begins peeling and crumbling from surfaces, it should be removed or sealed by a certified asbestos contractor. Consult your local health or environmental officials for proper handling and disposal procedures.

NITROGEN DIOXIDE

Nitrogen dioxide is a highly reactive and corrosive gas. Exposure can cause eye, nose, and throat irritation; it also has the potential to cause impaired lung function and increased respiratory infections in children, according to the EPA. Low-level exposure can cause problems for asthmatics and decreased lung function in people with chronic pulmonary disease and those with weakened immune systems or increased risk of respiratory infections. Concentrated exposure can lead to pulmonary edema.

WHERE IT LURKS It can be formed when combustion appliances, such as kerosene heaters and gas ranges, are not vented or when vented appliances are installed improperly. Welding and tobacco smoke also release this noxious gas.

HOW TO AVOID IT Proper installation of combustion appliances and ventilation systems are the best way to reduce exposure. Always open flues when fireplaces are in use. Choose woodstoves that are certified to meet Environmental Protection Agency standards. Never leave your car idling inside the garage.

PESTICIDES

Considered semi-volatile organic compounds (SVOCs) by the EPA, these can cause respiratory and skin irritation, coughing, and dizziness. Over the long term, they've been linked to central nervous system damage.

WHERE THEY LURK Floors, plants, pets, bottoms of shoes.

OW TO AVOID THEM Take another look at what you spray on pets and plants to ward off insects and pests. Be sure to apply flea powder and liquid pesticides outdoors and use more natural choices. Removing shoes indoors can help cut down on the amount of lawn fertilizer tracked inside.

PBDE'S (POLYBROMINATED DIPHENYL ETHERS OR FLAME RETARDANTS)

Animal research has shown links between flame retardants and thyroid, liver, and neurological disorders. Europe has already banned the use of certain formulations of PBDEs.

WHERE THEY LURK Mattresses, upholstery, electronics, polyurethane foam products (such as carpet padding).

HOW TO AVOID THEM Look for mattresses, upholstery, and carpets made from wool, a natural fire retardant. Or add a natural feather bed as a protective layer. When buying electronics, opt for ones made by manufacturers such as Apple, Dell, and Sony, which are phasing out certain PBDEs. Check the Environmental Working Group's website at www.ewg.org for more guidance.

FORMALDEHYDE

Considered a volatile organic compound (VOC), formaldehyde is a colorless, strong-smelling gas that can cause nausea and dizziness and, in severe cases, may harm the liver and kidneys.

WHERE IT LURKS Adhesives in furniture, flooring, cabinetry, and pressed-wood.

HOW TO AVOID IT Keep your home well ventilated. Antique pieces are also less likely to give off formaldehyde, a gas that dissipates from products significantly after five years.

RADON

Radon is an odorless, tasteless, invisible gas produced by the decay of naturally occurring uranium in the soil. It's unfortunately ubiquitous, and is the number one cause of lung cancer among nonsmokers, responsible for nearly 22,000 lung cancer deaths every year.

WHERE IT LURKS In the outdoor and indoor air of all kinds of buildings.

HOW TO AVOID IT Test your home with a radon test kit, available at home centers, by phone (1-800-SOSRADON [1-800-767-7236]), or online (www.sosradon.org/test-kits). If your home tests positive, click on your state at www.epa.gov/radon/whereyoulive for your Radon State Contact or call the Radon Fix-It Hotline at 1-800-644-6999.

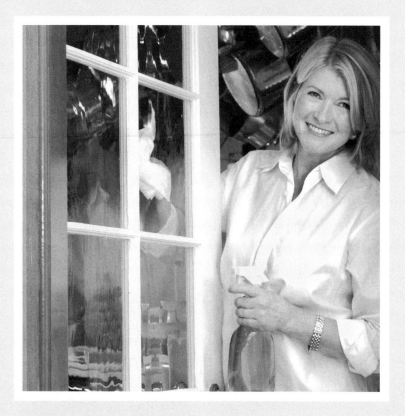

THE PLEASURE OF CLEANING

Believe it or not, I have always gotten a great deal of pleasure and satisfaction from cleaning and organizing. Sparkling-clean windows, no dust bunnies under beds and furniture, spotless sinks, shiny faucets, and clean kitchen floors—for me all are essential on a daily basis, and less difficult to attain and maintain than most of us realize. I actually like vacuuming, dusting, polishing, repairing, and sweeping. I have never called cleaning a chore—I refer to these tasks as "homekeeping." I never say, "I have to clean the basement"; instead I think of it as, "Today I am organizing my basement, getting the space into shape, finding a place for everything, and along the way washing the floor, dusting the shelves, and putting it all in order."

I have many pets living in my home, and they could pose a big problem if I wasn't a fastidious cleaner—but no one ever says my house smells of dog or cat or birds. I use unscented cleaning products, with no harsh chemicals or abrasives, and I try to find products that are organic and efficacious in terms of environmental safety.

I clean all the time—when I am finished preparing a meal, I wrap two damp rags around my clogs and skate around the kitchen (a trick I learned from my daughter). Any spots or crumbs are whisked away! And I don't let tasks pile up like dirty dishes in a sink. Everyone can function better, live better, and feel better in an orderly, organized, tidy environment. Remember, that the word "edit" does not only pertain to words, but can also apply to "neatening" up one's environment. Discarding extraneous stuff and getting rid of unnecessary clutter make a home look newer, fresher, and, ultimately, more inviting.

PART 2

HEALTHY LIVING INTO TOMORROW

CHAPTER 8   Healthy Living into the Future 302

CHAPTER 9   Healthy Caring 336

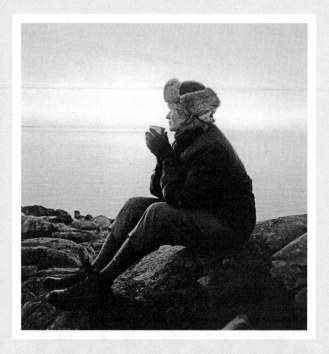

Healthy Living into the Future

PREPARE *for a healthier tomorrow* 304

SERVE *as your own wellness CEO* 307

REDUCE *risk factors* 311

FIGHT OFF *heart attack and stroke* 317

PROTECT *your bones and joints* 322

LOWER *your cancer risk* 330

MONITOR *vision and hearing* 334

I believe in preventive health and I try to live according to its principles. I know that the more vigilant I am about my care today, the healthier I'll be tomorrow. It requires discipline in making good choices each and every day: Do I reach for that pat of butter? Do I exercise or watch a movie? But you just learn to ask, Should I or shouldn't I?

Taking a preventive approach also requires making time in my busy schedule for doctors' visits when I'm well, not when I'm sick—mammograms, blood panels, flu shots, vision exams, nutritional consultations. Recently I had a bone density scan and my doctor said my bones looked stronger than two years ago! I was so pleased. And it was also concrete proof that all of that hard work pays off.

It's vitally important to stay on top of the information flow among all of your doctors. I chose to have one doctor who keeps all of my records. Every time I have a test, such as a mammogram, I have copies sent immediately to him. That way he has a full picture of my health, and he can factor it all in to his care. I also keep all my own records—you have to be your own health steward.

PREPARE *for a healthier tomorrow*

It's a fundamental principle of physics: a body at rest tends to stay at rest; a body in motion tends to keep in motion. How does physics relate to living healthily into your future? It means being proactive about your health and setting in motion as many preventive actions to avoid or minimize the onset of any chronic conditions as you can. Not years from now, but right now.

As we'll no doubt live longer, due to the increase in average life expectancy that we Americans enjoy, that benefit comes with a certain amount of responsibility. We're all aiming for not only quantity but quality of our greater number of years on this planet. The overall aim: to take good enough care of our bodies so that one part doesn't wear out before the others do.

What that comes down to is getting busy about taking the steps to prevent the major causes of age-related disability: diabetes, high blood pressure, elevated cholesterol/blood fats, heart attack, stroke, cancer, osteoarthritis, osteoporosis, and changes in your vision and hearing acuity. But more important, if diagnosed with one of these chronic conditions, is taking the necessary steps to slow the progression of that condition, not simply throwing your hands up in defeat. It doesn't mean living in a fantasy world or in a state of denial, but rather assuming a hands-on practical approach to taking care of yourself. Of course, you can't manage medical conditions all on your own, but you can in collaboration with your doctors. And once again, you make the first proactive move: consider yourself as "the boss of me" and work with your primary-care doctor to manage symptoms and any conditions. You are more than your diagnosis or a medical label; you are a living, breathing, moving person in charge of your life, so start living it that way!

FOLLOW A FEW NONNEGOTIABLE RULES

Despite the astonishing progress science makes every year in understanding the molecular basis for many diseases, no one has a crystal ball that can reveal your future health. But one message keeps emerging from the ongoing research into aging: what you do in the present has a huge impact on your health in the coming years.

We've learned that many chronic conditions—such as diabetes, heart disease, osteoporosis, arthritis, cancer, and depression—are closely tied to lifestyle, and can often be prevented, managed, or even reversed by healthy habits and behaviors. Start by taking these seven lifestyle commandments to heart:

1. STAY ACTIVE

Exercise boosts mood, relieves stress, strengthens the heart, improves circulation, builds muscle tone and bone strength, reduces body fat, decreases insulin blood levels, and reduces the risk of many cancers.

2. DRINK PLENTY OF WATER

Water helps flush wastes and toxins out of your system. Every time you swap in a glass of water for a soda, you help reduce your risk of diabetes, heart disease, and high blood pressure.

3. REDUCE YOUR STRESS LEVEL

Stress has a measurable impact on the body. Hormones and other chemicals released when you're under stress can impair immunity, disrupt blood sugar levels, increase levels of damaging blood fats, and in general overload the body's systems, raising your risk for depression, cancer, heart disease, stroke, diabetes, and lots of other conditions. There are many methods available for managing and reducing stress, including meditation and biofeedback.

4. EAT HEALTHFULLY

Shoot for seven to nine servings a day of fruits and vegetables; eat more whole grains, legumes, and fatty fish; cut back red meat; and watch portion sizes.

5. MAINTAIN A HEALTHY WEIGHT

Excess body fat not only stresses your joints, it undermines your general health. Overweight bodies produce excess insulin, which can increase inflammation—which in turn ups your odds for developing diabetes, heart disease, high blood pressure, and many cancers.

6. DON'T SMOKE

Smoking kills more people in the United States than alcohol, car accidents, suicide, AIDS, homicide, and illegal drugs combined, according to the National Cancer Institute. Fortunately, quitting has an immediate effect: those who quit before the age of 50 have half the risk of dying in the following 15 years than those who continue.

7. DRINK ALCOHOL MODERATELY

Women and anyone over age 65 should limit their alcohol intake to one glass per day; men under age 65 can have two glasses per day. If you're regularly drinking more than that—especially if you binge drink, which the Centers for Disease Control and Prevention classifies as drinking four or more drinks at one time—you can damage your health and increase your risk for accidents, injuries, and assault. Years of heavy drinking can lead to liver disease, heart disease, cancer, and pancreatitis.

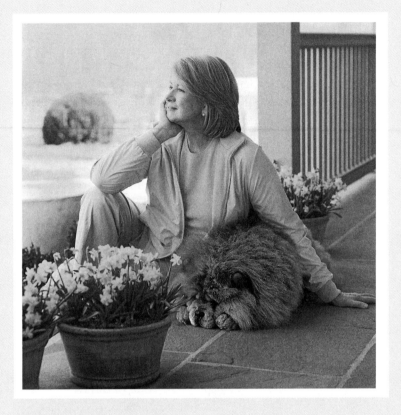

BE PROACTIVE

Living well is not a passive act. It is imperative to be engaged in taking care of ourselves. In addition to exercising and maintaining a varied and nutritious diet, one of the most important things I do for myself is to make sure I consult the right professionals at the right times. I try my best to schedule my routine doctor visits and age-appropriate medical tests for the entire year all at once, using the advice of my primary-care physician (very important to have one). That way, nothing gets forgotten and everything will be done when it should be. Get those appointments on your calendar now if you haven't already—and see how good it feels to take charge of your health.

SERVE *as your own wellness CEO*

You wouldn't put your career on autopilot, so why abdicate responsibility for your body? Longevity is really all about good management, and you should be handling your health like the vital business it is. Here's how to take charge.

FIND THE RIGHT PRACTITIONER FOR YOU

The older you get, the more new (or embarrassing, or mystifying) symptoms you'll develop. It's critical to have a doctor you can confide in and trust. Be honest: does your current physician fit the bill? If not, it's time to doctor-shop.

You should also consider switching to a geriatrician as you get older—they're clued in to many issues that your average family doctor won't be familiar with, and they tend to be up on the latest research about aging. But geriatricians can be hard to find, mainly owing to scarcity: there are only about 7,500 practicing in the United States to care for the 30 million people over age 65, according to the American Geriatrics Society. Here's how to find one:

CHECK WITH YOUR COMMUNITY HOSPITAL

Many have a geriatrics program, and most can at least refer you to one.

CALL A LOCAL ACADEMIC MEDICAL CENTER

Ask a hospital connected to a medical school for their geriatrics division, usually a subdivision of the department of internal medicine.

CALL A LOCAL MEDICAL SCHOOL

Ask for the department of internal medicine or family practice to obtain a list of recently graduated geriatricians in your area.

CONTACT YOUR LOCAL VETERANS HEALTH ADMINISTRATION

This government agency can offer referrals in your area.

ASK YOUR HMO

Motivated by recent government financial incentives, many HMOs are incorporating geriatrics practices into their offerings.

TALK TO YOUR CURRENT DOCTOR

He or she may keep up with developments in the field of aging and treating the elderly; if so, you may not need to switch at all.

MAKE YOUR VOICE HEARD

Many of us feel only a limited sense of empowerment or ease with our doctors. For example, you may be fine articulating a complaint at an office visit, but then feel hesitant to call between appointments for fear your question or problem is too trivial. In fact, it's the opposite: you should be giving your doctor ongoing feedback—it contributes to your overall care.

If a prescribed therapy isn't working after a few weeks, let your doctor know; it gives her the chance to refine or reconsider her decision. And if you're not happy with your doctor's proposed recommendations, you should speak up. You don't need to be confrontational; instead, ask, "Could you walk me through your thinking process so I can see how you got to this conclusion?"

You can also turn the tables: "Ask the doctor what he or she would do in your shoes," advises Dr. Gail Gazelle, assistant professor of medicine at Harvard Medical School and founder of one of the first physician-run patient advocacy practices, MD Can Help. "It's a critical question people are sometimes afraid to ask, but you should always ask it—whether it's your first, second, or ninth opinion." Often the doctor will answer with a very different course of action from what they've just advised for you, she says. "I've seen it both personally and professionally. It's a very powerful question."

It helps to ask for a road map at the end of an appointment. Find out how soon you should be seen again, what tests need to be scheduled, what should happen next, when you should expect results, and whom to call if you don't hear back.

HOW TO GET A SECOND OPINION

Here are two techniques to ensure you get the most complete medical picture:

1. Ask for a blind second opinion. "You want to get an opinion from a doctor who has no idea what any other doctor on the planet has to say about your condition," says Dr. Gazelle. "Be careful not to let it leak from your mouth. Let them decide on their own."

2. Go to a different institution. "It's tempting to just consult another doctor in the same department," says Dr. Gazelle, "but that's a mistake. Hospitals and group practices can be very set in their ways regarding the preferred way to treat a particular condition. This can be based on factors like whether the lead researcher in the area of expertise is based at that hospital, or whether a key medical device or procedure was invented by someone affiliated with the hospital, rather than being based on whether the treatment or procedure recommended is actually the best for that patient's unique medical situation."

QUESTION DRUG DOSAGES

Drug dosages are highly individual—no matter what you're told by the pharmacist or you've read in the *Physicians' Desk Reference*. Beyond factors like age and body weight, it appears that the speed with which a drug is metabolized by your body is influenced by genes in the liver and can vary from person to person. If you're concerned about side effects or have had unpleasant reactions to particular medications, ask your doctor if the drug comes in multiple strengths and whether you can start with the lowest dose. Keep in mind that a change in physical status (say, a weight loss of ten pounds or more) may affect your dosage, even with a medication you've taken for years. And whenever starting a new prescription, ask about possible side effects and interactions with any other drugs or supplements you're already taking.

SEE A SPECIALIST WHEN YOU NEED TO

There may be times when a difficult diagnosis or hard-to-treat chronic condition requires consulting a specialist. Your primary-care doctor can often provide the necessary referral, or you may find someone during your own research who is known for handling cases like yours. Specialists are often hard to access and appointments can be brief. You'll get the most out of your meeting by being well prepared and staying in control of the flow of information. Here's how:

BRING EVERYTHING YOU NEED
Create a folder and bring along your own patient record, containing:

☐ A list of all medications you're taking, by both brand and generic (chemical) names, along with dosages

☐ A list of your allergies and sensitivities to medications, foods, insects, or contrast dyes (used in medical imaging)

☐ An account of past major medical problems and surgeries you've had, complete with dates

☐ A photocopy of your most recent EKG (if you have heart problems or have had abnormal cardiogram results)

☐ A description of any consistently abnormal lab results you've had, even those that have been declared benign (for example, a minor degree of anemia, elevated liver function tests)

☐ Insurance information

☐ A durable power of attorney document, a living will, or advance directives

KEEP IN TOUCH WITH YOUR PRIMARY-CARE DOCTOR
Specialists are great at what they do—but you need someone who can see the big picture. Your primary-care physician (your internist or geriatrician) can be your ombudsman, a central source through whom all information can flow and specialty care can be coordinated.

STAY ON TOP OF YOUR MEDICAL RECORDS

Don't assume that all the details of your history will naturally find their way from your primary-care physician to the specialist. Ask for a copy of your physician's consultation request form (a note with a brief description of the reasons for the referral). After you meet with the specialist, ask him or her when and how information will be conveyed back to your doctor. If you're due to see your primary-care doctor quite soon, ask that the specialist call your doctor or jot down on a prescription pad the major findings and recommendations, to avoid delays.

Similarly, don't depend on a doctor or a hospital to keep your information; whenever you have blood work or a test (especially if it's not routine), get a copy for your own patient record. Keep physical or digital copies of X-rays, MRIs, CT scans, mammograms, and so on.

It's also important to have someone who can see the big picture. Patient advocates suggest you appoint a care gatekeeper—a doctor whom you ask to serve as the ultimate arbiter of your treatment. The older you get, the more doctors you'll have on your team, and it helps to elect a leader to avoid chaos and confusion.

Several online services offer a way to gather together all this information, in something known as an electronic Personal Health Record (PHR) or Electronic Health Record (EHR). Having your own PHR helps coordinate diagnoses, test results, and medication orders from your doctors. If you switch physicians, it can provide valuable continuity of care—and if you're ever rushed to the emergency room, it might be lifesaving. The downside is a risk of security breaches (they're rare, but not unheard of). Reduce your vulnerability by making sure the privacy policy gives you complete control over access, choosing a strong password, and not uploading sensitive information that could be viewed by employers or insurance companies.

Some computer-based sources to consider are Microsoft HealthVault, Mayo Clinic Health Manager, AARP Health Record, and WebMD Health Manager.

REDUCE *risk factors*

Thanks to the media, we hear about so many potential health threats these days—mercury in seafood! pesticides in our produce!—that it's easy to get overwhelmed and feel as if there's nothing you can do to protect yourself. In fact, the key risks to your health are well within your control and, even better, can all be managed by leading the kind of healthy lifestyle already described in chapters 1 through 7 of this book.

But there are some risk factors that you should take the time to understand more thoroughly. Experts agree that the "Big Three" human health risks that everyone needs to ward off are high blood pressure, high cholesterol, and type 2 diabetes because they predispose you to a host of other diseases and illnesses. The Big Three increase your odds of developing chronic conditions like heart disease and cancer, or suffering a devastating heart attack or stroke—any of which could rob your later years of independence and joy.

The good news is that while medical science originally thought that increases in blood pressure, cholesterol, and the onset of diabetes were just the inevitable effects of aging, we now know that's just not true. Dozens of studies have found that simple lifestyle changes can make a healthy difference, whether you're already in super shape or have had to start taking medications to control your blood pressure, cholesterol, or blood sugar.

It doesn't matter how old you are, either. Even those who make changes at age 65 can see prompt health benefits, according to a Medical University of South Carolina study that followed more than 15,000 volunteers for six years. You already know, from chapters 1 and 2, why maintaining healthy weight, eating well, and staying active will reduce your risk factors. On the following pages, you'll find information on each of the Big Three risk factors in detail so you can consider specific lifestyle changes to make if you're facing one of these issues.

REDUCE YOUR RISK OF HIGH BLOOD PRESSURE

High blood pressure, or hypertension, is known as the "silent killer" because it doesn't cause pain or any symptoms—until you suffer a heart attack or stroke (75 percent of heart attacks and strokes are at least partially caused by hypertension). Here's how it works: when the pressure inside your blood vessels is high, the force of the blood against the vessel walls damages them, encouraging the formation of calcium plaques (they're like scabs over a wound). Not only do those plaques end up gradually narrowing the inside of the vessels, possibly leading to a heart attack, but the extra pressure can also fracture those plaque buildups, breaking off stroke-causing clots. Hypertension is diagnosed when you have a blood pressure of 140/90 mmHG or higher.

With every birthday, your odds of developing high blood pressure inch upward. Some experts estimate that by age 55, nearly 90 percent of us will develop elevated blood pressure if we don't take preventive measures.[1] That statistic may sound fatalistic, but in fact, there are many ways to lower your blood pressure with simple lifestyle interventions.

In addition to the healthy lifestyle strategies discussed in chapters 1 through 5, consider the following to avoid trigger ingredients for high blood pressure:

REDUCE SODIUM

If you already have high blood pressure, or heart disease, it's particularly important to avoid excess salt. Too much sodium puts you at risk of congestive heart failure. It's a good idea, even if you don't have high blood pressure, to limit eating processed foods (where a large percentage of the sodium in American diets comes from). When cooking at home, opt for low-sodium condiments, and experiment with using herbs and lemon juice to brighten the flavors of food.

DRINK MODERATELY

Alcohol, in moderate amounts, can actually lower blood pressure. But consuming alcohol in higher amounts—more than one drink per day for women, or two per day for men—can raise blood pressure. If you already drink heavily, don't quit drinking cold turkey;

this drastic change can trigger high blood pressure for several days. Instead, seek the guidance of a doctor on how to taper off your drinking in a more moderate way.

AVOID HIGH-FRUCTOSE CORN SYRUP

If a package label lists high-fructose corn syrup (HFCS) near the top of the ingredient list, return the product to the grocery shelf. Cutting back on processed foods and beverages that contain HFCS, such as soda, may help prevent hypertension. Over the past twenty years, the rate of intake of fructose, which is twice as sweet as glucose, has risen 30 percent, directly paralleling the rate of obesity—and now, according to research at the University of Colorado Denver Health Sciences Center, it looks like fructose can affect your blood pressure as well.[2]

REDUCE YOUR RISK OF HIGH LEVELS OF CHOLESTEROL AND TRIGLYCERIDES

Decades ago, high levels of some forms of cholesterol and triglycerides were thought to be the blood equivalent of skin wrinkles—inevitable consequences of aging. But now we know that a healthy lifestyle can thwart most of these unhealthy changes, which happen to be the very same ones that up your risk for cardiovascular disease.

Your doctor will check your cholesterol and triglyceride levels at your annual exam. Your total cholesterol should be less than 200 mg/dL, and your triglycerides below 150 mg/dL. If you have no risk of heart disease, 100 mg/dL is considered optimal by the American Heart Association. Here's why these numbers matter. Your cholesterol is made up of two types of molecules: low-density lipoproteins (LDL) and high-density lipoproteins (HDL). These are often called "bad" and "good" cholesterol, respectively, because they work at cross-purposes. The LDL is made up of particles that can accumulate in artery walls, creating plaque that can form a stroke- or heart-attack–causing clot; the HDL molecules bind with the LDL particles and carry them away, reducing the risk of plaque and clots. When triglyceride levels rise, they become the building blocks of LDL, contributing to plaque buildup. The good news is that it's never too late to start improving your numbers—and decreasing your risk for heart attack or stroke—with a healthy lifestyle.

DIETARY CHOLESTEROL VS. BLOOD CHOLESTEROL

There's a distinction between dietary cholesterol—the kind you eat—and blood cholesterol, which exists in every cell of your body. The latter, produced in the liver and other organs, regulates metabolism and hormones. This precious substance gets transported around the bloodstream via LDL and HDL. Dietary cholesterol, meanwhile, is found in eggs and other animal proteins. The amount you ingest has less of an impact on cardiovascular health than you might think. In fact, the biggest culprit behind elevated LDL "bad" cholesterol is in saturated fat, found in meats and high-fat dairy foods. Trans fats, such as hydrogenated oils, also raise LDL levels. While cholesterol found in food such as eggs and shellfish can bump up LDL counts in some people, saturated fats are a much bigger danger, so they should be kept to a minimum.

FOODS TO FIGHT HEART DISEASE

Too much cholesterol in the blood can cause atherosclerosis, a type of heart disease. Research supports that eating whole foods over processed choices will limit your risks. The following five foods are particularly heart-healthy.

WHOLE GRAINS	Try for six daily servings of whole grains. Rich in a cholesterol-lowering fiber called beta-glucan, oats appear particularly powerful in protecting against heart disease. Try cooking up hot cereal from steel-cut oats (higher in phytochemicals than the rolled variety). Also, regularly incorporate brown rice, quinoa, and barley into your diet.
OILY FISH	Canned or fresh, oily fish such as wild salmon contains a wealth of omega-3 fatty acids, which help to improve triglyceride levels, stabilize heartbeat, lower blood pressure, curb heart-harming inflammation, and reduce stroke risk. Aim for two to seven servings a week.
NUTS	Crack open a walnut shell and you'll find plenty of plant sterols, compounds that help stop your gut from absorbing cholesterol. A source of blood-clot–preventing omega-3s, walnuts also nourish your heart with vitamin E, fiber, potassium, and protein. For better heart health, eat a handful of walnuts, almonds, cashews, or pistachios about five times a week.
OLIVE OIL	With its abundance of polyphenols (antioxidants that may prevent heart trouble by keeping LDL, or "bad," cholesterol from oxidizing), healthy fats, and vitamin E, olive oil is your heart-healthiest option for sautéing veggies or dressing salads. Choose the extra-virgin variety, which contains more polyphenols.
BEANS	Beans boost heart health by supplying magnesium, which helps to keep blood pressure in check, and folate, which decreases levels of homocysteine (an amino acid that raises heart-disease risk when it occurs at elevated levels). Include black, red, or adzuki beans in your repertoire; research suggests that darker beans deliver more antioxidants.

REDUCE YOUR RISK OF DIABETES

Type 2 diabetes is a one-two punch: it's a diagnosis of a disease but also a risk factor for other conditions such as heart attack, stroke, blindness, nerve pain, memory problems, Alzheimer's disease, and dementia. Furthermore, type 2 diabetes (the most common type among adults) is a strong predictor of functional decline, or the inability to do everyday activities and live independently.

Fortunately, lifestyle changes can prevent, delay, and in some cases reverse the disease, which results when the pancreas doesn't make enough insulin or your body develops insulin resistance. Ultimately, excess glucose builds up in your bloodstream, which damages vital organs, nerves, and blood vessels. If unchecked, the disease can be fatal.

According to the Centers for Disease Control and Prevention, the biggest factor in preventing type 2 diabetes is maintaining a healthy weight. Women who have a body mass index (BMI) between 18.5 and 24.9—considered to be normal—are 78 percent less likely to contract type 2 diabetes; men with the same BMI are 70 percent less likely. Integrating other positive lifestyle choices, such as a healthy diet, exercise, not smoking, and limiting alcohol consumption, will further reduce the risks.

Even if you've been diagnosed with type 2 diabetes (which has no cure), there's still hope. Research has shown that patients can keep the disease in remission, without the aid of medications, through diet and exercise. Taking preventive steps to fight off the disease will improve your health, regardless of your current risks.

GO FLEXITARIAN

Diet fads may come and go, but scientists have consistently found that people who eat plant-based foods tend to consume fewer calories, weigh less, and have lower cholesterol than meat-eaters. This doesn't mean, however, that you need to become a strict vegetarian to gain the benefits of this regimen. In fact, adopting a flexitarian diet—eating mostly vegetables, and moderate amounts of fish, poultry, and meat—can help you lose weight and improve overall health. As its name implies, this approach to eating is very flexible. You can adopt a "vegetarian till dinner" policy, or simply abstain from meat or animal products one day per week and still accrue modest benefits. Try using meat and highly caloric animal products such as cheese as flavor accents in your meals, rather than as the main attraction. You may find that you enjoy these ingredients even more in moderation.

TESTING FOR PREDIABETES

Type 2 diabetes is almost always preceded by a condition called "prediabetes"—blood glucose levels that are higher than normal but not yet high enough to be diagnosed as diabetes. Almost 80 million people in the United States have prediabetes, and the most common symptoms include feeling hungrier or thirstier than normal, going to the bathroom more frequently, feeling more tired than usual, unexplained weight loss, and blurred vision. Since diabetes develops so gradually, however, you may not experience any symptoms at all, or brush aside any that you do have. As a result, you may already be incurring long-term damage to the body, especially the heart and circulatory system.

Your doctor can test your blood glucose to determine whether you're prediabetic. If you do receive a diagnosis, it's important to remember that a positive test result is not necessarily destiny. Research has conclusively shown that people with prediabetes can prevent type 2 diabetes by eating healthfully, being physically active, and managing their weight. To determine your risk, your doctor can administer one or several of the following tests:

TEST	HOW IT WORKS	RISK FACTOR
HEMOGLOBIN A1C TEST	This simple blood test measures average glucose over a period of 2 to 3 months. It's frequently used to test whether diabetes is under control, but can also be used to test for prediabetes.	NORMAL: Less than 5.7% PREDIABETES: Between 5.7% and 6.5% DIABETES: Greater than 6.5%
FASTING PLASMA GLUCOSE TEST (FPG)	Your blood is assessed for elevated blood glucose after an overnight fast.	NORMAL: Less than 100 mg/dL PREDIABETES: Between 100 mg/dL and 126 mg/dL DIABETES: Greater than 126 mg/dL
ORAL GLUCOSE TOLERANCE TEST (OGTT)	An initial blood sample is taken after an overnight fast. Then you're given a high-sugar liquid to drink. Blood glucose levels are measured several times over a period of three hours.	NORMAL: Less than 140 mg/dL PREDIABETES: Between 140 mg/dL and 200 mg/dL DIABETES: Greater than 200 mg/dL

FIGHT OFF *heart attack and stroke*

The previous sections showed you how to reduce your risk factors for all kinds of chronic illness, including cardiovascular ones like heart attack and stroke. Here's what doctors and researchers know today about how to avoid these largely preventable conditions.

HEART DISEASE

RECOGNIZE YOUR RISK FACTORS

In addition to the Big Three (see page 311), women face gender-specific risk factors that play a big role in the development of heart disease. Talk to your doctor if you experience any of these:

Metabolic syndrome: the combination of three of the five signs—fat around your abdomen, high blood pressure, high blood sugar, high triglycerides, and low HDL cholesterol.

Mental stress and depression: Depressed women had a 30 percent higher risk of stroke in the Nurses' Health Study. Depression makes it difficult to maintain a healthy lifestyle (depressed people are more likely to be overweight, smoke, and skip regular exercise) and follow recommended treatment. Antidepressants may be linked to stroke risk.

Smoking: The nicotine in smoke is believed to cause heart disease by increasing blood pressure and heart rate and damaging cells that line coronary arteries.

Low levels of estrogen: Women's estrogen levels fall after menopause, which may pose a significant risk factor for developing cardiovascular disease in the smaller blood vessels. Yet use of hormone replacement therapy is linked to increased risk of heart disease.

SEE YOUR DENTIST

Good dental hygiene may reduce your risk of heart attack, stroke, and other cardiovascular problems by at least one third, according to a recent study—especially in women.[3] The link? Inflammation of the gums allows bacteria to enter the bloodstream.

CHECK YOUR PULSE

A postmenopausal woman's resting pulse rate is a good measurement of her heart attack odds, regardless of other factors including smoking and alcohol consumption, according to one study based on data from the Women's Health Initiative (WHI). Women with the highest resting heart rate—more than 76 beats per minute—were significantly more likely to experience a coronary event than those with a resting heart rate of 62 beats per minute or less. So take your pulse periodically, and if yours seems high, check in with your doctor. In the meantime, increase your workouts; regular exercise lowers your resting pulse rate.

CONSIDER A DAILY ASPIRIN

Low-dose aspirin therapy may help prevent a first heart attack or stroke among diabetics who also have an elevated risk for heart disease, according to a joint statement of the American College of Cardiology Foundation, the American Diabetes Association, and the American Heart Association. Overall evidence suggests that benefits are likely to exceed any downsides. Consult your doctor regarding whether or not you should take aspirin as a preventive measure.

DON'T LET GENDER AFFECT YOUR TREATMENT

Recent research in France found that women were 57 percent less likely than men to undergo angiography, a procedure that identifies blocked arteries. Men were also 72 percent more likely to receive clot-busting drugs and 24 percent more likely to undergo angioplasty, a procedure to reopen a blocked artery.[4] Women were also more likely than men to die during their initial hospital stay and within a month of having a heart attack, so this is literally a life-or-death matter. If there aren't any clear reasons not to, women should be treated with all recommended strategies—including invasive ones.

KNOW THE SIGNS OF A HEART ATTACK

More women than men die of heart disease each year. That may be because women tend to experience some different symptoms from men, which they often don't recognize as signaling a heart attack. Instead of the classic crushing pain, women are more likely to experience vague symptoms such as these:

- Neck, jaw, shoulder, upper back, or abdominal discomfort
- Shortness of breath
- Nausea or vomiting
- Sweating
- Lightheadedness or dizziness
- Unusual fatigue

If you have these symptoms or think you're having a heart attack, call 911 or have someone drive you to a local emergency room. Don't let the ER staff turn you away (some don't even realize that women's symptoms are different from men's). Instead, insist on being tested. Medical staff will listen to your heart and lung sounds with a stethoscope, and you'll likely be given an electrocardiogram (ECG). Samples of your blood may be taken, to test for the presence of certain heart enzymes that slowly leak out into your blood if your heart has been damaged by a heart attack. Additional tests could include a chest X-ray, an echocardiogram, and/or coronary catheterization (angiogram).

STROKE

There are two kinds of strokes: in 90 percent of strokes, a clot gets loose in your bloodstream and stops the flow of blood and oxygen through the brain; in the other, rarer type, a weakened blood vessel ruptures and spills blood into brain tissue, damaging it. Strokes kill or alter the lives of older men and women more than any other health problem. By far the most important thing you can do to reduce your risk for stroke is to lower your blood pressure (see tips in Reduce Your Risk of High Blood Pressure, page 312). But there are many other things you can also do in an effort to minimize your stroke odds:[5]

UNDERSTAND THE RISKS OF MINOR STROKES

If you've had one of the symptoms listed on page 320, but it went away, you may have had a ministroke, called a transient ischemic attack (TIA). These occur when a blood clot temporarily clogs an artery and blocks blood flow to the brain. These minor strokes don't typically cause permanent harm, but you must seek medical attention because they are a major sign that you're at risk for another, more serious stroke. Check with your doctor promptly or go to the emergency room if you experience a possible stroke symptom.

DON'T FRY YOUR FOOD

Choosing omega-3–rich fatty fish is a smart move to reduce your risk of many diseases, including stroke, but the way you cook may make all the difference. According to a study in the journal Neurology, frying fish causes a loss of these beneficial fatty acids. Shoot for the American Heart Association's recommendations—two or more 3-ounce servings per week—but poach, bake, or roast rather than fry.

MUFFLE TRAFFIC NOISE

If you live near a busy intersection, consider soundproofing your home. The noises generated by road traffic may increase the risk of stroke in people age 65 and older. Danish researchers found that for every 10-decibel increase in noise, the risk of having a stroke increased 27 percent overall for those aged 65 and over. Previous research had linked traffic noise with increased blood pressure and risk of heart attacks. This study adds to the accumulating evidence that traffic noise may cause a range of cardiovascular diseases.[6]

Noise is a stress and can disturb sleep, which results in increases in blood pressure and heart rate. The older you get, the more fragmented sleep becomes, making you more susceptible to the sounds outside your bedroom. Find ways to insulate your home from noise pollution.

KNOW THE SIGNS OF A STROKE

The symptoms of a stroke are similar in men and women; they should never be ignored. If you or someone you are with experiences any of the following, call 911 and ask for an ambulance equipped for advanced life support. Every moment counts, because delay increases the potential for damage and disability from a stroke.

- **Sudden numbness or weakness** of the face, arm, or leg, especially on one side of the body

- **Sudden confusion**, or trouble speaking or understanding

- **Sudden trouble seeing** in one or both eyes

- **Sudden trouble walking,** or dizziness, loss of balance, or coordination

- **Sudden, severe headache** with no known cause

RECOGNIZE CHRONIC INFLAMMATION

Inflammation is one of your body's natural defense mechanisms, and you have some first-hand experience with it if you've ever experienced redness, swelling, heat, and pain after an injury. But more and more research is finding that chronic inflammation may be at the bottom of everything from wrinkles to Alzheimer's.

HOW INFLAMMATION WORKS Certain cells and chemicals of the immune system are mobilized in response to trauma, to heal damage and protect organs. As you recover, the system calms down and the signs of inflammation resolve.

This response to an injury is healthy. With age, however, certain inflammatory proteins, known as cytokines, rise and persist in the bloodstream. This chronic inflammation is a problem. Think of it this way: if your body is revved up to fight something and finds nothing, serious damage to normal tissue may result. That's the mechanism researchers suspect is behind many chronic conditions.

HOW CAN YOU FIGHT BACK? The healthy lifestyle choices described throughout this book are effective in both lowering inflammation and reducing your risk for chronic conditions. In addition, you can make a concerted effort to reduce and manage your stress levels and keep your gums healthy (gum disease is a source of cytokines, among other harmful substances that may raise your risk of heart disease and other inflammatory conditions). Also, you can get tested: ask your doctor for a blood test that measures levels of the inflammatory C-reactive protein (CRP) and lipoprotein-associated phospholipidase A2 (LP-PLA2), to assess your risk and the impact of your lifestyle choices. The correlation between high CRP and heart disease is not well understood.

PREPARING FOR A HOSPITAL STAY

It's never pleasant to check in to the hospital, whether you're there for a day for testing or a week or two for surgery and recovery, but the whole experience can go a lot more smoothly if you're prepared. This list is a good start; for more tips and tactics for your stay, download the booklet "Don't Leave the Hospital Sicker Than You Went In!" by Dr. Gail Gazelle, available at www.mdcanhelp.com/onlinestore and the Discharge Preparation Checklist at www.caretransitions.org/documents/checklist/pdf.

ARRIVE WITH . . .

☐ Your patient record (see Bring Everything You Need, page 309)

☐ A list with your doctors' names and contact information

☐ Glasses, contact lenses, hearing aids (with extra batteries), dentures

☐ Cell phone, charger, and phone numbers of key family members or caregivers (check the hospital's policy on other electronic items before you pack your laptop, tablet, portable DVD player, or MP3 player, and be sure that these electronics can be kept secure when you're not in your room)

☐ Socks and slippers (hospital floors are heavily trafficked places and not always clean)

☐ Bathrobe, cardigan, or zip-front sweatshirt

☐ Notebook and pen to note questions you need to ask the doctor or nurse

LEAVE WITH . . .

☐ Directions for follow-up care. Know which doctors you're seeing, why you're seeing them, and when.

☐ A list of pending tests, when to expect the results, and whom to call to find out their status.

☐ The name and phone number of the person to contact if problems arise.

☐ Copies of your discharge instructions and the summary to be given to your follow-up doctors. (Request a copy of the summary as well, and keep it in your patient record folder.)

☐ An idea of what, if any, symptoms to expect and when to call the doctor. There are some potentially disturbing symptoms that are normal after surgery, such as a headache after a lumbar puncture or coughing blood after a bronchoscopy. Knowing what to expect and what to be concerned about can save a lot of anxiety.

☐ The right medications. Check any new prescriptions and compare with what you're currently taking. Your prescription or a dosage may be changed when you're in the hospital; make sure it matches what you have at home or what you think you should be taking.

PROTECT *your bones and joints*

Bones and joints constitute your body's scaffolding system. Protecting both the support (bone) and the hinges (joints) is crucial because these are the basis for your mobility and help you live longer independently. Here's how to safeguard both:

YOUR BONES

Stooped-over posture is a telltale sign of fragility and age. None of us wants to find ourselves in that compromising position, but 10 million Americans have osteoporosis, the bone disease that results from a loss of bone density—and many of them don't even know it. Women are more prone to osteoporosis than men, with an estimated 8 million women affected by it, versus 2 million men, according to the National Osteoporosis Foundation.

Bones become less dense over time, particularly in the weight-bearing areas of the body—the hips, wrists, and spine. Doctors aren't sure why these spots are the first to lose density, but if you fall, you're most likely to break or fracture bones in one of these three areas. Significant bone density loss puts you at high risk for fractures. A bone fracture likely won't kill you, but the disability it brings can decrease your mobility, reduce your independence, and impact your quality of life.

While some risk factors for the disease (low body weight, early menopause, being white or Asian) may be inherited and beyond your control, for the most part osteoporosis is preventable. If caught early enough, it can be arrested and even reversed. If you have a family history of osteoporosis, take these steps to lower your odds of developing it:

GET ENOUGH CALCIUM

If you're over 50, you need to take in about 1,200 mg of calcium (from foods, supplements, or a combination of both) every day. (See Calcium-Rich Foods, page 37.)

GET ENOUGH VITAMIN D

Eat foods such as vitamin D–fortified milk, fatty fish (such as salmon, tuna, mackerel), fish liver oil, and egg yolks. You need 800 to 1,000 IU daily. Since it can be difficult to get enough vitamin D through food alone, talk to your doctor about whether you should take supplements.

DON'T FORGET VITAMIN K

Found mainly in leafy green vegetables (broccoli, Brussels sprouts, dark green lettuce, collard greens, or kale), this vitamin likely plays an important role in calcium regulation and bone formation. Low levels of circulating vitamin K have been linked with low bone density, and supplementation with vitamin K shows improvements in bone health. A report from the Nurses' Health Study suggests that women who get at least 110 micrograms of vitamin K a day are 30 percent less likely to break a hip than women who get less. It was found that eating one serving of a green leafy vegetable per day cut the risk of hip fracture in half, when compared with eating just one serving a week.[7]

MIND YOUR MAGNESIUM

Half of your body's supply of magnesium is found in bones, and research has shown that this mineral is vital to keeping your skeleton strong. Find it in halibut, dark leafy greens, beans, peas, nuts, seeds, and whole grains.

GET THE RIGHT VITAMIN A

Long associated with good vision, vitamin A is also important to bone formation and maintenance. But not all vitamin A is good: too much preformed vitamin A (also known as retinol, found in many supplements) can promote fractures. Check the label on your multivitamin supplement; all or the majority of its vitamin A should be in the form of beta-carotene, a vitamin A precursor, which does not increase your fracture risk.

CUT BACK ON CAFFEINE

There is some evidence that drinking a lot of coffee—four or more cups per day—can increase your risk of fracture, because caffeine tends to promote calcium excretion in urine. The Framingham Osteoporosis Study has found that older women who drink colas, but not other carbonated beverages, every day have significantly lower bone mineral density in the hip than those who drink it less than once a month, possibly due to cola's high levels of caffeine and phosphorous, a known bone weakener.[8]

BE ACTIVE

Aim to exercise for at least 30 minutes most days of the week. Regular physical activity burns abdominal fat—that is, belly fat—which may have a damaging effect on bone health. Researchers did imaging studies on fifty premenopausal women with a mean BMI of 30. Results revealed that women with more belly fat had decreased bone density. Fat on the hips or total body fat did not have the same impact on bones.

QUIT SMOKING

Smoking doubles your risk of osteoporotic fractures. While the precise mechanism is unclear, research has shown that smoking harms the cells responsible for building new bone. Smoking, or the chemicals contained in cigarette smoke, may also decrease your body's ability to absorb calcium. And for women, smoking may block estrogen's protective effect on bones. Quitting can help limit further bone loss, as well as improve your cardiac, lung, and circulatory health.

WEIGHT-TRAIN TO AVOID A FALL

It's important to maintain and build body strength because it means you're less likely to lose your balance and fall. Weight training also builds bone; working muscles tug on the bones they connect to, and this "stress" increases bone density. (For exercises you can do at home, see Chapter 2. For more on how to prevent falls, see pages 262–265.)

LIMIT YOUR ALCOHOL INTAKE

You should keep consumption to one or two drinks at most per day; any more raises your risk of losing bone and increases the likelihood of a fall.

KNOW THE SIGNS OF OSTEOPOROSIS

After age 50, a broken bone is not just a broken bone—it's a potential symptom of osteoporosis. Here are some other subtle signs of this bone-thinning disease.

BREAK YOUR WRIST?

Ask your doctor to evaluate you for osteoporosis. According to a study in the *Journal of Bone and Joint Surgery*, postmenopausal women who broke a wrist were less likely to be evaluated for osteoporosis than those who broke a hip or their spine. But a wrist fracture should be as big a red flag for osteoporosis as the other breaks.

BAD HOT FLASHES?

You may have lower-than-average bone density. The conclusion of a study published in the journal *Menopause,* which analyzed data from 2,213 women between the ages of 42 and 52 who were participating in the Study of Women's Health Across the Nation, found that postmenopausal women with symptoms of hot flashes had lower lumbar and total hip bone density than those who didn't suffer from hot flashes. If you're experiencing hot flashes, ask your doctor to assess your osteoporosis risk.

LIVING WITH OSTEOPOROSIS

Even if you've been diagnosed with osteoporosis, there are plenty of ways to help keep your condition from worsening. Stay healthy by doing the following:

EXERCISE OUTDOORS

Sunlight helps your skin convert pre-vitamin D to its active state.

LIMIT SATURATED FAT

According to the National Osteoporosis Foundation, consuming too much saturated fat, typically found in red meat and animal by-products, can lead to a high level of homocysteine, a chemical in the body known to decrease bone mass.

SWITCH TO GREEN TEA

A cup of tea contains phytochemicals that can stimulate bone formation and help slow its breakdown. In a study, certain green tea components boosted an enzyme that promotes bone growth and blocked the activity of cells that weaken bones.

CONSULT YOUR DOCTOR

There are specific medications available for osteoporosis; your doctor can decide if they're right for you.

REPORT EVEN MILD DEPRESSION

A study published in the *Archives of Internal Medicine* found that premenopausal women with major depressive disorder (MDD) had less bone mass than did their nondepressed peers. In fact, the level of bone loss was as high as that associated with more commonly recognized risk factors for osteoporosis, including smoking and low calcium intake.

CONSIDER SUPPLEMENTS FOR BONE SUPPORT

If you have trouble getting enough calcium in your diet (see page 37), you may need to take a supplement. Talk to your doctor about the amount and type you need, as well as about vitamin D, which your body needs to absorb calcium.

CALCIUM

The two most widely available supplements, calcium citrate and calcium carbonate, are equally well absorbed by the body. Calcium carbonate is less expensive and supplies more elemental calcium than citrate (40 percent vs. 21 percent); the carbonate form is best absorbed when taken with a meal, while citrate can be taken any time of day.

VITAMIN D

The Institute of Medicine (IOM) now recommends 600 IU of vitamin D every day for most healthy adults under age 71, and 800 IU for healthy people age 71 and older. This is an increase from previous recommendations that cited 200 to 400 IU per day for healthy adults under age 71 and 600 IU per day for those aged 71 and older.

ABOUT PROTEIN AND BONE HEALTH

Your body needs protein to build healthy bones. But as your body digests protein, it releases acids into the bloodstream, which the body neutralizes by drawing calcium from the bones. Following a high-protein diet for a few weeks probably won't have much effect on bone strength. Doing it for a long time, though, could weaken your bones. In the Nurses' Health Study, women who ate more than 95 grams of protein a day were 20 percent more likely to have broken a wrist over a twelve-year period, when compared with those who ate an average amount of protein (less than 68 grams a day). This area of research is still controversial, and findings have not been consistent. To be safe, moderate your protein intake.

STRENGTHEN BONES WITH EXERCISE

Regular exercise is key to both prevention and treatment of osteoporosis. Weight-bearing activities, such as walking, hiking, and aerobics classes, strengthen bones by making them produce more cells. Alternating high-impact and low-impact activities can help you keep active without injury.

LOW-IMPACT ACTIVITIES	HIGH-IMPACT ACTIVITIES
Cycling	Walking
Swimming	Running, jogging
Spinning	Hiking
Kayaking	Jumping rope
Elliptical training machine	Calisthenics, such as jumping jacks
Cross-country ski machine	Racquet sports
Rowing machine	Nordic walking (with poles)
Upper body ergometer	
Stair climber	
Yoga	
Pilates	
Tai chi	
Gardening	

FIND A FITNESS MENTOR

If you're finding it difficult to motivate yourself to get out and exercise, you may benefit from taking a class or working with a personal trainer. Almost every community has a gym that offers classes and trainers to help structure an exercise program. In urban areas, many personal trainers even teach classes in parks during the summer months. Working with a trainer for 30 to 60 minutes, several times a week, is a great way to stick to a program and stay in shape.

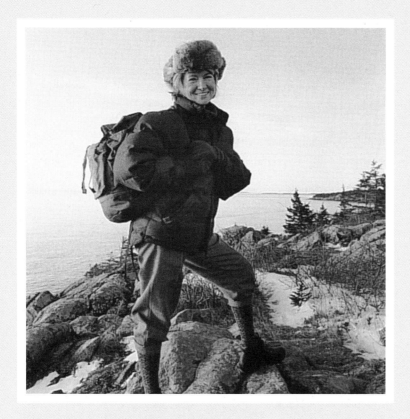

ENJOY YOUR EXERCISE

Invigorated, healthy, strong, and accomplished—there's nothing like the sense of well-being that comes with exercising. If you are having trouble getting motivated, it's genuinely helpful to remind yourself of how good you'll feel when you're finished. The key to sticking with a regimen is finding something you love to do. For me, because nature is so important to me, one of those activities is hiking. I've been fortunate enough to hike all over the world, but one of the most special places to me is close to home, Maine's Acadia National Park. It's my habit to get out early, to savor the quiet beauty and the early-morning light. Then I'm back home with the whole day ahead of me.

YOUR JOINTS

Pain and stiffness from cartilage-compromised joints don't have to be your reality, yet one in two Americans will be diagnosed with osteoarthritis (OA) during their lifetime. Your risk steps up after age 45, and women are at a higher risk than men. The disease's hallmark is the breakdown of the protective shock absorbers that cushion the ends of bones. These pads of cartilage simply wear, tear, and disintegrate away, leaving you with joint pain, swelling, and stiffness.

Certain factors may predispose you to OA, including a family history, previous joint injury, being overweight, or repetitive overuse from a work or sports activity. Take these steps to lower your odds of developing the disease:

MAINTAIN A HEALTHY BODY WEIGHT

Extra weight stresses joints, especially in the hip, knee, ankle, and foot, and may increase the likelihood of damaging cartilage in the lower joints, which can result in arthritis.

AVOID REPETITIVE MOTIONS

Too many uninterrupted repetitions of an activity or motion can wear away the cartilage at the end of bones. Find ways to modify your activities, take breaks, and learn strategies to avoid periods of repetitive stress to your joints.

EXERCISE MODERATELY

Studies show that strengthening your muscles reduces your risk of arthritis because muscles take some of the load off joints. However, don't overdo it. According to a study presented at the Radiological Society of North America, MRI exams revealed that light exercisers had the healthiest knee cartilage among all exercise levels; that is, patients with minimal strength training had healthier cartilage than patients with either no strength training or frequent strength training. Moderate strength training and flexibility moves support joints without risking damage to the cartilage.

FOCUS ON YOUR QUADS

The quadriceps, the muscles located in your upper thighs, are the largest muscles of your body. When they are toned and strong, they relieve much of the stress on your knees; stress and strain can injure the cells that help maintain normal cartilage, known as chondrocytes. Smart moves to strengthen quadriceps include squats, seated knee extensions, and step-ups (using a sturdy bench or stair).

DISH UP THE VITAMIN D

Vitamin D is crucial to bone health, and bone strength comes into play with arthritis. As cartilage strives to repair itself after injury, the process triggers bone remodeling—the loss or addition of bone cells. A Boston University study of 221 arthritis patients found an association between blood levels of vitamin D and knee and muscle pain; the lower the levels of vitamin D, the greater the pain reported. And the older you are, the harder it is to convert and absorb vitamin D from the sun. Sunlight is the best source of vitamin D (15 minutes daily exposure is the recommended dose). Other sources include supplements, fatty fish such as salmon, fortified whole-grain cereals, and egg yolks. Still other research from the Iowa Women's Health study suggests that greater vitamin D intake may be linked to a lower risk of developing rheumatoid arthritis, the second most common form of arthritis.

LIVING WITH ARTHRITIS

Joint pain can limit everyday activities and simple comfort for perfectly healthy people of every age. Thankfully, there are a number of natural, effective approaches to help you stay mobile and reduce pain.

CONSULT YOUR DOCTOR

Your doctor will help you figure out if medication is right for you and suggest different exercises and devices for you to try until you find what works (as the symptoms of arthritis vary greatly from person to person).

STAY ACTIVE

Regular exercise protects and stabilizes joints, nourishes cartilage, and increases range of motion. Exercising can also lead to weight loss, which tends to be beneficial. Every pound of extra weight you carry translates into three additional pounds of pressure on your knees and hips, so losing even a few pounds can take a significant load off those hardworking hinges. Start with low-intensity activities that don't aggravate your joints; ask your health-care practitioner, a physical therapist, or a personal trainer what kinds of exercise would help you most. In general, fitness routines for those with joint pain, like most fitness programs, include flexibility, weight training, and cardio exercises. Listen to your body, and don't try to work through the pain. Try resting for several minutes when your pain is at its peak. Then, slowly ease back into your activity. Or take your workout to the water: exercising in the buoyancy of water can cushion the impact from exercise.

GIVE YOUR JOINTS SOME EXTRA CUSHIONING

Consider using shoe inserts or splints.

REVAMP YOUR DIET

An inflammation-fighting diet can pay healthy dividends for your joints. Omega-3 fatty acids and monounsaturated fats like canola and olive oils soothe inflammation. Sources of omega-3s include salmon, walnuts, flaxseed, and fortified eggs. The antioxidants in fruits and vegetables fight free radicals, the extraneous molecules that have been shown to contribute to inflammation. Eat a rainbow of produce to get a range of antioxidants (see page 50). Vitamin D protects against hip arthritis, according to a 1999 study published in the journal *Arthritis & Rheumatism*. Fortified milk and breakfast cereals are good sources of vitamin D, as are tuna, salmon, and mackerel. Avoid partially hydrogenated oils and vegetable oils high in polyunsaturates, which trigger inflammation and can exacerbate joint pain.

USE HOT OR COLD PACKS

They can ease stiffness, swelling, and pain.

TRY ACUPUNCTURE

This technique of traditional Chinese medicine may provide pain relief and improve function for people with arthritis. In one study by the National Center for Complementary and Alternative Medicine, those who received acupuncture to treat knee arthritis had a 40 percent decrease in pain and nearly 40 percent improvement in function compared with those who got a "sham" acupuncture session or counseling.

LOWER *your cancer risk*

"The Big C" is probably one of your biggest fears about aging, and with good reason: despite President Richard Nixon's declaration of war on cancer in 1971, the battle is far from over. Cancers that involve the breasts, lungs, skin, colon, and rectum are the ones most commonly diagnosed in women of nearly every racial and ethnic group, while prostate, colon, skin, and lung cancers top the list for men.

Despite how widespread cancer is, many of us still don't understand exactly what it is or why it can be so deadly. Basically, cancer is your own cells running amok—they multiply and divide without ceasing, as normal cells would. In the process, cancer cells co-opt valuable body resources, such as the blood supply, oxygen, and nutrients, thus literally starving other cells. And the older you are, the longer your cells have been dividing and the greater the odds that some mistakes have occurred in those serial divisions.

The good news is that scientists have found preventive steps that will reduce your risk of developing cancer. It's difficult to generalize about this large group of diseases, but the National Cancer Institute (NCI) estimates that as many as one third of common cancers could be prevented just by adopting a healthy lifestyle. To do your part, note the steps below. Also, don't ignore early warning signs—a lump, a sore that won't heal, a change in energy, a feeling of being "off." When it comes to cancer, it's better to be safe than sorry. Whether or not you have a family history of a specific cancer, take these steps to lower your odds of developing it:

EAT A CANCER-FIGHTING DIET

That means low in fat, with plenty of whole grains, legumes, and fruits and vegetables; limit your intake of red meat and processed or preserved meats, eat more fish, and reduce your intake of animal fat.

QUIT SMOKING

If you've tried to quit before and failed, keep trying. It's never too late to quit, and your body will benefit almost immediately.

GET REGULAR SCREENING TESTS

Schedule clinical exams, mammograms, and colonoscopies. (See chart on pages 188–189.)

EXERCISE

Regular activity helps maintain a healthy weight. Exercise also helps your muscles become more efficient users of insulin (the hormone that helps cells absorb glucose from food). This lowers blood insulin, blood glucose, and production of free radicals, all of which play a role in development of cancer. More specifically, exercise is associated with a decreased risk of breast and colon cancers.

SUPPLEMENTS THAT MAY FIGHT BREAST CANCER

One in eight American women will be diagnosed with breast cancer during her life. And the risk of developing breast cancer increases with age. Talk to your doctor about whether adding one of the following supplements makes sense for you:

VITAMINS C AND E

Breast cancer patients who used antioxidants (vitamin E, vitamin C, multivitamins) had an 18 percent reduction in their mortality risk, and the risk for recurrence was decreased by 22 percent.[9] This study may allay concerns that supplements might reduce the efficacy of cancer treatments and increase the risk of mortality; see where your doctor stands on this issue.

FISH OIL CAPSULES

Postmenopausal women who took fish oil supplements with high levels of the omega-3 fatty acids EPA and DHA had a 32 percent reduced risk of invasive ductal breast cancer.

VITAMIN D

Researchers at the Mount Vernon Cancer Centre in Middlesex, England, recommend that women with breast cancer be tested for vitamin D levels and offered supplements, if necessary. Breast cancer cells have vitamin D receptors, and when these receptors are activated by vitamin D, a series of molecular changes are triggered that can slow cell growth and cause cells to die. Even if it does not have a direct effect on the tumor, vitamin D is needed to maintain the bone health of women with breast cancer. That's especially important given the increasing use of aromatase inhibitors, which carry an increased risk of bone loss.

GET MORE OUT OF YOUR MAMMOGRAM

Don't stop hormone therapy. Some doctors recommend that women on hormone replacement therapy (HRT) cease the therapy one to two months before having a mammogram because the HRT makes breasts denser and harder to read on mammography, leading to more falsely abnormal results. But new research suggests that women should not stop HRT before a screening. Most women over 50 have low breast densities to start with, say the researchers, and the magnitude of the increase with HRT is small. What's more, stopping therapy is likely to bring on a recurrence of symptoms in women, with no convincing evidence of improved screening accuracy. Instead, the researchers recommend that health-care providers should alert their HRT patients that they might require additional evaluation.

Time your mammograms. If you're still getting periods, schedule your mammogram during the first week of your cycle. A new study in *Radiology* found that accuracy may be better during that time—possibly because breasts are less dense then. Researchers examined 387,218 mammograms from women aged 35 to 54 who got the screenings from 1996 through 2007; the number of true positive findings was highest in those who had the mammograms the first week of their cycle. Having a mammogram then raised the chance of catching the cancer 7 to 13 percentage points.[10]

PRACTICE REGULAR BREAST SELF EXAMS

Annual mammograms and clinical examinations (performed by a health-care provider) offer one of the best early detections for breast cancer. However, performing monthly breast self exams (BSE) will help you notice if anything looks or feels amiss, in which case you should immediately consult your doctor. If you're still menstruating, the best time for a BSE is when your breasts are least swollen, such as a few days after your period. For postmenopausal women, choose a day, such as the beginning of the month, to perform the examination. (If you happen to be taking hormones, consult your physician on when to perform a BSE.) Check with your doctor immediately if you notice changes in your breast tissue, such as swelling, nipple abnormalities (pain, redness, scaliness, turning inward), skin irritation, dimpling, discharge (other than breast milk), or if you find a lump or abnormality in performing the following breast exam.

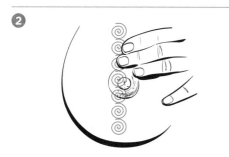

Lay on your back, with your right arm tucked under your head. This position allows breast tissue to spread over the chest wall, making it easier to detect changes.

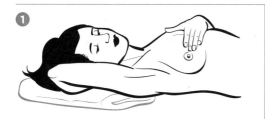

With the pads of the three middle fingers of your left hand, feel for lumps in the right breast by using overlapping, circular movements to feel the breast tissue. Before progressing to the next spot, circle with three levels of pressure: light pressure for tissue closest to the skin; medium pressure for deeper tissue; and firm pressure to feel tissue closest to the rib cage and chest.

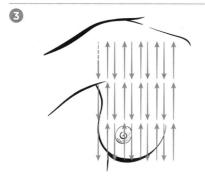

Drag your fingers in an up and down motion, starting just under your armpit and moving across the breast to the middle of the chest bone. Make sure to move across the entire length of the breast, from ribs to collarbone. Repeat steps 1 through 3 for the left breast.

STOCK UP ON POWER FOODS

Many factors play into cancer prevention, but mounting evidence suggests that eating a healthy, plant-based diet (such as the Mediterranean diet, page 29) may be one of your best defenses. Although eating a variety of foods is best for overall health, the following fruits and vegetables have shown promise as cancer fighters.

CRUCIFEROUS VEGETABLES

This family of vegetables—which include broccoli, cauliflower, kale, cabbage, and Brussels sprouts, among others—contain compounds called isothiocyanates (ITCs), which may protect against colon, stomach, prostate, and respiratory cancers. The phytochemicals in crucifers may also stimulate enzymes that help the body detoxify carcinogens before they harm cells.

LEAFY GREEN VEGETABLES

Leafy greens, such as Swiss chard, collards, and spinach, are an excellent source of antioxidants called carotenoids, which fight cell-damaging free radicals. Additionally, these vegetables are packed with folate, a B-complex vitamin shown to reduce the risks of breast and lung cancers.

BERRIES

The flavonoids in all berries counter cell damage and reduce risk of cancer. Each berry contains a different collection of flavonoids, so it's good to eat a variety. Blueberries, blackberries, raspberries, and strawberries contain several anthocyanins—potent antioxidants—that help to reduce inflammation and could curb cancer cell growth.

ONIONS AND GARLIC

More than just flavoring agents, the organosulfides that onions and garlic contain are powerful antioxidants. In large population studies, the more onions and garlic consumed, the lower the risk of colon, breast, prostate, and other cancers.

TOMATO

Lycopene, which gives tomatoes their orange and red colors, is associated with lower risk of prostate, cervical, skin, breast, and lung cancers. Cooked tomatoes contain two to eight times more lycopene than raw because the carotenoid is tightly bound with the tomato's cell walls; heat breaks down those walls, releasing more lycopene for absorption and use by the body. Good sources of lycopene include sautéed fresh tomatoes, canned tomatoes, jarred salsa, spaghetti sauce, tomato paste, and tomato soup.

MONITOR *vision and hearing*

Hearing and sight are your social senses—the ones that connect you to the world. Protecting these should be a top priority.

YOUR VISION

The triple threat to vision is cataracts, glaucoma, and macular degeneration (see pages 204–207). Caught early, any progression can be slowed dramatically, ensuring years of good vision. Take these steps to lower your odds of developing them:

QUIT SMOKING

Early-stage age-related macular degeneration (AMD) appears to be related to modifiable risk factors, including smoking and low levels of high-density lipoprotein (HDL, or "good" cholesterol), according to the Beaver Dam Offspring Study.

WATCH BLOOD SUGAR AND BLOOD PRESSURE LEVELS

High levels of either are damaging to the delicate blood vessels in the eye.

EAT A DIET RICH IN FRUITS, VEGETABLES, AND FATTY FISH

Results from the Carotenoids in Age-Related Eye Disease study of 1,808 women (aged 55 to 86) living in Iowa, Wisconsin, and Oregon indicate that eating a healthy diet more strongly related to the lower occurrence of nuclear cataracts than any other modifiable risk factor or protective factor studied. In the Women's Health Study, eating dark-meat fish, such as tuna, salmon, trout, and sardines, may reduce the risk for developing AMD; women who ate one serving per week were 42 percent less likely to be diagnosed with AMD compared with women who ate the fish less than once a month.

WEAR EYE PROTECTION

Goggles are essential during any activity that could injure your eyes, such as mowing the lawn or operating heavy machinery. Also, wear sunglasses whenever outside. Chronic overexposure to UV radiation increases your risk of both cataracts and macular degeneration. If you wear contacts, consider getting a prescription for UV-protective lenses. As UV damage to your eyes is cumulative, overexposure to the sun's rays can lead to harmful changes in the cornea, conjunctiva, and lens, including cataracts. A study reported in *Investigative Ophthalmology & Visual Science* found that UV-blocking contact lenses can reduce or eliminate the effects of the sun's harmful UV radiation, especially UVB.

USE CAUTION WITH ANTIDEPRESSANTS

Seniors who take SSRI antidepressants may increase their risk of developing cataracts by about 15 percent.[11] The apparent increased risk is associated only with current, not past, drug use, and mainly with three drugs: Luvox (fluvoxamine), Effexor (venlafaxine), and Paxil (paroxetine). The eye's lens has serotonin receptors, and animal studies have shown that excess serotonin can make the lens opaque and lead to cataract formation. Talk to your doctor if you take one of these SSRIs.

YOUR HEARING

Hearing does decline with the years, but keeping your ears healthy (having a regular checkup for wax accumulation) and protecting your ears from loud noises both go a long way toward helping you maintain acute hearing ability.[12] In addition, doing the following will help you maintain good hearing:

DON'T IGNORE HEARING LOSS

Nearly two-thirds of adults 70 and older suffer from hearing loss, yet only a fraction use hearing aids. Researchers from Johns Hopkins School of Medicine note that there's a general perception that hearing loss is not significant, but besides isolating you socially, hearing loss is associated with incipient dementia, falls, and poorer cognitive functioning. Talk to your doctor as soon as you notice any changes.

INCREASE FOLIC ACID

In a Dutch study of 728 older men and women, those who got 800 mg of folic acid a day had less hearing loss after three years than those who didn't. A bowl of split pea soup, a glass of orange juice, some spinach, or a slice of whole-grain bread are all good sources of folic acid.

STABILIZE BLOOD SUGAR

When University of Maryland researchers compared the blood-sugar levels and hearing acuity of over 1,600 men and women, they found that those with diabetes were 30 percent more likely to have hearing loss than nondiabetics. High blood sugar damages tiny nerves and blood vessels in the ears. Monitor your blood sugar if you have diabetes.

CHECK MEDICATION

Both prescription and nonprescription medications may damage ears and cause hearing loss. These include antibiotics such as erythromycin, vancomycin, tetracycline, gentamicin, and streptomycin. Check with your doctor if you notice changes.

STEER CLEAR OF EXCESS SODIUM

Reducing your salt intake can help lower your odds for Ménière's disease, an inner-ear disorder that affects balance and hearing. Fluid retention in the delicate tissues of the inner ear, caused by excess salt, may alter pressure in your ear and cause these problems. Read labels—packaged entrées and canned soups and vegetables contain much more sodium that you need—and look for no-salt versions of your pantry staples. Rinse canned beans before using them to remove sodium, or cook dried beans.

KEEP MOVING

Exercise improves the flow of blood to every cell in your body, including the delicate hair cells inside your ears that help you hear. But skip the headphones. Even at moderate volume, using headphones may result in hearing loss or pose a safety hazard.

USE EARPLUGS

Keep earplugs within arm's reach—in your home, in the car, in your purse, or in your briefcase, and pop them in whenever you encounter loud noise. This will help to protect against hearing loss from loud music, construction, lawn mowers, even hair dryers. Cotton balls or wadded tissue won't cut it—foam earplugs block up to 32 decibels of noise; cotton, only 7 decibels. Many smart phones will accept a decibel meter application (check out Decibel Deluxe or Pico Brothers decibel meter), so you can assess the loudness of a noise and take appropriate action to save your hearing.

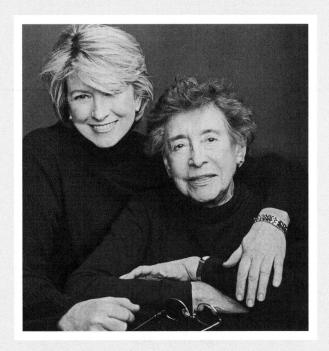

CHAPTER 9

Healthy Caring

BE *prepared* 338

ADDRESS *family matters* 345

KNOW *when to hire help* 349

FIGURE OUT *housing* 352

INFORM *yourself about insurance* 360

OPTIMIZE *quality of life* 362

PREPARE *for the end* 368

My maternal and paternal families never sent an elder to a "home." There was always time and space to provide living quarters for "Grandma." But we were lucky, with longevity on our side, with good health and strong physiques. And we were a large enough family to be able to share time with the grandparents, to be inclusive and accommodating.

Many families today still find ways to care for elders at home. There is stress inherent in such serious work, which is usually done while also raising children, taking care of spouses, and going to a demanding job; it is exhausting and difficult. Some seem to take on the added burden—and it is a burden—gracefully: living quarters are created, conversation is encouraged, and holidays and meals are enjoyed together.

Other families look for options outside the home, such as an assisted living center, where care is provided and a stimulating environment is available. More and more of these centers are being built, and if well run, affordable, and ambitious in daily programmed activities, they can be the answer for us as a nation facing the "silver tsunami."

When does the shift from caregiver to caretaker occur? That has to do with many factors, but the reality is the shift happens. Plans have to be discussed and made. Finances have to be in order, living quarters decided upon, caregivers designated. My friends and I joke about turning my farm into such a place for all of us. There is plenty to do, the neighborhood is amenable, and there is room to live comfortably. Those are the things, after all, that everyone needs.

BE *prepared*

So many of us are now living life as the peanut butter of our sandwich generation—"stuck" between raising our own children and caring for aging parents. In fact, it's more a question of *when* than *if,* as the American population over age 75 continues to grow. There are 42 million of us acting as caregivers for loved ones today; that number is sure to grow.

Caregiving is the ultimate in multitasking: you may be getting your kid off to school one moment, helping your father put his shoes on in the next, all the while rehearsing what you'll say at a department meeting later on. The competing demands of the generation ahead and the one behind can put a strain on your time and attention, as well as drain your finances. There's no course on caregiving, nor is there some magic gene that switches on when the time comes to help you out. Instead, you have to learn on the fly: finances, insurance, in-home care, second opinions, Medicare, Medicaid, hospice, and funeral planning. As caregiver, it's likely you'll be the executive in charge of decisions for your elder. It's undeniably a difficult job, but it provides a chance to help and support your parent, partner, or elder, just as that person once nurtured you. Through it all, you have to care for yourself so you can continue in your various day-to-day roles of child, parent, friend, colleague, neighbor, and more, with grace, dignity, and energy.

Medical advances have meant that people who would have been felled by a massive heart attack or a stroke now often survive, and instead die gradually, incrementally, from conditions that steal life by degrees—due to slow killers such as congestive heart failure, Alzheimer's, Parkinson's, diabetes, lung disease, and a host of others. As a result, death is becoming less an event and more of a process. And because this process takes time—months, even years—patients need help along the way. Most of the help will come from family members. In some capacity, each of us will be tapped to be a caregiver, perhaps short-term for a relative recovering from surgery, or long-term for a parent suffering from dementia or another debilitating condition. That means we have to be prepared; think of this chapter as your road map to providing such care. Regardless of where you are on the aging spectrum, the information that follows can help you plan effectively—for your parents, when it's your turn to be the caregiver, and for yourself, so that you can assist your own eventual caregivers in making myriad important late-life-stage decisions.

DISCUSS THE OPTIONS

"What I hear time and time again from caregivers and families involved with the care of a loved one in declining mental or physical health is, 'I was so unprepared.' Learn from their mistakes and start your caregiving preparations early," says Carol Bradley Bursack, founder of MindingOurElders (www.mindingourelders.com), a website that provides caregiving information and caregiver support. "No one wants to think about it beforehand, but when you're in the middle of a crisis, you simply won't have time for big-picture planning," she adds.

One of the first steps is to get information about your elders' wishes and desires about where they want to live, medical interventions to undertake (or not), and any funeral arrangements. If you start early, when life is calm and your aging loved one is still relatively healthy, you'll have much more productive conversations than when you're in a crisis because your mother has suffered a stroke or your aging aunt has taken a fall.

For some families, these talks are awkward or just plain difficult. Though it may be tempting to put them off, don't. You may have to work up to an initial conversation, or to repeat the same one again, giving everyone time between talks to think about the issues that have been raised.

Many times, it's the elders who put off the conversation—"There's time for that later," they'll say. For your part, be persistent and bring up the topic until the conversation begins. "I tell families all the time that they shouldn't have The Talk, they should have The Talks, because you need to cover a lot of issues," says Bradley Bursack. Plan on discussing the following subjects sooner rather than later: financial matters, end-of-life paperwork, health insurance, housing options, and driving.

One way to get the ball rolling on the needed long-term planning for your elders' future is to make an appointment with a financial planner who specializes in this field. An Internet search for "retirement financial planners" or even "longevity financial planners" will give you a wide variety of options. Tag along with them to the appointment, and don't be surprised if you discover there are things you should be doing, even at your age. Based on your elders' predicted longevity, any current conditions that are likely to progress, plus their risk of being diagnosed with a condition or disease from family history, your longevity planner can help crystallize important issues: how much to set aside for future care, whether to invest in long-term care insurance (which covers the costs of assisted living), the pros and cons of continuing a life insurance policy as well as how to invest their current nest egg. Advance planning may help you avoid a money meltdown later.

REVIEW FINANCES

When discussing health care with an elder, finances are a good place to start. Figuring out the money picture may be an easier conversation to have, since it's basically about bookkeeping and organization, rather than a charged subject like end-of-life care. If your family doesn't feel comfortable discussing money, you can still have a productive talk without going into specific amounts. Here are the questions to ask:

1. **IS THE POWER-OF-ATTORNEY PAPERWORK, BOTH MEDICAL AND FINANCIAL, IN PLACE?**
Who is the agent (the person named in the Power of Attorney document)? If it's someone outside the family, get contact information.

2. **WHERE DOES YOUR ELDER KEEP FINANCIAL RECORDS?**
If records are in a safe or locked file cabinet, appoint one person (typically a family member) to know the location of the keys or the combination on the lock, or place this information in a sealed, marked envelope, kept in a safe place.

3. **WHAT'S YOUR ELDER'S INCOME?**
How much annual income does he or she earn from pension(s), dividends, Social Security, disability, or alimony payments?

4. **WHAT'S THE CONTACT INFORMATION FOR THE ACCOUNTANT, TAX PREPARER, OR FINANCIAL PLANNER?**
Collect all of their contact information in one place.

5. **WHAT BANKS OR OTHER FINANCIAL INSTITUTIONS, SUCH AS AN INVESTMENT PLANNING FIRM, DOES THE ELDER USE?**
Write down contact information and list all account numbers and types.

6. **HOW MUCH ARE CURRENT MONTHLY EXPENSES?**
Include any mortgage, loan, car, or credit card payments; gas and electric bills; cable fees; taxes; medical care costs; and the cost of a housekeeper or gardener. Assessing your elder's financial health and balancing it against anticipated cost increases may help you decide whether the loved one should move in with you or apply for assisted living.

7. **HOW ARE BILLS USUALLY PAID?**
Online or paper checks? Which accounts are used?

Once you've gathered this financial information, place it in a binder or a file folder and make sure all family members involved in the elder's care know where it is.

GET END-OF-LIFE PAPERWORK IN ORDER

Asking your elder about how he or she wants to die may sound morbid, but it's time to adopt a more pragmatic point of view about end-of-life issues. Think of it this way: you and your elder have planned for potential emergencies by buying home insurance so you don't face financial ruin due to a fire or a tornado. You invest in life insurance so that loved ones left behind are cared for. In the same way, you can help your elders plan a good death by making sure they have advance directives in place.

Once you've talked through your elder's wishes, you'll need two separate types of advance directives.

HEALTH-CARE PROXY

This document allows your elder to name someone he or she trusts to make decisions about medical care when the elder cannot. (In many states, this person is authorized to speak for the patient any time the patient is unable to make a health decision, not only about end-of-life decisions.)

LIVING WILL

This document puts your elder's wishes about medical treatment in writing, so that if he or she can't communicate, his or her wishes are followed. A living will can be very detailed, with specifics about treatment desired should your elder become seriously or terminally ill, but it does not name a health-care proxy to make decisions for that elder.

You'll also want to make sure your elder has

- Appropriate resuscitation orders

- A signed and duly witnessed, up-to-date last will and testament

One way to start the paperwork process for power of attorney and advance directives is to make your own appointment and invite your parent. Tell your parent that you're going to the estate lawyer (or financial planner) to get your paperwork in order and ask if he or she wants to come. Once your relative's paperwork is completed, put it in a safe place. Again, make sure any caregivers involved know the location of the documents or have their own copies.

CONSIDER HEALTH INSURANCE OPTIONS

"You want to have this conversation sooner rather than later, just to make sure your parents are adequately covered," says Richard Nix, president of Agingcare.com, a website community for caregivers. "If they don't have the right policies in place, their life savings—your inheritance—could easily be spent paying for assisted living or a home health aide." Here are some questions to ask:

1. ARE THEY ON MEDICARE? MEDICAID?
   Individuals 65 and older are eligible for Medicare, while Medicaid eligibility is purely income based. Your elder may qualify for both.

2. WHAT IS THEIR INSURANCE COMPANY AND WHAT IS THE POLICY?
   Make sure you understand the details of their health coverage. Also find out if they have adequate life insurance coverage.

3. DO THEY HAVE A LONG-TERM-CARE INSURANCE POLICY?
   This is especially important if there is a history of long-term, high-care conditions such as dementia in the family. Agingcare.com offers an organizing checklist so you can keep all these details in one place. Make sure that all relevant family members have their own copies, or know where this information is kept.

RESPECT END-OF-LIFE WISHES

"This one is probably the hardest conversation to have, simply because as a society we don't really talk about death," says geriatric care manager Linda Packer. Try easing into the conversation by relating an anecdote about a friend: "When Jane's mom died, Jane discovered she had no idea whether there was a family plot." Then segue into how you don't know what your parents' wishes are and you'd like to hear more about them. Getting their preferences in writing may be helpful if family members are likely to disagree, Packer notes.

ADVANCE PLANNING PAPERWORK: WHAT EVERYONE NEEDS—AT ANY AGE

Use the chart on this and the following page to make sure you have all the appropriate paperwork in place for your elder and, while you're at it, for yourself. You can obtain these forms from a doctor, the local health department, the state department on aging, or a lawyer. Computer software packages are also available to help you create many of these documents yourself.

Once you've taken care of the paperwork, remember, don't let the documents do all the talking. Have conversations with all the stakeholders (family members, doctors) now, so everyone understands these plans before they're needed. It may be a good idea to write down explicit instructions: "X will be involved in decisions about my care; and the following family members will not." Include the directions with other advance directives. Finally, keep the directives updated; medical circumstances or wishes may change over time, and paperwork should be kept current to reflect new considerations.

DOCUMENT	DO YOU NEED A LAWYER?	DON'T FORGET
DURABLE POWER OF ATTORNEY (POA) Empowers a designated person to make medical decisions on your behalf (say, if you are in a coma or under anesthesia).	Lawyer optional; make sure to have a suitable witness (must be at least 18 years old) sign the document.	• Consider separate POAs—one for health care and one for finances (allowing a designated person to make bank transactions, sign Social Security checks, or write routine checks). • Give your health-care POA the written right to interpret your living will in case any uncertainty should arise about your care. • Get a HIPAA release to gain access to your elder's health records and physicians.

(CONTINUED ON NEXT PAGE)

DOCUMENT	DO YOU NEED A LAWYER?	DON'T FORGET
HEALTH-CARE PROXY A person who will make health-care decisions for you, should you not be able to (your proxy can be the same person to whom you grant durable power of attorney).	No lawyer needed, but a witness must sign the document.	• Inform your proxy that he or she has been chosen. • Update your proxy if your wishes have changed. • Consider naming an alternate in case something happens to your first choice.
LIVING WILL A description of how end-of-life care should be managed. This document takes effect when you are terminally ill.	Lawyer optional; witness signatures necessary.	• Consider making decisions about use of pain relief, antibiotics, hydration, nutrition, life support, surgery, and resuscitation. • Tell your physician and family about your desires, and give them a copy of the document.
DO NOT RESUSCITATE (DNR) ORDER A type of advance directive that instructs health-care professionals not to perform CPR or other lifesaving procedures, such as intubation.	No lawyer needed, but two witnesses must sign the document. This order can also be incorporated into a living will.	• Consider creating two DNR orders—one for a hospital/nursing home setting and one for an out-of-hospital setting to cover treatment by EMTs.
PHYSICIAN ORDERS FOR LIFE-SUSTAINING TREATMENT (POLST) Complements other directives with more specific instructions on the use of breathing and feeding tubes, mechanical respirators, and antibiotics.	Document signed by patient and doctor (the document may also be signed by another medical practitioner, such as a nurse practitioner or even a social worker).	• Currently 14 states have POLST programs, and 16 more are considering them. Be sure to check whether your state recognizes the POLST as legal.

ADDRESS *family matters*

In most families, there's at least one child who's likely to become the point person or chief caregiver for an ailing parent. It may be the person who lives nearby, or the one who's always had the closest relationship with the parent. In one study, Cornell University gerontologist Karl Pillemer interviewed 1,200 older people and found that most of them were very clear about which child they'd prefer as a caregiver. So it may be a choice that's made for you, but there's still plenty to discuss.

DECIDE HOW TO DELEGATE CARE

If you have siblings, suggest a meeting to discuss your parents' care—even if Mom and Dad are healthy and currently don't need any help. It's important to talk about all aspects of the process: who will take charge of the caregiving, who could possibly be a caregiver when the primary caregiver has an emergency or another commitment, who has a house that a parent could move into. Talking through the roles you may play in the future is important because, no matter how adult you are, the roles you played growing up come to the fore. Don't assume the oldest child will do the caretaking, or that the baby of the family can't be held responsible. At the same time, recognize that family dynamics are extremely powerful, and it can be difficult to change tendencies that are decades old. Here's a good ground rule: if a family member wants to be able to weigh in on what the solution to an elder's care should be when problems arise, then that person should have to participate in the process leading up to it.

At this meeting (or series of meetings), aim to assemble a list of everyone's strengths and weaknesses, and how much or how often each would be able to pitch in. This can help put together your family-caring safety net. One sibling may have the temperament or skills to deal with bureaucracy. Another may be a natural nurturer, or live in a community with excellent senior programs.

Caretaking affects your whole family and your whole life, whether you want it to or not. But many caregivers are deeply grateful for the chance to give back to the parents who raised them. When considering this added responsibility, you need to be able to concentrate on all of your other roles, too. Make a plan that takes into account the dignity of your elder, honors your marriage or other relationships, allows for the demands of being a parent, and values the sanity of the caregiver. And if that plan stops working, make another one.[1]

BALANCING WORK AND CAREGIVING

Whether you continue to work while caregiving is a personal and financial decision. Many caregivers simply don't have the discretionary income to support an elder and also support a child, so they continue to work, at least part time. Before making any drastic change, set up an appointment with your company's human resources director to discuss what your company can do for you in this situation. If you work for a company that has fifty or more employees, you're eligible under the federal Family and Medical Leave Act of 1993 to take up to twelve weeks of unpaid leave per year to care for a sick family member, and you're guaranteed not to lose your job or your health insurance during that time.

Some larger companies also offer basic eldercare benefits, which may include unpaid leaves of absence, eldercare flexible spending accounts, elder daycare or backup elder care. Even if your company doesn't offer specific eldercare benefits, it may have programs that will make your life easier, such as flexible work arrangements, job sharing, telecommuting, or a shortened work week.

DEALING WITH PARENTS WHO "DON'T NEED HELP"

Recognize that your elders may see you as mounting a hostile takeover when you sign on to be their caregiver. For some seniors, the loss of independence and choice is not something they want to face, so your offers of help get pushed away. It's critical to be very strategic in getting your elder to accept help. Here are some key points:[2]

- Timing and location are important. You don't want to confront your elders during a family dinner or holiday get-together. Instead, choose a quiet location where you can be alone, such as your place or theirs.

- Start talking about how you feel. Try, "I worry about you more than ever these days. Can I tell you why I'm worrying so much?"

- Present a cost-benefit analysis. If your elder is the pragmatic type, crunching numbers or making a list of pros and cons of moving in with a child or into a retirement community may seal the deal.

- Consult a geriatric care manager (GCM); he or she can give you advice and help your elder see things from an objective point of view (see page 349 for more information). Broach the topic by saying that you would like to hire a professional to do an evaluation. Then, reassure your elder: "If you agree, we can look at what she recommends to see what makes sense, okay?"

BUILD YOUR SKILLS

If you're the one who's most likely to be tapped to help with caregiving, you can prepare yourself by learning new skills. Do you know CPR? How to read a blood pressure gauge? The proper way to lift someone without hurting your back? How to make nutritious meals for a person on chemo? How to file a Medicare claim? The Family Caregiver Alliance provides an online overview of the skills caregivers need for frail, elderly people or individuals with chronic conditions (learn more at www.caregiver.org).

Taking classes for caregivers before you need the skills also gives you a preview of what will be required of you, which is a valuable lesson in itself. Often such classes are offered for little or no money. Here are some examples:

THE AMERICAN RED CROSS sells an instructional DVD and reference guide on caregiving; go to www.redcross.org.

THE ALZHEIMER'S ASSOCIATION offers classes for caregivers; for more information, visit www.alz.org.

POWERFUL TOOLS FOR CAREGIVERS (PTC) is a six-week course offered in many communities. The lessons deal with stress, guilt, communication, decision-making, depression, and increasing your self-confidence as a caregiver, among other topics. You can search for classes in your area at www.powerfultoolsforcaregivers.org.

CAREGIVING.COM offers free webinars for caregivers. The offerings change over time. Check it out at www.caregiving.com/caregiving-webinars.

VIDEOCAREGIVING presents streaming videos of people coping with real-life caretaking situations, such as moving a stroke patient from bed. It also offers video tips on how to prevent infection at home, how to prevent and deal with falls, and more. Their website is www.videocaregiving.org/caregiving.php.

CAREGIVING 101, sponsored by the National Family Caregivers Association and the National Alliance for Caregiving, is a guide to help beginning caregivers get their bearings. There's also an active message board community: www.familycaregiving101.org.

RESOLVE DISAGREEMENTS

In an ideal scenario, family members would unite and rally around an ailing parent, older sibling, or other relative, with each party contributing equally so that no one person bears the brunt of caregiving. And then there's the reality. No matter how old you are, this situation can throw you back to your childhood years—and childhood scripts: Who's the good one? Who's the prodigal son or daughter? Who gets away with everything? In many cases, siblings can cause more problems than an aging parent.[3] In fact, research at Cornell University has found that the issue that causes the most conflict among siblings is caring for an aging parent. If members of your family are squabbling, you need to set up a meeting to air grievances, discuss the needs of the ailing elder, and decide together how you're going to solve these problems. Here's how to proceed:

INVITE EVERYONE TO THE TABLE

Be sure to include the elder (if she or he is up to it) and a doctor or nurse who knows the elder's case.

ASK AN OBJECTIVE THIRD PARTY TO RUN THE MEETING

You can turn to a geriatric care manager, a social worker, a psychotherapist trained in family counseling, someone from your place of worship, or a mediator. Mediators can be found at www.eldercaremediators.com.

COUNTER EXCUSES FOR NOT PITCHING IN

If you're the primary caregiver, there may come a time when you get more excuses than offers of help from your relatives. Instead of getting angry, offer alternatives. For example, if you hear, "I live too far away," then suggest planning a vacation to the patient's city to give you a break for a few days, or contributing money toward the cost of care. If the excuse is "I don't have the money," suggest other ways to help, such as taking on bookkeeping tasks, calling insurance companies, making inventories of valuables, or organizing paperwork. If you hear, "I can't stand seeing Mom/Dad that way," suggest performing behind-the-scenes tasks, such as making home repairs, picking up prescriptions, or grocery shopping.

SET AN AGENDA

Be sure an agenda is mutually agreed upon ahead of time. Topics could include the latest report from the patient's physician, regular care needs of the elder (daily, weekly, monthly), roles that each person can take on, costs of care, needs of the primary caregiver, feelings about the illness/condition, and the origin of any discord.

ASK SOMEONE TO TAKE NOTES

Or you can tape-record the meeting. Afterward, send everyone a summary of what was discussed and what the resolutions are.

SET UP A TIME TO MEET AGAIN

Following the meeting, create a shared family calendar online to help distribute duties. Give those involved access to the elder's schedule and updates on his or her condition. You can do this on your own (Google Calendar and Google Documents make it easy to share schedules and other paperwork with the click of a button) or check out the free online calendar at www.lotsahelpinghands.com.

KNOW *when to hire help*

The first rule of caretaking is that you accept that you cannot do it all by yourself. "You need to be able to ask for help and ask for it early on in the process, not once you're overwhelmed and burned out," says Joan Griffiths Vega, facilitator of an Alzheimer's caregiver group and group teacher for caregiver stress relief at the Mount Sinai School of Medicine. Focus on getting help for as many of the tasks of daily care (paying bills, handling insurance, driving to doctors' appointments, bathing, shopping) as you can, so you can focus on your crucial role as child, spouse, and parent. Here are some options for available help.

GERIATRIC CARE MANAGERS

This health and human services specialist is trained to aid families who are caring for older relatives. A geriatric care manager (GCM) should have extensive knowledge of the local resources available to you, whether it's aging, caregiving, or family or personal issues. Unfortunately, they're expensive; Medicare doesn't cover their fees, and most long-term health-care policies don't, either. But the right GCM can be worth the investment, especially if you're giving care from a distance. The geriatric care manager should be trained in a number of related fields, such as care management, nursing, gerontology, psychology, physical therapy, occupational therapy, or social work. You may consider hiring a GCM on a one-time or short-term basis, such as for the first few weeks after a health crisis. Hiring a GCM as a short-term consultant can help you get your priorities straight if you're unsure about how to set up an elder's care. To find a good GCM:

ASK FOR REFERENCES

Get referrals from former clients who share your same situation, and talk with them about how the GCM handled things. A good GCM will customize her services to meet the needs and concerns of the family.

CHECK CREDENTIALS

There is no single organization that certifies GCMs. Some may be credentialed by the National Association of Social Workers, others by the National Academy of Certified Care Managers or the Commission for Case Managers. Make sure they are members of the National Association of Professional Geriatric Care Managers (NAPGCM).

CHECK COMMUNITY RESOURCES

Many states and cities have local agencies that employ geriatric social workers who can make a house call and acquaint you with local resources. It may be free if your elder is eligible. Find these agencies through www.eldercare.gov.

ASSESS THEIR RESOURCES

You want someone who can solve any problem. "Your GCM should have a wide referral network, so, for example, she could find a podiatrist to make a house call so your mother can walk without pain," says Linda Packer of the Prime Life Network. Ask the prospective GCM about his or her expertise in medical insurance, palliative care, finding a nutrition and exercise specialist, adult day care, and your elder's specific needs. Many GCMs are independent contractors, but managers can also be found through agencies, such as the National Association of Professional Geriatric Care Managers, at www.caremanager.org.

UNDERSTAND THE SERVICES OFFERED

Be specific about what services they will provide as well as on-call availability. "The best ones are available 24/7," Packer adds. Be sure to ask about fees and extra charges, such as phone calls or car mileage.

TROUBLESHOOT

If you anticipate that your elder will resist the idea of a GCM, tell the GCM ahead of time. You can arrange for a low-key, no-commitment meeting. "Gaining trust early is essential to making a smooth transition," Packer says.

HOME HEALTH AIDES

Home health aides are an invaluable part of a caregiving team. Their role can range from providing short-term relief for primary caregivers, to a larger, daily role in helping an elder stay at home for as long as possible. If you have a GCM, she may have suggestions on home health aides to hire. You can also ask your elder's doctor for the names of local agencies. "The biggest consideration in a health aide, besides adequate training, is personality," says Carol Bradley Bursack of MindingOurElders. "You want someone who gets along with and shares interests with your elder."

The advantage to hiring through an agency is that the aide will likely be trained specifically for elder care issues. For example, if your elder is prone to falling, you can hire someone trained in fall prevention. There's also more built-in accountability, since an agency will have to vouch that their aides are reliable, honest, and can be depended upon to care for specific medical conditions. For more information, visit the National Association for Home Care and Hospice (www.nahc.org).

If you prefer not to use an agency (and your elder doesn't have major health issues), you might find someone in your elder's life who could provide good companionship. Someone at your elder's place of worship, a loyal housekeeper, or family friend might be a good option. The advantage to this route is that your elder may already have a strong bond with the person and will find their company pleasurable. For a directory of home aides and other direct-care workers, visit www.directcareclearinghouse.org.

VOLUNTEERS

Not all helpers require compensation, which is a relief in the current economy. If you're specifically looking for companionship for your elder, consider finding helping hands by doing the following:

Call a guidance counselor at your local high school. Many schools require students to accumulate hours of community service before they graduate. Find a student who will visit your elder for an afternoon or evening so you can get things done around the house. Depending on your situation, they could even "eldersit" so you can get some errands done.

Swap services with other caregivers. Alternate weeks of caring for two elders at once so you get an afternoon free. Your elders may also benefit from the opportunity to socialize with a peer.

Contact local volunteer groups. Generally, these are healthy seniors who are available to visit or "eldersit." Or check out a free program from the AARP, called Create the Good, at www.createthegood.org. Once you register, you can create a posting of the type of volunteer you need.

Get in touch with your local religious center. Many synagogues and churches have a corps of volunteers ready to help. Your church may offer a program called the Stephen Ministry, through which trained laypeople offer spiritual guidance, companionship, counseling, and support. Find out more at www.stephenministry.org.

FIGURE OUT *housing*

The ability to feel at home can be deeply symbolic as we age. Whether it's remaining in one's own home, living with family members, or moving to an assisted-living facility, it's a balancing act to make sure your elder can live safely and at the level of independence he or she wants and can handle.

STAY IN THE HOME

There are many concrete benefits to keeping your elder in his or her home as long as possible. "If someone can live safely at home, not only are costs reduced but family relationships are enhanced, because everyone knows that the beloved senior is happy and safe," says Andrew Carle, assistant professor and founding director of the Program in Assisted Living/Senior Housing Administration at George Mason University, in Fairfax, Virginia. If staying put is what your elder wants, make sure his or her home poses minimal danger (see Chapter 7 for a room-by-room guide to preventing falls and other problems).

INVESTIGATE HOME MODIFICATION SERVICES

These websites can help you assess what would have to be done to help your parents stay put and stay safe:

- **Environmentalgeriatrics.com** provides lots of basic tips to make a home more elder-friendly.
- **Thiscaringhome.org** offers tips on how to handle family members with dementia or Alzheimer's disease.
- **Homemods.org** offers a checklist for safety assessment from the National Resource Center on Supportive Housing and Home Modification. Another good checklist is available at www.rebuildingtogether.org/resource/age-in-place-checklist.
- **Easterseals.com** links to low-cost ideas for making your home more accessible, as well as a home-safety checklist to download.
- **Pva.org** offers information for those with mobility challenges from the Paralyzed Veterans of America; they also offer services from a team of accessible-design architects.
- **Eldercare.gov** can direct you to a local area agency on aging for possible financial assistance to defray the costs of modifying an existing home.

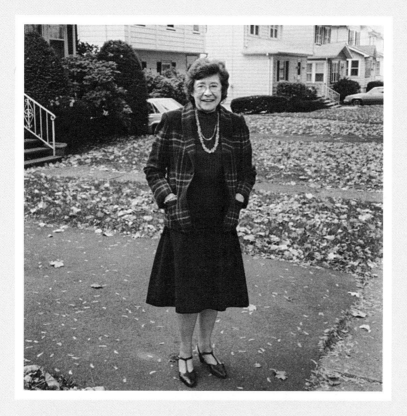

ENGAGED IN LIVING

Here's my mother, Martha Kostyra or "Big Martha," outside
our family home on Elm Place in Nutley, New Jersey, in the
early 1980s. She lived there for many years, but as happens
with everyone fortunate enough to enjoy a long life, there
came a time when she needed some assistance with daily
activities. At that point, she was lucky to live in an apartment
and share my sister's home. She had the stimulation of the
grandchildren and the convenience of her own car, which she
drove herself into her nineties—she was even the chauffeur to
her much younger friends. She remained actively and happily
engaged in living until the very end.

INVEST IN SAFETY TECHNOLOGY

A wide range of new technology offerings can give you and your elders peace of mind as they stay put. Consider the following:

AT-HOME MONITORING

The most basic monitors are pendants that can be worn around the neck and activated with the push of a button, such as Philips Lifeline (www.lifelinesys.com). Pushing the button connects the elder to a center that contacts emergency medical personnel. If it is an emergency (or if the client does not respond after the button is activated), the call center calls 911. This system also features a fall-detection feature for an extra fee.

Other systems offer customized sensors that can be tuned to a client's daily habits. GrandCare (www.grandcare.com) sets up sensors that can detect when the front door or window is opened, how often the fridge is opened, or when the client goes to bed and gets up in the morning. More customizable monitoring is available, and designated family members can get e-mail alerts.

"OUT AND ABOUT" MONITORING

Some services can keep seniors safer when they're out of the house. The ActiveCare Personal Assistance Link (www.activecare.com) and MobileHelp (www.mobilehelpnow.com) are hand-held cell-phone-like devices that can detect if a client has fallen. A push of the button activates the GPS feature so the client can be located. A help button can connect the user to a call center for assistance. The Wellcore Personal Emergency Response System (www.wellcore.com) features a pedometer-like device that can detect whether an elder person has fallen and issues an alert to a call center, as well as to caregivers, even if the elder is unconscious.

"NANA" TECHNOLOGY

This term, a play on the word "nanotechnology," covers equipment that can help seniors live safely and independently. There are good devices for reminding someone to take their medications, such as those available at www.managemypills.com; or monitoring services for those with diabetes (www.ideallifeonline.com), who need to keep tabs on their weight and glucose levels. A walking shoe with GPS, available from Aetrex Worldwide (www.navistargpsshoe.com), lets you track your elder and locate the person if he or she gets lost—especially crucial if your elder suffers from Alzheimer's disease.

CONSIDER GIFTING THE HOME

Even though your parent wants to stay in the home, it may make sense for him or her to go ahead and gift the property to you and/or your siblings. You'll both save on taxes—and your parent can retain the right of use and occupancy for his or her life, according to the Financial Planners of America. Here's how it works: Currently, the IRS allows a parent to make nontaxable gifts of up to $13,000 a year, or up to $1 million during a lifetime. If the parent gifts the property, it prevents future appreciation of that asset before the parent's death. The recipient pays no inheritance taxes on it because it was a gift. Say, your elder "gifts" the house to you when it has a market value of $1 million. If the property is worth $3 million when you die, that's $200,000 less to be taxed against your estate.

MOVING IN WITH FAMILY

Another option to consider is having your parent or parents move in with you; or having you (and your family) move in with them. Of course, this is not a solution that's tailor-made for all families, but if it's something you're seriously considering, ask yourself the following:

HOW DO I HONESTLY FEEL ABOUT THIS?

If having your parents move into your house gives you a sense of being invaded, this feeling will probably get worse, not better, as time goes on. The same goes if visiting your parents' home makes you feel like a powerless kid again. All parties involved should have respect for one another.

HOW DO I OR MY PARENTS FEEL ABOUT MY BEING THE POTENTIAL INTERLOPER IN THE HOUSE OR VICE VERSA?

Will you be able to handle the fact that it's "their" house? Will they be able to handle being the second-in-command in yours? Will you each have a voice in making household agreements? Ideally, you're creating a household of equals.

HOW WILL WE HANDLE THE FINANCES?

Who pays how much for what? Get the money stuff settled before you merge, to sidestep any monetary misunderstandings.

IS THERE ENOUGH ROOM FOR EVERYONE TO HAVE A DESIRED LEVEL OF PRIVACY?

Even though you're living together, each member of the family deserves some room of their own. Lack of privacy will try everyone's feelings—elders, adults, and children.

HOW MUCH OF MY/THEIR STUFF CAN BE ACCOMMODATED IN THE NEW SPACE?

What happens to the belongings that don't fit? If you have items that you can't part with, you may want to consider a storage facility.

CONSIDER RESIDENTIAL FACILITY OPTIONS

If you and your elder decide that there's a need to leave the home, be prepared to do a lot of research, as this is a very big decision and represents a significant financial outlay. There are many types of residential options for seniors—some allowing for great independence and some offering round-the-clock living and nursing assistance. Following is a list of options. You and your elder will need to evaluate which is right.

ACTIVE ADULT HOUSING

These communities of freestanding homes are designed for those over age 55.

Best for: Independent adults who can live without assistance.

For more information:
www.seniorhousingnet.com

NICHE HOUSING

Also called affinity communities, these have a specific focus, such as being religion-based, or geared toward artists, gardeners, LGBT communities, RVers, or even nudists. The Burbank Senior Artists Colony in California; Rainbow Vision in Santa Fe, New Mexico; and Kendal, a university community in Ithaca, New York, are three popular examples.

Best for: Those able to live independently who want to share common interests.

For more information: Search online for communities of interest groups.

ELDER COHOUSING

In these relatively new arrangements, a group of elders owns a property cooperatively and live in condos or attached houses. They usually have a communal space for weekly dinners, an outdoor space, and other amenities, like a media room or fitness center. Some are seniors-only; others are multigenerational. Oakcreek Cohousing Community in Stillwater, Oklahoma, and Silver Sage Village in Boulder, Colorado, are at the forefront of this trend.

Best for: Active seniors who enjoy communal living.

For more information: The Cohousing Association of the United States and the National Cohousing Conference, both at www.cohousing.org.

GREENHOUSE PROJECTS

These group homes provide intimate nursing for six to ten residents. There are more than a hundred Greenhouses in twenty-seven states, including California, Texas, Florida, Arizona, New York, and Ohio.

Best for: Someone who needs ongoing care but wants a more intimate alternative than an institutional-style nursing home.

For more information:
www.thegreenhouseproject.org

VILLAGE MODEL

These communities spring up when a naturally occurring pocket of seniors (like Beacon Hill Village in Boston, founded in 2001) decides to organize into a more official elder-focused neighborhood. There are more than sixty such village models nationwide, with another six hundred in development.

Best for: Active adults who want to live in a community tailored to their needs.

For more information: The Village to Village Network, www.vtvnetwork.org.

CONTINUING CARE RETIREMENT COMMUNITIES (CCRC)

These facilities offer a spectrum of options, from independent living to nursing care. A CCRC can accommodate the changing needs of residents, who might start out living independently, often in apartment-style units, but later require an assisted living arrangement with more intensive levels of care offered as needed. The big advantage is that your loved one moves from his or her home only once, and then is transitioned into higher levels of care at the same facility. Make sure the CCRC is accredited by CARF-CCAC, an organization that was formed when the Commission on Accreditation of Rehabilitation Facilities acquired the Continuing Care Accreditation Commission in 2003. Accreditation is voluntary.

Best for: Someone who wants to make the move while he or she is still able-bodied, then add on greater levels of care.

For more information: Commission on Accreditation of Rehabilitation Facilities offers a directory of CCRCs by area at www.carf.org.

ASSISTED LIVING FACILITIES (ALF)

Also called residential care, board and care, adult living, personal care, supported care, or congregate care, these facilities can be part of a retirement home or a senior housing complex or be stand-alone operations. The federal government does not regulate assisted living facilities, so definitions and services may vary from state to state. In general, ALFs may provide housekeeping services, activities, security, and transportation, as well as basic health care. Residents can cook for themselves or not, as they desire. Make sure the facility is close enough to family and friends so they can visit, and that it's near diversions such as shopping malls, movie theaters, and parks. Check the social, spiritual, and recreational activities offered.

Best for: Someone in need of social interaction and having trouble with mobility.

For more information:

- U.S. Administration on Aging Eldercare Locator (www.eldercare.gov)

- Assisted Living Federation of America (www.alfa.org)

- American Seniors Housing Association (www.seniorshousing.org)

- Leading Age (www.leadingage.org)

- National Center for Assisted Living (www.ncal.org)

SKILLED NURSING FACILITIES (SNF)

This is the term that's fast replacing *nursing home*. You may hear these facilities referred to as "sniffs," from the acronym SNF; they're also called custodial care or long-term-care facilities. Typically, about half of the residents at a SNF are short-term acute patients (such as those recovering from major surgery or a catastrophic bone fracture); the other half are people who require twenty-four-hour skilled nursing care. These facilities are licensed by individual states and are regulated by the federal government.

Best for: An elderly person recovering from major surgery or declining health owing to Alzheimer's disease.

For more information: Access a directory at www.skillednursingfacilities.org, and obtain info on Medicare- and Medicaid-certified nursing homes at www.medicare.gov/NHcompare/home.asp.

MEMORY CARE PROGRAMS

These are typically subunits of SNFs or other residential care facilities. They are organized to meet the needs of those with dementia.

Best for: Those with Alzheimer's or memory issues.

For more information: Contact Alzheimer's Association at www.alz.org.

HOW TO ASSESS A CAREGIVING FACILITY

Here's how to determine whether a potential living facility will be a safe and happy fit for your loved one.

REVIEW STATE LICENSING REPORTS

Each state licenses these communities through different departments, but most require facilities to post in a visible location the name, address, and phone number of the licensing organization. Alternatively, any management staff member (including the marketing person) should be able to provide this. State long-term-care ombudsmen also check on assisted care and nursing home facilities, which are required to post this contact information and/or provide it upon request. Take down all the contact information and ask the appropriate departments to provide licensing reports or information about any complaints filed.

Many states now also provide licensing reports online, as well as any complaints received and their outcome. It is not unusual to find minor and easily corrected deficiencies on a survey—for example, a thermometer missing from the refrigerator. Deficiencies of concern would include anything related to staffing, background checks, or resident safety. And walk away if the community has ever been fined or temporarily lost its license—that would be an indicator of a major deficiency.[4]

CONTACT A LOCAL GERIATRIC CASE MANAGER

He or she may have information and opinions on local facilities.

EVALUATE SAFETY AND LIVING CONDITIONS

Get a sense of how old the facility is, how long the operator has been in charge of the facility (you're looking for experience), and the overall financial health of the facility. The age of the facility is most relevant in terms of whether it is current enough to include sprinklers and fire safety construction. Newer buildings are required to have both sprinklers and firewalls, which prevent the fire from spreading to other parts of the building. Older buildings may have been grandfathered out of these requirements. Steer clear of a community that doesn't, at a minimum, have a spinkler system.[5]

PAY ATTENTION TO WHAT YOU FIRST SEE AND SMELL

These are signs of the quality of overall management. Age of a facility is not the most important indicator. An older community might be clean, lively, and look almost new, while a three-year-old community could be dirty, worn, or smell bad.[6]

MEET WITH THE ADMINISTRATOR

At the end of the day, a community and its staff will be a reflection of the person in charge. If the director is unwilling or says he or she is too busy to meet with you and answer all your questions, it is probably not a place you would want to live. Ask if the administrator can provide the tour. If he or she doesn't know his own building, staff members' names, or worse, the names of the residents you pass in the hallway, it's a bad sign.[7]

INTERACT WITH THE PEOPLE DOING THE DAY-TO-DAY CARING

Ask about their certification (most positions are described in state licensing standards, but the point is, you should be comfortable asking). And be sure to ask, "How long have you worked here?" A high turnover rate may be a sign of poor management; some nursing homes use temporary workers. Staff turnover is typically in the 50 percent range or more, so if you find a community where a number of core staff have been employed for at least three to five years, it's a positive sign.[8]

VISIT AT DIFFERENT TIMES OF THE DAY

You want to get a sense of what care is like at night or during the weekend, when staff numbers are reduced, instead of during standard visiting hours. Try to visit at least once unannounced, so you get an authentic sense of the place. Visit at meal times, and try the food.

GET A COPY OF THE MONTHLY ACTIVITY SCHEDULE

You're looking for activities that provide intellectual, physical, social, and spiritual engagement. The calendar should also include activities both within and outside of the community.

INFORM *yourself about insurance*

The longer we live, the more we depend on different types of insurance. You'll profit from taking time to become familiar with your own policies as well as those of your elder. Here's how to start:

GET EDUCATED

Many caregiving associations and websites have information about senior insurance options and coverage. Several offer seminars so you can learn more about how to file claims, dispute decisions, and make your policy work better for your loved ones, as well as for you when you will need it in the future.

A financial planner can help you understand your benefits, and make sure you're receiving all the services to which you're entitled. A geriatric care manager can offer insight and advice on your elder's health-care options. (See page 349.)

REVIEW MEDICARE SUPPLEMENTAL INSURANCE

Everyone is eligible for Medicare when they turn 65, but it's not automatic—you'll need to apply for it. Medicare doesn't come even close to paying for all of a senior's medical bills, so you should seriously consider a policy that fills the gap left by the deductibles and uncovered services. These "medigap" policies are sold by private companies and offer big advantages if you need a lot of medical services. The time to enroll in an Advantage or medigap program is during the first six months after you turn 65, and annually near year-end thereafter. You won't be refused coverage, there is no waiting period for benefits to start, and premiums won't be increased as a result of new or worsening health problems. For more information, visit www.medicare.gov/medigap. Or download an easy-to-understand document, "Choosing a Medigap Policy," at www.medicare.gov/Publications/Pubs/pdf/02110.pdf. You can also call your state insurance department or your state health insurance assistance program.

INVESTIGATE LONG-TERM-CARE POLICIES

Policies that provide for long-term care in later years are mainly applied to covering assisted living and home care beyond the little that Medicare covers. Find out more at National Clearinghouse for Long-Term Care Information, www.longtermcare.gov.

REVISIT YOUR LIFE INSURANCE POLICY

Your elder's needs regarding life insurance change with time. If your elder is in good health and/or has substantial savings, there may be no need for this added expense, which comes with increasingly pricey premiums as the years pass. On the other hand, if your elder has ongoing medical problems that could wipe out his or her savings, it may be worth your while to explore. A financial planner, accountant, or tax lawyer can help elucidate the issues for your specific case.

MEDICARE VS. MEDICAID: WHAT'S THE DIFFERENCE?

	MEDICAID	MEDICARE
ORIGINAL INTENT OF PROGRAM	To pay for medical care for poor and low-income people.	To reimburse medical costs in the final years of life. (Prior to this law, when you retired, you lost employer-provided insurance; Medicare was designed to make up the deficit.)
WHO FUNDS IT	State and federal dollars, but services vary from state to state.	Since it is funded solely by the federal government, benefits are uniform among states.
WHEN AND HOW YOU GET IT	You must apply and meet certain income requirements; no age requirement.	If you sign up, you're in once you turn 65, or younger if you're disabled or have end-stage kidney disease.
EXTENT OF MEDICAL COVERAGE	Basic physician and hospital services and some medications; coverage varies by state.	Depending on what you qualify for, Medicare covers hospitalization, skilled nursing, hospice, drug costs, and home health care, as well as compensates doctor care and medical equipment.
COVERAGE OF LONG-TERM CARE	Yes; program is a primary payer for long-term care.	No; program is designed to pay only for short-stay services, such as rehabilitation after a hip fracture or hospitalization after an acute illness.
FYI	This is a federally funded program, but benefits and eligibility vary by state.	If you don't sign up when you turn 65 or after you stop working, Part B and D premiums may have a penalty.
FOR MORE INFO	www.cms.gov/home/medicaid.asp	www.medicare.gov

OPTIMIZE *quality of life*

Caregiving certainly includes providing clean sheets and healthy meals, but remember to nurture your elder's spirits as well. Your parents are your parents no matter what losses they incur from age or disease. Never forget who it is you are caring for. These are adults with a legacy, a life well lived. Honoring that legacy can help you care more thoughtfully, and make the experience more positive and rewarding for both of you.

KEEP YOUR ELDER ENGAGED

Most people feel more satisfied when their days have purpose. There are plenty of strategies for helping your elder feel loved, needed, and engaged in daily life.

GET OUT AND ABOUT

Discover the resources in your own community. Many art museums have special hours and programs for those who are wheelchair bound or suffering from dementia. "There are even ballroom dancing programs for people with dementia and their caregivers, and singing and musical events for caregivers and their elders," says Amy Trommer, of the Alzheimer's Association, New York City Chapter. Check out websites devoted to your elder's condition, or contact local museums, art galleries, or dance academies. Elders need companionship and conversation. They can get it by attending religious services, going out for meals, visiting local museums or malls, or taking walks in the park (in a wheelchair, if necessary). Adult day care may offer stimulating company for your elder, and some downtime for you. And remember to invite local volunteers to visit your elder at home (see page 351 for tips on finding volunteers).

INCLUDE YOUR ELDER IN DAILY ACTIVITIES

"People need to feel a sense of purpose, a reason to live, so giving them a mission is good," says Carol Bradley Bursack. Asking the elder to help fold clothes, garden, prepare dinner, or even look out for the mail delivery will make him or her feel more vital and valued. Your elder may accomplish the task in a longer time or less efficiently than you would be able to, but that does not diminish the power of being asked to contribute.

PLAN AROUND THEIR PLEASURES

Acknowledging a preference (your dad's love for jazz or your mom's birdwatching) and being recognized in this way is extremely gratifying to elders. It's another way you can express your love and caring, too. If you can't ask your elder directly, ask other family members to name the elder's favorite music, movies, meals, and other accessible pleasures.

DISPLAY MEANINGFUL MEMENTOS

Cluster family photographs, artwork, or travel souvenirs near the spot where your elder usually sits. The display will make a great conversation starter for grandkids or other visitors. A small bulletin board studded with family photos or notes is a good item for a bedside at home or in a hospital.

TAP INTO YOUR ELDER'S INTERESTS

Look at the skills your elder has developed over his or her lifetime. They will reveal what your elder might enjoy and want to learn more about in his or her twilight years. Perhaps these interests involve something artistic such as painting or music, or sports like swimming or bowling. Try helping your elder find outlets for his or her interests with seniors' groups, churches, or community organizations. Or, better yet, participate with your elder in these activities and both of you may gain meaningful memories together.

PROVIDE A SACRED SPACE

If your elder has moved in with you or into a care facility, he or she will likely feel displaced and miss being independent. Helping to decorate your elder's new home, whether it be a single room or an apartment, with meaningful objects from his or her past can help create a peaceful oasis where your elder feels safe. Consider arranging your elder's bedroom in a similar way to his or her former room, and hang family pictures and meaningful tokens on the walls. If your elder has a pet, provide a space where the animal will feel comfortable and offer good companionship.

READ TO YOUR ELDER—OR LET HER OR HIM READ TO YOU

Reading aloud—from a book, a magazine, or the newspaper—is diverting and educational. It also gives the elder (if he or she can still see to read) an important role in the family. At gatherings, have family members read or recite favorite poems.

TRADE PLACES

This exercise is a helpful way to refresh your perspective when you're feeling frustrated by your elder's demands: "Mentally step into your elder's reality, and try to understand their underlying emotional needs," advises Amy Trommer, of the Alzheimer's Association. "The list of needs may involve things like inclusion, a sense of identity, attachment, love, comfort, and occupation." Once you have a better understanding of what your elder is experiencing, talk about those challenges or frustrations if possible, to get some guidance and direction. "Try to understand that anger on the part of your loved one may not be directed at you, but may arise due to their frustration from being sick or unable to articulate their needs," Trommer adds.

ELDER PASTIME PLEASURES

If your elder is unable to participate in his or her old favorite pastimes, or unable to communicate preferences to you now, start by thinking of activities or outings that would stimulate one of his or her senses.

TO STIMULATE THE SENSE OF . . .	TRY . . .
SMELL	• Cooking a favorite dish and reminiscing about it • Buying a bunch of preferred flowers to display nearby • Burning a scented candle • Visiting a botanical garden during prime blossom times (cherry, rose, peony) • Going to the beach • Sitting outside at different times of the day—when the lawn is being mowed or just after a rainstorm
SIGHT	• Watching a parade or attending a street fair • Visiting a zoo, aquarium, or nature center • Tuning in to beloved classic movies and watching them together • Watching a favorite sport on TV • Serving colorful foods at most meals • Looking through family photo albums or scrapbooks • Asking about the significance of a memento your elder treasures
TOUCH	• Performing gentle massage or hiring someone to perform a rubdown • Sitting and holding hands with your elder • Encouraging every visitor to give the elder a hug • Hiring someone for a Reiki or acupuncture session • Making sure that blankets or wraps are soft
HEARING	• Playing favorite music or going to a concert • Taking an outing to a wilderness area to enjoy birdsong, wind in the trees, or children playing • Turning on a radio show; talking about the memories it evokes
TASTE	• Cooking up a favorite meal; discussing why it's such a favorite • Using fresh herbs to perk up a dish • Adding a sprig of mint to a glass of water • Squeezing a fresh lemon or lime over vegetables or sliced fruit

PREVENT CAREGIVER FATIGUE

As a caregiver, you have a responsibility to keep yourself healthy, well rested, well fed, and relaxed. "You can only care for another person as well as you care for yourself," notes Joan Griffiths Vega, who leads a mindfulness-based stress-reduction class at Mount Sinai. "Many caregivers become so focused on the patient that they disregard their own needs." The result is a state of psychological and physical crisis that is known as "caregiver fatigue" or "caregiver burnout."

"Caregivers often describe feeling stressed out, anxious, and isolated," Vega explains. "They also complain of not being able to eat or sleep, having no energy, and worrying all the time." Other signs of burnout include anger, depression, constant worrying, irritability, lack of focus, and inability to concentrate.

Part of the problem is that caregivers may feel as if they don't have any boundaries between their on-duty and off-duty hours. "Especially when it comes to dementia, no matter how much you give, more is still needed," Vega says. "And even if you do carve out your boundaries—taking time to do something for yourself, whether it's exercise, a nap, or catching up with a friend—often your mind is still on your caregiving. This lack of rest for the mind may be just as damaging as not actually taking the break."

STOP—AND UNDERSTAND NEGATIVE EMOTIONS

"It's normal to experience grief, anger, sadness, frustration, and many other negative emotions [when caring for a loved one]," says Amy Trommer, of the Alzheimer's Association. "Understand that many of these emotions result from the changes that occur with your elder. It's not them, it's the disease." But keeping these emotions bottled up inside you, denying them or being ashamed of them, will only hurt your health. Be sure to talk about your feelings, whether it's with your doctor, therapist, or caregiving group. One helpful technique, she notes, comes from researcher Jon Kabat-Zinn, founder of the Stress Reduction Clinic at the University of Massachusetts. The STOP acronym represents a way to ease stress and improve mood:

S Stop

T Take a breath

O Observe

P Proceed

FIND RESOURCES TO HELP YOU AVOID BURNOUT

Whether you want to talk it out or just be by yourself, there are a range of options for care-takers to take care of their mental and emotional health.

MEDITATION

"Most caregivers I've talked to say, 'I don't have the time to meditate,'" says Joan Griffiths Vega. "But I counter, 'You spend at least ten minutes a day worrying, so why not use that ten minutes more constructively?'" Meditation is a proven way of reducing stress, because most stress results from obsessing over worrying thoughts, while meditation teaches you to observe your thoughts, even the distressing ones, as temporary phenomena.

Vega's meditation mode of choice is Jon Kabat-Zinn's Mindfulness-Based Stress Reduction (MBSR). "It takes about eight weeks to master, and trains you to stop and observe what's happening around you and within you, so that you can respond pragmatically instead of reacting emotionally."

SUPPORT GROUPS

The best support for a caregiver is another caregiver, especially someone dealing with the same illness or condition, say researchers at Cornell University. In most support groups, facilitators carefully screen each member before admission. The intent is that the members of the group support and help one another, so individuals are chosen with the overall group dynamic in mind.

REGULAR GETAWAYS

Plan a mini-vacation—for a day, a weekend, a week, if you can manage it—at least every six weeks to six months. Set up your support system so that when you're away, you can mentally detach and not worry. Most important, lay down the law about phone calls or e-mails: you can be reached, but only in an emergency. This is time for you to rest and rejuvenate.

FRIENDS

You may feel as if you don't have the energy to socialize, but staying linked to your friends is vital. These are the people who keep you in touch with who you were before you became a caregiver. It is all too easy to lose your identity, especially as the needs of your elder increase. If you can't get together for a meal, tea, or a walk, ask your friends to send you something funny or something that made them think of you—a favorite song, news of an exhibition of your favorite artist, a nutty piece of news or YouTube video— anything to take yourself out of the present for a moment. A recommendation for a funny movie, an absorbing book, or a distracting TV series can boost your spirits and make you feel cared for.[9]

DON'T NEGLECT YOUR OWN HEALTH

If you're accompanying your elder to appointments, you may be sick of doctors' waiting rooms. However, it's important not to neglect your own health. It's especially vital that you don't skip routine screening tests such as mammograms. And pay attention to everyday aches: constant worry about an elder (or finances) can exacerbate body aches and pains; try soothing them through alternative approaches such as acupuncture, acupressure, or Chinese medicine. Here are some more suggestions for staying in good shape while also caregiving.

STAY PHYSICAL

Find an activity that you enjoy, one that you can do regularly. Not only will it help you control stress levels but regular aerobic exercise can help protect you from Alzheimer's, heart disease, even falls. For ideas, see Chapter 2. If you've never done yoga or tai chi, you may find these practices soothing and meditative; they're helpful for restoring balance, both physical and emotional.

FEED YOURSELF WELL

Fresh vegetables and fruits, whole grains, and lean protein will keep up your energy—and spirits. Minimize your intake of caffeine and sugar; the buzz they bring is quickly followed by a crash, and that roller coaster isn't good for your stamina or your mood. Take the time to sit down to a meal. If possible, set the table with nice china and glassware. Light a candle. You may not feel particularly hungry, but the very act of setting a lovely table nourishes your spirit. Consider consulting a nutritionist for advice on keeping yourself healthy through diet. (See Chapter 1.)

GIVE YOURSELF A DAILY TREAT

For your health and mental balance, you need to give yourself permission to revel in at least one pleasurable activity a day. You might:

- Go for a walk outside.
- Putter in the garden.
- Read for an hour, undisturbed.
- Call a friend.
- Have coffee with a friend.
- Do yoga (or other exercise).
- Meditate.

- Go window-shopping.
- Sit in a park and feed the birds.
- Drop into a museum or art gallery.
- Schedule a manicure or massage.
- Knit, scrapbook, or do some other craft project that you enjoy.

PREPARE *for the end*

Your final task as a caregiver is possibly the most daunting: to ease your elder through this last stage of life. It starts with a conversation about how he or she would like to handle the death. How you talk about death is highly personal and individual, but if your elder is not bringing up the topic, you certainly should.

To start the conversation, you might say, "I'm sad about what's happening to you. Can we talk about this?" or "I'm sorry about your bad news [or recent diagnosis], do you want to talk about it?" Your elder's response will guide you: if he or she changes the subject, it's not the right time for a discussion and you may have to keep trying.

Once you've had an initial conversation, more are sure to follow. You want to have a good idea of what your elder wants in the way of a memorial, funeral services, and burial. "It's not unusual for elders to talk a lot about their wishes for burial or cremation, or even their funeral service," notes geriatric psychiatry social worker Ella Jolly, from the Mount Sinai School of Medicine in New York City. "It's uppermost in their mind and talking it through can be very comforting to them." In fact, "talking openly about death may even prove to be a relief for the two of you. Aside from working out the practical details of a funeral or memorial, being able to express your mutual love, admiration, and appreciation may enrich your experience of this final life transition."

OFFERING SUPPORT

KEEP THE LINES OF COMMUNICATION OPEN

Make sure your elder isn't isolated in his or her final days. Visits from friends and family may decrease as death approaches, out of a sense of preserving the elder's privacy and dignity. But your loved one may very well want to talk, make amends, and say last good-byes. "This can be a time of great closeness and compassion," says geriatric case manager Linda Packer, "both for the elder and the family." At the very least, listen to your elder, ask questions about his or her life, and hear who your elder really is and was.

Find out the most meaningful moment, the challenges, the joys and the sorrows of your elder's life.

Don't hesitate to ask: "Is there anything you want to say to me?" and "Is there something you want to hear from me?" Packer suggests.

HELP MAKE AMENDS

When facing death, many elders feel the need to come to resolution on unfinished business in their lives. It could be an estranged sibling, a relative who's having troubles, an apology that is owed, or some other worry.

You can help by letting your elder know you're available to help take care of these personal matters, by getting in contact with the sibling (or helping your elder make contact), making sure that the relative will get proper help, or mailing that note of apology.

INVITE IN A SPIRITUAL COUNSELOR

Many hospices offer counseling through a trained minister, pastor, or rabbi. Even if your religions don't match, or your elder isn't particularly religious, talking with a spiritual counselor can help you and your elder get some perspective on the process. "A clergy person can start the difficult conversations, such as, 'Are you struggling with wanting to stop trying so hard to live?' or 'Are you worried about letting yourself or someone else down by dying?'" These are important conversations to have, notes Carol Bradley Bursack. "They are openings to letting all parties know that the elder is ready to go and the family is ready to let go."

CONSIDER A VIGIL

Many religions have rituals surrounding dying that can be very comforting, even if the elder isn't particularly religious. Roman Catholicism includes the Anointing of the Sick and Last Rites. Protestant churches also practice anointing before death. For Jewish people, a prayer of confession known as the Vidui is recited. In the Muslim tradition, reciting the Kalimas reaffirms the commitment to Allah. Buddhists recite mantras and scriptures to help the dying person achieve peace.

Find out more about religious rituals or how to create your own vigil from the Sacred Dying Foundation (www.sacreddying.org), a non-profit educational organization whose mission is to change the way our culture deals with death and dying.

TAKE COMFORT FROM DEATH

The slow, inevitable decline of today's old age and death does have an upside, notes social worker Jolly: "A family that has participated in and contributed to a comfortable, pain-free death actually transforms this sad event into something else." Of course, you'll grieve and feel the loss of your loved one, but as the grief subsides, you can feel good about a job well done and take pride and have a sense of accomplishment.

HELP YOUR ELDER WITH GRIEF

Grief doesn't only happen with death; often the process of dying also involves grieving, for that life you love that is ebbing away. A therapist, social worker, spiritual counselor, or hospice worker can help with your feelings of grief. Consider having a group session with family members and your elder; if you're having difficulty with your feelings, chances are they are, too.

To make sure that you get the help you need, you should ask questions, such as the following:

- What is your helping style?

- Do you give guidance or do you prefer not to give suggestions?

- Can you give me an example of a technique that you've found useful in counseling?

"When your elder finally dies after getting weaker for weeks (or months, or years), you should expect a mix of feelings," says Carol Bradley Bursack. Don't feel guilty if you feel relief on some level. "Of course, you'll grieve for the loss of that elder, but you may also feel relief for not having to act as a caregiver anymore," she explains. "It's very common, yet caregivers somehow feel that this is wrong; it's perfectly normal."

CONSIDER YOUR ELDER'S COMFORT

There is no official definition of a "good" death, but certainly, ensuring that your elder is comfortable and pain-free during the process can help. That's where palliative and hospice care services come in. The difference between these terms lies in the prognosis. Hospice is a service that relieves the symptoms for someone who's at or near the end of life. Palliative care takes a similar approach, but it's for people still actively fighting their illness or who expect to live with that illness for a long time.

PALLIATIVE CARE

WHAT IT IS Care that is focused on improving the quality of life when someone is facing a serious chronic illness, such as MS, Alzheimer's, Parkinson's, arthritis, cancer, or ulcerative colitis. Pain relief and symptom management are certainly part of palliative care, but so are facilitating communication among family members and the medical team, as well as clarifying the goals of care.

WHEN TO REQUEST IT All too often, doctors seem to be focused on the cure, while the family's—and the patient's—goals may be very different. Palliative care can bring all views into alignment. It can be requested from the time of diagnosis and can be provided along with curative treatment. It is appropriate for anyone, at any point in a serious illness, and it can be provided at the same time as treatment that is meant to prolong life. You don't have to have a terminal diagnosis or a life expectancy of six months to receive this care. Technically, a doctor must order palliative care, in much the same way that medication or a course of treatment must originate from a doctor's orders.

WHERE TO GET IT You can get palliative care in a hospital, but not all hospitals have palliative care programs; this may be a consideration in choosing a hospital, so speak to your doctor. Care can also be provided on an outpatient basis and in your home.

HOW TO PAY FOR IT Most insurance plans cover all or part of palliative care treatment received in a hospital. Depending on the situation, drugs, medical supplies, and equipment may also be covered. Medicare and Medicaid also cover palliative care costs.

FOR MORE INFORMATION Visit the website www.palliativecare.org.

HOSPICE CARE

WHAT IT IS Hospice care is appropriate if your loved one has been given a terminal diagnosis and will no longer be seeking curative treatment. According to the Medicare definition, hospice is for someone who has a life expectancy of six months or less. The medical emphasis shifts from curing to caring, with focus on relieving symptoms (much like palliative care) and with emotional and household support for the patient.

WHEN TO REQUEST IT Your doctor will "prescribe" hospice and should bring up the topic at the appropriate time. However, you can also start the conversation about hospice timing.

WHERE TO GET IT Hospice care is provided in the home, in a nursing home, in the hospital, or in a hospice residence.

HOW TO PAY FOR IT Medicaid covers all services, medications, and equipment related to the patient's illness, including physician and nursing services, home health aides, and medical equipment and supplies, as well as spiritual, dietary, and other counseling services. Many private health insurance policies also offer hospice coverage and benefits. In general, Medicare, Medicaid, and private insurers do not pay for anything unrelated to the hospice diagnosis, however. So if, for example, the hospice patient has high blood pressure in addition to terminal cancer, the high blood pressure costs would not fall under hospice coverage.

FOR MORE INFORMATION For a hospice in your area, see www.nhpco.org.

CALLING THE FUNERAL HOME

You or your geriatric care manager should call the funeral home and give them the doctor's number. The funeral home must have verbal confirmation that a death certificate will be signed within twenty-four hours, before they will retrieve the body. The doctor will sign the death certificate. If hospice is involved, they will call the funeral home if these arrangements have been made ahead of time. Otherwise, the designated family member must call the funeral home so that the funeral home can call hospice to sign the death certificate.

CELEBRATE A LIFE WELL LIVED

Honoring your elder's passing may take many forms, and with some thoughtful planning, it can be an occasion for celebration and joy rather than prolonged grief. As Faith Moore writes in her book, *Celebrating a Life: Planning Memorial Services and Other Creative Remembrances*, if you have the opportunity beforehand, ask your elder: "How do you want to be remembered? What best symbolizes who you are?"

If your elder wanted a memorial service, schedule it anywhere from a few days to months after death. Your elder's wishes may guide you on how to structure the event, what music to choose, and what photos to project. Even if your elder didn't want a formal service, your family and elder's friends may need closure. In this case, consider organizing a less formal gathering to share memories. Remember, it takes time to process grief and you may not feel ready to talk about your loss or hold an event immediately.

In addition to a gathering, many families create keepsakes—booklets of the elder featuring photos from his or her lifetime, a brief timeline of major milestones (marriages, births, promotions), and favorite quotes and poems. Another option is to arrange to have a bench with a memorial plaque placed in a park, at the beach, or at another spot where your elder liked to visit; this also provides a peaceful spot to sit and remember a loved one in a location he or she liked best.

Beyond these physical remembrances, some families choose to set up a memorial fund or charitable giving drive in their elder's name. Donations go to support community organizations, specific charities, universities, or hospitals. Most families choose to support a cause their elder cared deeply about, such as a specific health issue, the environment, or education. Giving drives can be organized directly with local charities, while memorial funds are often set up through nonprofit community foundations; to find one in your area, visit the Council on Foundations (www.cof.org).

However you choose to commemorate your elder, the goal should be to acknowledge the person's strengths and values in a way that feels like a fitting tribute to his or her singular life.

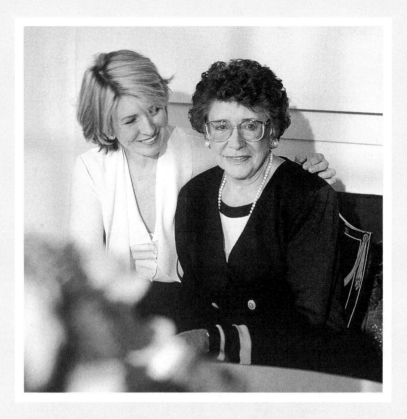

LESSONS FROM MY MOTHER

Up until the very end of her life, my mother, Big Martha, paid attention to the details of her daily life: she wrote down her appointments, she faithfully went to her hairstylist and colorist, she put out an outfit to wear each day, she got dressed up every week to go to church. She kept her driver's license current so that she would be able to drive her friends to church or doctor's appointments. I think staying up with these little things made a big difference in how long she lived and how well she lived. She felt competent, needed, and vital. It kept her optimism and spirits up, which in turn reinforced her motivation to care for herself. That's a big lesson: no one is going to do it for you; you are in control of how you live every day.

RESOURCES

Listed below are organizations mentioned throughout the book that have helpful information on aging and caregiving.

GENERAL

AMERICAN ASSOCIATION OF RETIRED PERSONS (AARP)
601 E Street, NW
Washington, DC 20049
888-687-2277
www.aarp.org
Information and services for seniors

DEPARTMENT OF HEALTH AND HUMAN SERVICES ADMINISTRATION ON AGING
1 Massachusetts Avenue, NW
Washington, DC 20001
202-619-0724
www.aoa.gov
Government information and resources on aging

MARTHA STEWART CENTER FOR LIVING AT MOUNT SINAI
1440 Madison Avenue
The Mount Sinai
Medical Center
New York, NY 10029
212-659-8552
www.mountsinai.org
Outpatient clinic specializing in geriatric care and services

NATIONAL INSTITUTE ON AGING
Building 31, Room 5C27
31 Center Drive, MSC 2292
Bethesda, MD 20892
800-222-2225
www.nia.nih.gov
Research and information on health and aging

U.S. FOOD AND DRUG ADMINISTRATION
10903 New Hampshire Avenue
Silver Spring, MD 20993
888-463-6332
www.fda.gov
Information on medications and medical devices

CHAPTER 1: HEALTHY EATING

THE ACADEMY OF NUTRITION AND DIETETICS
(formerly The American Dietetic Association)
120 South Riverside Plaza
Suite 2000
Chicago, IL 60606-6995
800-877-1600
www.eatright.org
Nutritional advice and information

BLUE ZONES PROJECT
www.bluezones.com
Details on the study of the places where people live the longest and healthiest

NATIONAL HEART & LUNG INSTITUTE BODY MASS INDEX CALCULATOR
www.nhlbisupport.com/bmi
Tools to calculate your Body Mass Index (BMI), which is a measure of body fat based on height and weight

USDA MYPLATE
USDA Center for Nutrition Policy and Promotion
3101 Park Center Drive
Alexandria, VA 22302-1594
www.choosemyplate.gov
Nutrition guidelines and information

CHAPTER 2: HEALTHY FITNESS

AMERICAN COUNCIL ON FITNESS
4851 Paramount Drive
San Diego, CA 92123
888-825-3636
www.acefitness.org
Exercise tutorials, workouts, and other fitness information

ARTHRITIS FOUNDATION
P.O. Box 7669
Atlanta, GA 30357-0669
800-283-7800
www.arthritis.org
Information on arthritis

THE COMPLETE GUIDE TO THE ALEXANDER TECHNIQUE
www.alexandertechnique.com
Information on this practice to adjust body postures and relieve stresses

FALL STOP . . . MOVE STRONG
www.fallstop.net
Education and exercise program to prevent falls and promote fitness

INQUIRING MIND
www.inquiringmind.com
Information on meditation, plus lists of groups and retreats

IYENGAR YOGA INSTITUTE OF NEW YORK
150 W. 22nd Street,
11th Floor
New York, NY 10011
212-691-9642
www.iyengarnyc.org
Iyengar yoga workshops in New York City

PILATES-RING.NET
www.pilates-ring.net
Information on the exercise of pilates, its techniques, and equipment

THE WALKING SITE
www.thewalkingsite.com
Information on walking for fitness

YMCA OF THE USA
101 N. Wacker Drive
Chicago, IL 60606
800-872-9622
www.ymca.net
Fitness, recreation, and other programs

CHAPTER 3: HEALTHY BRAIN

ACADEMY OF AMERICAN POETS
75 Maiden Lane, Suite 901
New York, NY 10038
212-274-0343
www.poets.org
"Poem a Day" program, poems, and essays

INDEPENDENT MEDITATION CENTER GUIDE
www.gosit.org
Meditation-center location finder

OPEN CULTURE
www.openculture.com
Free online courses, videos, and language lessons

RICK HANSON
www.rickhanson.net
Articles and class listings on brain science and personal growth

CHAPTER 4: HEALTHY OUTLOOK

ACCESSIBLE TRAVEL AND LEISURE
www.accessibletravel.co.uk
Specializes in barrier-free vacations for those who have trouble with stairs or with walking in general

ELDERCARE
800-677-1116
www.eldercare.gov
A public service of the Department of Health and Human Services, U.S. Administration on Aging, with information on services for older adults and their families. Locates services for seniors, plus fact sheets and brochures, caregiver information

ELDERTREKS
800-741-7956
www.eldertreks.com
Adventure-travel company for people age 50 and over

EXPERIENCE CORPS
601 E Street, NW
Washington, DC 20049
202-434-6400
www.experiencecorps.org
Community service opportunities for seniors

GET OLDER ADULTS ONLINE (GOAL)
202-436-4313
www.TheProjectGoal.org
Promotes the adoption of broadband services by older adults

THE INTERGENERATIONAL CENTER AT TEMPLE UNIVERSITY
1700 N. Broad Street
Room 412
Philadelphia, PA 19122
www.comingofage.org
Community service opportunities for seniors

THE NATIONAL CENTER FOR CREATIVE AGING
4125 Albemarle Street, NW
Washington, DC 20016-2105
202-895-9456
www.creativeaging.org
Information on arts programs for seniors

PROJECT ENHANCE
2208 2nd Avenue
Seattle, WA 98121
206-448-5725
www.projectenhance.org
Offers community health programs for older adults across the country

OLDER ADULTS TECHNOLOGY SERVICES (OATS)
168 7th Street, Suite 3A
Brooklyn, NY 11215
718-360-1707
www.oats.org
Training and support for older adults in using technology

THE SLOAN CENTER ON AGING & WORK AT BOSTON COLLEGE
140 Commonwealth Avenue
Chestnut Hill, MA 02467
617-552-9195
www.bc.edu/research/agingandwork
Compiles research and reports on quality of employment for older workers

THE SOCIETY FOR ACCESSIBLE TRAVEL & HOSPITALITY IN NEW YORK CITY
347 5th Avenue
Suite 605
New York, NY 10016
www.sath.org
Referrals to travel agents who can handle—and meet—most special needs.

STORYCORPS
80 Hanson Place
2nd Floor
Brooklyn, NY 11217
646-723-7020 (office)
800-850-4406 (to make reservations to record)
www.storycorps.org
Records and archives oral histories

CHAPTER 5: HEALTHY LIVING EVERY DAY

AMERICAN SOCIETY FOR THE ALEXANDER TECHNIQUE
P.O. Box 2307
Dayton, OH 45401-2307
800-473-0620
www.alexandertech.com
Physical education to improve posture and mobility; certified-teacher locator

MAYO CLINIC
200 First Street SW
Rochester, MN 55905
507-284-2511
www.mayoclinic.org
Information on healthy living, medical conditions, and diseases

MY MEDICINE RECORD
www.fda.gov/drugs/resourcesforyou/ucm079489
Download a free record to help you keep track of your medicines

NATIONAL ACADEMY OF MEDICAL ACUPUNCTURE
1970 E. Grand Avenue
Suite 330
El Segundo, CA 90245
310-364-0193
www.medicalacupuncture.org
Database of acupuncture physicians, acupuncture information, and FAQs

NORTH AMERICAN MENOPAUSE SOCIETY
5900 Landerbrook Drive
Suite 390
Mayfield Heights, OH 44124
440-442-7550
www.menopause.org
Information on menopause and hormone therapy

PILL CARD
www.ahrq.gov/qual/pillcard/pillcard.html
Download a free pill card to help keep track of medicines and when to take them

CHAPTER 6: HEALTHY LOOKS

AMERICAN ACADEMY OF DERMATOLOGY
866-503-7546
www.aad.org
Information on skin conditions

SKIN CANCER FOUNDATION
149 Madison Avenue
Suite 901
New York, NY 10016
212-725-5176
www.skincancer.org
Devoted to the education, prevention, detection, and treatment of skin cancer

CHAPTER 7: HEALTHY HOME

ELECTRICAL SAFETY FOUNDATION INTERNATIONAL
1300 North 17th Street
Suite 1752
Rosslyn, VA 22209
703-841-3229
www.esfi.org
Information on home electrical systems and safety

ENVIRONMENTAL PROTECTION AGENCY
Ariel Rios Building
1200 Pennsylvania Avenue, NW
Washington, DC 20460
202-272-0167
www.epa.gov
Resources and information on green living, health and safety, and healthy home environments (e.g., mold, radon, indoor air quality)

FALL STOP . . . MOVE STRONG
www.fallstop.net
A fall-prevention and strengthening program, with class listings and DVD instruction

NATIONAL RADON PROGRAM SERVICES
www.sosradon.org
Resources and information on radon, testing, and techniques to reduce radon levels in homes

PET PARTNERS
(formerly Delta Society)
www.deltasociety.org
Pet therapy resources

U.S. CONSUMER PRODUCTS SAFETY COMMISSION
4330 East West Highway
Bethesda, MD 20814
800-638-2772
www.cpsc.gov
Information on product safety and recalls

CHAPTER 8: HEALTHY LIVING INTO THE FUTURE

AMERICAN CANCER SOCIETY
250 Williams Street NW
Atlanta, GA 30303
800-227-2345
www.cancer.org
Cancer information and resources, local service locator

AMERICAN HEART ASSOCIATION
7272 Greenville Avenue
Dallas, TX 75231
800-242-8721
www.heart.org
Resources for heart health, information on heart disease, caregiver resources

CENTERS FOR DISEASE CONTROL AND PREVENTION
1600 Clifton Road
Atlanta, GA 30333
800-232-4636
www.cdc.gov/features/osteoarthritisplan
Information and resources on arthritis

COMMONWEALTH FUND
www.whynotthebest.org
Tracks performance of health-care organizations on regional, state, and national levels

DOCFINDER
www.docboard.org
Database of all licensing background and disciplinary information of physicians and other health-care practitioners

GEORGE MASON UNIVERSITY PROGRAM IN SENIOR HOUSING ADMINISTRATION
703-993-9131
http://seniorhousing.gmu.edu
Undergraduate and graduate curriculum devoted to senior housing, with articles and other resources

NATIONAL OSTEOPOROSIS FOUNDATION
1150 17th Street, NW
Suite 850
Washington, DC 20036
800-231-4222
www.nof.org
Osteoporosis information and resources, health-care provider directory

CHAPTER 9: HEALTHY CARING

THE ADMINISTRATION ON AGING (AOA)
202-619-0724
www.aoa.gov
Part of the Department of Health and Human Services, this federal agency provides resources for home- and community-based long-term care

AGINGCARE.COM
720 Goodlette Road North
4th Floor
Naples, FL 34102
239-594-3222
Caregiver support and information on senior living and elder care

THE ALZHEIMER'S ASSOCIATION
225 N. Michigan Avenue
17th Floor
Chicago, IL 60601-7633
800-272-3900
www.alz.org
Helpline for information and support, education, and training for caregivers

AMERICAN ASSOCIATION OF DAILY MONEY MANAGERS
174 Crestview Drive
Bellefonte, PA 16823
877-326-5991
www.aadmm.com
Lists professionals who can help with an elder's finances, bill-paying, and bookkeeping

BENEFITSCHECKUP
(National Center for Benefits Outreach and Enrollment)
www.benefitscheckup.org
Federal, state, and private benefits locator, and application help

CARING FROM A DISTANCE
4125 Albemarle Street, NW
Washington, DC 20016
www.cfad.org
An organization for those trying to coordinate the care of a loved one who lives far away. Includes service directories, links to resources, and an option to store health records

CENTER FOR MINDFULNESS
University of Massachusetts Medical School
55 Lake Avenue North
Worcester, MA 01655
508-856-2656
www.umassmed.edu/cfm/home/index.aspx
Resources and training in mindfulness-based stress reduction (MBSR)

CENTERS FOR MEDICARE AND MEDICAID SERVICES
7500 Security Boulevard
Baltimore, MD 21244
877-267-2323
www.cms.gov
www.medicare.gov
www.medicaid.gov
Information on Medicare and Medicaid coverage, eligibility, and enrollment; resource locator

CHILDREN OF AGING PARENTS (CAPS)
800-227-7294
www.caps4caregivers.org
A national listing of support groups, elder-care training seminars educational webinars, and links to helpful organizations and agencies, both national and local

FAMILY CAREGIVER ALLIANCE
785 Market Street, Suite 750
San Francisco, CA 94103
800-445-8106
www.caregiver.org
Caregiving information and advice, workshops and online seminars

HOSPICEDIRECTORY.ORG
800-854-3402
Hospice care locator

LOTSA HELPING HANDS
34 Washington Street
Suite 310
Wellesley Hills, MA 02481
www.lotsahelpinghands.com
Create a personalized web site to coordinate caregiving with friends and relatives

MEDICARE RIGHTS CENTER
520 Eighth Avenue
North Wing, 3rd Floor
New York, NY 10018
800-333-4114
www.medicarerights.org
Information on Medicare coverage

MINDING OUR ELDERS
www.mindingourelders.com
Articles and information on caregiving

THE NATIONAL ACADEMY OF ELDER LAW ATTORNEYS, INC.
1577 Spring Hill Road
Suite 220
Vienna, VA 22182
703-942-5711
www.naela.org
Directory of elder-law attorneys

NATIONAL ALLIANCE FOR CAREGIVING
4720 Montgomery Lane
Bethesda, MD 20814
www.caregiving.org
A nonprofit coalition of national organizations focusing on issues of family caregiving

NATIONAL ASSOCIATION FOR HOME CARE AND HOSPICE
228 Seventh Street, SE
Washington, DC 20003
202-547-7424
www.nahc.org
Information on home care and hospice, hospice agency directory

NATIONAL ASSOCIATION OF AREA AGENCIES ON AGING
1730 Rhode Island Avenue, NW
Suite 1200
Washington, DC 20036
202-872-0888
www.n4a.org
A one-stop web site to get a sense of the local services in your community, such as meal services, adult daycare, in-home health aides, caregiver counseling, and support

NATIONAL ASSOCIATION OF SKILLED NURSING FACILITIES
866-333-6002
Skillednursingfacilities.org
Directory of nursing homes, plus articles and information

NATIONAL CLEARINGHOUSE FOR LONG-TERM CARE INFORMATION
Administration on Aging
Washington, DC 20201
202-619-0724
www.longtermcare.gov
Information and resources for planning long-term care

NATIONAL FAMILY CARE-GIVER SUPPORT PROGRAM
www.aoa.gov/AoARoot/AoA_Programs/HCLTC/Caregiver/index.aspx
Federal program that funds local agencies on aging and local and community service providers to support family caregivers

NATIONAL RESPITE NETWORK
4016 Oxford Street
Annandale, VA 22003
703-256-2084
http://archrespite.org/national-respite-coalition/lifespan-respite-task-force
Lists local organizations that provide a respite to caregiv-ers, from in-home babysitting to transportation and home repair help

PACE (PROGRAMS OF ALL-INCLUSIVE CARE)
801 North Fairfax Street
Suite 309
Alexandria, VA 22314
703-535-1565
www.npaonline.org
Services to help seniors live independently by providing community-based care to those who would otherwise be placed in a nursing home

PROFESSIONAL GERIATRIC CARE MANAGERS
3275 West Ina Road
Suite 130
Tuscon, AZ 85741
520-881-8008
www.caremanager.org
Information on care manage-ment, care manager locator

SACRED DYING FOUNDATION
P.O. Box 210328
San Francisco, CA 94121
415-585-9455
www.sacreddying.org
Information on spiritual end-of-life rituals

SENIORHOUSINGNET.COM
910 Hamilton Avenue
6th Floor
Campbell, CA 95008
Senior living locator, infor-mation and tools for finding senior care

NOTES

CHAPTER 1

1. Ogden, Cynthia L., and Margaret D. Carroll. "Prevalence of Overweight, Obesity, and Extreme Obesity Among Adults: United States, Trends 1960–1962 Through 2007–2008," Centers for Disease Control and Prevention, 2012 report.

2. Rickman, Joy C., et al. "Nutritional Comparison of Fresh, Frozen, and Canned Fruits and Vegetables," *Journal of the Science of Food and Agriculture* 87 (2007): 87–994.

3. Covington, Maggie G. "Omega-3 Fatty Acids," *American Family Physician*, Volume 70, no. 1 (2004): 133–39.

4. "The Sunny Side of Eggs," *UC Berkeley Wellness Letter* (March 2008).

5. Cappuccio, Francesco P., and Chen Ji. "Less Salt and Less Risk of Stroke," *Stroke* 43 (2012) 1195–1196.

6. Food and Nutrition Board, Institute of Medicine, National Academies. "Dietary Reference Intakes (DRIs): Estimated Average Requirements."

7. Jana Klauer, M.D., physician with an expertise in nutrition and metabolism, and a Martha Stewart Center for Living at Mount Sinai board member.

8. Ibid.

9. Pollock, Norman, et al. "Adolescent Fiber Consumption Is Associated with Visceral Fat and Inflammatory Markers," *The Journal of Clinical Endocrinology & Metabolism* (August 2012): E1451–7.

CHAPTER 2

1. Berry, Jarett D., et al. "Lifetime Risks for Cardiovascular Disease Mortality by Cardiorespiratory Fitness Levels Measured at Ages 45, 55, and 65 Years in Men," *Journal of the American College of Cardiology* 57, no. 15 (2011): 1604–1610.

2. "Fall Prevention: 6 Tips to Prevent Falls," *Mayo Clinic Healthy Aging* (July 2010): 1–2.

3. Franklin, Deborah. "How Hospital Gardens Help Patients Heal" (published in print as "Nature That Nurtures"), *Scientific American,* 306 (March 2012): 24–25.

4. Ibid.

5. "Talking of Walking in Three Easy Pieces," *Harvard Health Letter,* Harvard Health Publications, Harvard Medical School (March 2011).

6. Villareal, Dennis, et al. "Bone Mineral Density Response to Caloric Restriction-Induced Weight Loss or Exercise-Induced Weight Loss," *Archives of Internal Medicine* (2006).

7. Talanian, Jason, et al. "Two Weeks of High-Intensity Aerobic Interval Training Increases the Capacity for Fat Oxidation During Exercise in Women," *Journal of Applied Physiology* (December 2007).

8. Sung, B. H., et al. "A002: Effectiveness of Various Relaxation Techniques in Lowering Blood Pressure Associated with Mental Stress," *American Journal of Hypertension*, 13 (April 2000).

9. Ibid.

10. Wang, C., J. P. Collet, and J. Lau. "The Effect of Tai Chi on Health Outcomes in Patients with Chronic Conditions: A Systematic Review," *Archives of Internal Medicine* (2004): 493–501.

11. Mangione, Kathleen Kline, et al. "Improving Physical Function and Performance with Progressive Resistance Strength Training in Older Adults," *The Cochrane Review*, vol. 90, no. 12 (December 2010): 1711–15.

12. Nagamatsu, Lindsay S., et al. "Resistance Training Promotes Cognitive and Functional Brain Plasticity in Seniors with Probable Mild Cognitive Impairment," *Archives of Internal Medicine* 172, no. 8 (2012): 666–668.

CHAPTER 3

1. Middleton, Laura E., and Kristine Yaffe. "Promising Strategies for the Prevention of Dementia," *Archives of Neurology*, vol. 66, no. 10 (2009): 1210–15.

2. Hall, C.B., et al. "Cognitive Activities Delay Onset of Memory Decline in Persons Who Develop Dementia," *Neurology* 73, no. 5 (2009): 356–361.

3. Schaie, K. Warner. "Intellectual Development in Adulthood," *Handbook of the Psychology of Aging*, 4th ed., San Diego Academic Press (1996): 266–86.

4. Schaefer, Ernst J., et al. "Plasma Phosphatidylcholine Docasahexaenoic Acid Content and Risk of Dementia and Alzheimer Disease," *Archive of Neurology* 63, no. 11 (2006): 1545–1550.

5. Morris, M.C., et al. "Associations of Vegetable and Fruit Consumption with Age-Related Cognitive Change," *Neurology* 67, no. 8 (2006): 1370–1376.

6. Kang, J.H., et al. "Fruit and Vegetable Consumption and Cognitive Decline in Aging Women," *Neurology* 57, no. 5 (2005): 713–720.

7. Commenges, D., et al. "Intake of Flavonoids and Risk of Dementia," *European Journal of Epidemiology* 16, no. 4 (2000): 357–363.

8. Larsson, Susanna C. "Chocolate Consumption and Risk of Stroke in Women," *Journal of the American College of Cardiology* 58, no. 17 (2011): 1828–1829.

9. Suhr, J.A., et al. "The Relation of Hydration Status to Declarative Memory and Working Memory in Older Adults," *Journal of Nutrition, Health and Aging* 14, no. 10 (2010): 840–843.

10. Andrade, Jacklie. "What Does Doodling Do?," *Journal of Applied Cognitive Psychology*, vol. 24, no. 1, (January 2010): 100–06.

11. Cynthia Green, Ph.D., assistant clinical professor of psychiatry at the Mount Sinai Medical Center.

12. Ibid.

13. Ibid.

14. Ibid.

15. Rick Hanson, Ph.D., author of *Buddha's Brain: The Practical Neuroscience of Happiness, Love, and Wisdom*.

16. Cynthia Green, Ph.D.

CHAPTER 4

1. Levy, Becca R., et al. "Longevity Increased by Positive Self-Perceptions of Aging," *Journal of Personality and Social Psychology* 83, no. 2 (2002): 261–270.

2. Tindle, Hilary A., et al. "Optimism, Cynical Hostility, and Incident Coronary Heart Disease and Mortality in the Women's Health Initiative," *Circulation* 120, no. 8 (2009): 656–662.

3. Stone, Arthur A., et al. "A Snapshot of the Age Distribution of Psychological Well-Being in the United States," *Proceedings of the National Academy of Sciences*, vol. 107, no. 22 (June 2010): 9985–9990.

4. Jackson, Joshua J., et al. "What Do Conscientious People Do? Development and Validation of the Behavioral Indicators of Conscientiousness (BIC)," *Journal of Research in Personality* (August 2010): 501–11.

5. Musick, Marc A., and John Wilson. *Volunteers: A Social Profile*, Bloomington: Indiana University Press, 2007.

6. Vallerand, Robert J. "The Role of Passion in Sustainable Psychological Well-Being," *Psychology of Well-Being: Theory, Research and Practice*, vol. 2, no. 1 (March 2012).

7. Ibid.

8. Giles, Lynne C., et al. "Effect of Social Networks on 10 Year Survival in Very Old Australians," *Journal of Epidemiol Community Health* 59 (2004): 574–579.

9. The Pew Internet and American Life Project: www.pewinternet.org.

10. Ong, Anthony, C. S. Bergeman, and Steven M. Moker. "Resilience Comes of Age: Defining Features in Later Adulthood," *The Journal of Personality*, vol. 77, no. 6 (December 2009): 1777–1804.

11. *Body & Soul* (September 2008).

12. Dennis Popeo, M.D., attending psychiatrist at the NYU Langone Medical Center.

13. Ibid.

14. Ibid.

CHAPTER 5

1. Srikanthan, Preethi, et al. "Waist-Hip-Ratio as a Predictor of All-Cause Mortality in High-Functioning Older Adults," *Annals of Epidemiology* 19, no. 10 (2009): 724–731.

2. Jana Klauer, M.D., physician with an expertise in nutrition and metabolism, and a Martha Stewart Center for Living at Mount Sinai board member.

3. Maroon, J.C., and J.W. Bost. "Omega-3 Fatty Acids as an Anti-Inflammatory," *Surgical Neurology* 65, no. 4 (2006): 326–331.

4. Little, Paul, et al. "Randomised Controlled Trial of Alexander Technique Lessons, Exercise, and Massage for Chronic and Recurrent Back Pain," *British Medical Journal* 42, no. 12 (2008): 965–968.

5. Jana Klauer, M.D.

6. Ibid.

7. Buysse, Daniel J., et al. "Efficacy of Brief Behavioral Treatment for Chronic Insomnia in Older Adults," *Archives of Internal Medicine* 171, no. 10 (2011): 887–895.

8. Jana Klauer, M.D.

9. Meydani, Simin N., et al. "Vitamin E and Respiratory Tract Infections in Elderly Nursing Home Residents," *Journal of the American Medical Association* 292, no. 7 (2004): 828–836.

10. Sita Chokhavatia, M.D., associate professor of medicine at the Mount Sinai School of Medicine.

11. DiSilvestro, Robert A., et al. "Anti-Heartburn Effects of Fenugreek Fiber Product," *Phytotherapy Research*, vol. 25, no. 1 (January 2011): 88–91.

12. Michael A. Palese, M.D., associate professor of urology and director of Minimally Invasive Surgery at the Mount Sinai Medical Center.

CHAPTER 6

1. Gerald Imber, M.D., plastic surgeon and author of *The Youth Corridor*.

2. Ibid.

3. Catherine Orentreich, M.D., dermatologist, professor of dermatology at the New York University School of Medicine.

4. Ibid.

CHAPTER 7

1. Rantz, Marilyn. "Evaluation of Aging in Place Model with Home Care Services and Registered Nurse Care Coordination in Senior Housing," *Nursing Outlook*, vol. 59, no. 1 (January–Febuary 2011): 37–46.

2. Runyan, C.W., and C. Casteel (editors). *The State of Home Safety in America*, 2nd edition (Washington, DC: Home Safety Council, 2004).

3. Fear, Josh. *Stuff Happens: Unused Things Cluttering Up Our Homes* (Canberra: The Australia Institute, 2008).

4. Ibid.

5. Papinchak, Heather L., et al. "Effectiveness of Houseplants in Reducing the Indoor Air Pollutant Ozone," *HortTechnology* 19, no. 2 (2009): 286–290.

6. Ibid.

7. Gammack, Julie K., and Julie M. Burke. "Natural Light Exposure Improves Subjective Sleep Quality in Nursing Home Residents," *Journal of the AMDA* 10, no. 6 (2009): 440–441.

8. Centers for Disease Control and Prevention. "Unintentional Non-Fire-Related Carbon Monoxide Exposures—United States, 2001–2003," *Morbidity and Mortality Weekly Report* 54, no. 2 (2005): 36–39.

CHAPTER 8

1. "What Are High Blood Pressure and Prehypertension?" National Heart Lung and Blood Institute, www.nhlbi.com; "Staying Attuned to Blood Pressure," *Harvard Women's Health Watch,* Harvard Health Publications, Harvard Medical School (August 2009).

2. Jalal, D. I., et al. "Increased Fructose Associates with Elevated Blood Pressure," *Journal of the American Society of Nephrology* 21, no. 9 (2010): 1543–1549.

3. Brown, Timothy, *Health Economics* (September 2010).

4. Sinha, Seema S., and Jennifer A. Tremmel. "Sex Differences in Acute Coronary Syndrome," *Symposium in Cardiac and Vascular Medicine*, 2007 Yearbook, Ch. 6, www.sis.org/docs/2007Yearbook_Ch6.pdf.

5. Christine Chang, M.D., associate professor of geriatrics and palliative care at the Martha Stewart Center for Living at Mount Sinai.

6. Sorensen, Mette, et al. "Road Traffic Noise and Stroke," *European Heart Journal* 33, no. 21 (2010).

7. Feskanich, Diane, et al. "Vitamin K Intake and Hip Fractures in Women: A Prospective Study," *American Journal of Clinical Nutrition* 69, no. 1 (1999): 74–79.

8. Tucker, K. L., et al. "Colas, but Not Other Carbonated Beverages, Are Associated with Low Bone Mineral Density in Older Women," *American Society for Clinical Nutrition* 84, no. 4 (2006): 936–942.

9. Nelson, Roxanne. "Vitamin Supplements Beneficial in Patients with Breast Cancer," *Cancer Epidemiology, Biomarkers & Prevention* (December 2010): www.medscape.com.

10. Miglioretti, Diana L., et al. "Accuracy of Screening Mammography Varies by Week of Menstrual Cycle," *Radiology* 258 (2011): 372–379.

11. Etminan, Mahyar. "Antidepressants Linked to Cataract Fisk; Parkinson's Drug May Cause Corneal Damage," *Ophthalmology* (June 2010).

12. Christine Chang, M.D.

CHAPTER 9

1. Carol Bradley Bursack, author of *Minding Our Elders: Caregivers Share Their Personal Stories* and founder of mindingourelders.com.

2. Ibid.

3. Linda Packer, MSW, LSCW, geriatric care manager and founder of Prime Life Network.

4. Andrew Carle, MHSA, assistant professor and founding director of the Program in Assisted Living/Senior Housing Administration at George Mason University.

5. Ibid.

6. Ibid.

7. Ibid.

8. Ibid.

9. Carol Bradley Bursack.

SUGGESTED READING

Agronin, Marc. *How We Age: A Doctor's Journey into the Heart of Growing Old.* Da Capo Press, 2011.

Arnold, Elizabeth. *Creating the Good Will: The Most Comprehensive Guide to Both the Financial and Emotional Sides of Passing On Your Legacy.* Portfolio Trade, 2006.

Bateson, Mary Catherine. *Composing a Further Life: The Age of Active Wisdom.* Knopf, 2010.

Beer, Kenneth. *Palm Beach Perfect Skin.* MDPublish.com, 2006.

Buettner, Dan. *The Blue Zones: Lessons for Living Longer from the People Who've Lived the Longest.* National Geographic, 2008.

Davich, Victor. *8 Minute Meditation: Quiet Your Mind. Change Your Life.* Perigee Trade, 2004.

Editors of *Whole Living* Magazine. *Power Foods: 150 Delicious Recipes with the Healthiest Ingredients.* Clarkson Potter, 2010.

Gunaratana, Bhante. *Mindfulness in Plain English.* Wisdom Publications, 1991.

Hanson, Rick, and Richard Mendius. *Buddha's Brain: The Practical Neuroscience of Happiness, Love, and Wisdom.* New Harbinger Publications, 2009.

Hartmann, Thom. *Walking Your Blues Away: How to Heal the Mind and Create Emotional Well-Being.* Park Street Press, 2006.

Imber, Gerald. *The Youth Corridor: A Renowned Plastic Surgeon's Revolutionary Program for Maintenance, Rejuvenation, and Timeless Beauty.* William Morrow, 1997.

Kabat-Zinn, Jon. *Coming to Our Senses: Healing Ourselves and the World Through Mindfulness.* Hyperion, 2005.

——. *Full Catastrophe Living: Using the Wisdom of Your Body and Mind to Face Stress, Pain, and Illness.* Delacorte Press, 1990.

Stewart, Martha. *Martha Stewart's Homekeeping Handbook: The Essential Guide to Caring for Everything in Your Home.* Clarkson Potter, 2006.

Taylor, Dan. *The Parent Care Conversation: Six Strategies for Dealing with the Emotional and Financial Challenges of Aging Parents.* Penguin, 2006.

ACKNOWLEDGMENTS

A book this lengthy and full of practical information requires a small army of people to produce it. In this case, the small army's command central is the Special Projects Group at Martha Stewart Living Omnimedia, headed by Editorial Director Ellen Morrissey and Editorial and Brand Director Eric A. Pike. They and the very talented team of editors in the group—Evelyn Battaglia, Amy Conway, Susanne Ruppert, Stephanie Fletcher, and Kelsey Mirando—worked tirelessly "in the trenches" to ensure that this book is as clear and accurate and useful as can be. They are fortunate to work with an equally talented team of art and design directors, including Gillian MacLeod and Jessi Blackham, who made this book look as striking as it does, collaborating at various points in the process with Deb Wood, Michele Outland, William van Roden, and Jennifer Wagner. John Myers, Anna Ross, and Alison Vanek managed the voluminous illustrations and photographs found throughout these pages. I am so grateful to photographer John Dolan for the lovely cover portrait (and to Matthew Axe for his art direction of the photograph), and to all of the photographers whose work appears within (a complete list appears on page 390), as well as to Remie Geoffroi for his illustrations. Denise Clappi and her team of imaging specialists, particularly Spyridon Ginis, are also to thank for their fine work throughout. Thank you to Gael Towey, former Chief Creative Officer at MSLO, for her contributions, as well as to my longtime publicist Susan Magrino and Kelly Galvin at SMA and to MSLO's internal corporate communications team for helping this book reach the widest possible audience.

Alex Postman, former editor in chief of *Whole Living*, logged many long hours putting the text into good working order, collaborating with Stephanie Young and Virginia Sole-Smith along the way. Christine Cyr Clisset offered invaluable assistance editing the manuscript; researcher Karen Bruno helped to confirm the accuracy of much of the reporting. We are grateful as well to Nanette Maxim and Amber Muriello.

This is my seventy-seventh book with Clarkson Potter/Publishers, a division of Random House, and I am so grateful for all that they have done for this and the seventy-six that preceded it. I am especially indebted to the hardworking team behind this very important book, including Angelin Borsics, Emma Brodie, Doris Cooper, Erica Gelbard, Carla Gorgy, Derek Gullino, Pam Krauss, Linnea Knollmueller, Maya Mavjee, Mark McCauslin, Anna Mintz, Donna Passannante, Marysarah Quinn, Jane Treuhaft, and Kate Tyler.

The book began as my pledge to the Clinton Global Health Initiative at their annual assembly in 2007. I wanted to write a book that would address the growing needs of our growing population of seniors, in this country and around the world. So I thank former President Clinton and everyone else at the CGHI for inspiring me to compile all of this information into one accessible, easy-to-use volume.

Finally, I thank everyone who has devoted his or her life's work to the subjects covered within these pages. Without their ongoing research and scholarship, we would not be able to provide you with this comprehensive and very valuable resource. For that, I am truly grateful and appreciative.

CREDITS

WILLIAM ABRANOWICZ 282 (top and bottom right), 283, 306

LUCAS ALLEN 221

SANG AN 55 (bottom right), 60 top right, 61 (bottom right), 291

CHRISTOPHER BAKER 202

JIM BASTARDO 271

ROLAND BELLO 60 (bottom left)

FERNANDO BENGOECHEA 282 (top left)

ANITA CALERO 51

EARL CARTER 180

PAUL COSTELLO 81, 105

REED DAVIS 61 (top left), 276 (bottom right)

JOHN DOLAN 163, 173

TODD EBERLE 302, 327

ANDREW ECCLES 171, 226

BRYAN GARDNER 49, 52, 56 (bottom right), 63 (top right), 135

REMIE GEOFFROI illustrations 82, 87-89, 94-97, 100-104, 112-115, 118-120, 241, 332

HELOISE GOODMAN 74

RAYMOND HOM 42, 54 (top right), 58 (top left and bottom right), 59 (top right and bottom left), 62 (bottom left), 247, 274 (bottom right), 278 (top and bottom right)

MATTHEW HRANEK 275 (bottom left), 285

JOHN HUBA 16 (bottom left), 108, 111, 116

LISA HUBBARD 55 (top left), 58 (top right), 272 (top left, bottom right), 273 (bottom left and right)

DITTE ISAGER 258, 272 (top right)

DEVON JARVIS 45

JOHN KERNICK 62 (top right)

YUNHEE KIM 56 (bottom left)

ANDERS KRUSBERG 10, 16 (top left and right)

FREDERIC LAGRANGE 2, 72, 85, 133

ANNIE LEIBOVITZ 336

VANESSA LENZ 160, 298

DAVID LOFTUS 54 (top left)

STEVEN MCDONALD 275 (top and bottom right)

JAMES MERRELL 274 (top right)

ELLIE MILLER 60 (bottom right), 277 (right), 279 (right)

JOHNNY MILLER 53 (top left and bottom right), 56 (top left and right), 58 (bottom left), 59 (bottom right), 61 (top right), 63 (top left), 64, 272 (bottom left), 273 (top left and right), 286–287

MIKE MOORE/STRINGER/COURTESY OF GETTY IMAGES 139

LAURA MOSS 276 (bottom left)

MARCUS NILSSON 55 (top right), 59 (top left)

VICTORIA PEARSON 26, 126, 238, 275 (top left)

JASON PENNEY 277 (left)

GRANT PETERSON 373

ERIC PIASECKI 276 (top left and right), 279 (left)

ROBERT POLIDORI 122

CON POULOS 53 (bottom left), 61 (bottom left)

DAVID PRINCE 274 (top and bottom left), 278 (bottom left)

JOSE MANUEL PICAYO RIVERA 63 (bottom right)

EMILY KATE ROEMER 54 (bottom left and right)

ANDERS SCHONNEMANN 62 (top left)

KEVIN SHARKEY 79

MARTHA STEWART 157

COURTESY OF MARTHA STEWART 16 (middle left, middle right, and bottom right) 130, 153, 167, 353

KIRSTEN STRECKER 53 (top right)

CLIVE STREETER 63 (bottom left)

PERTRINA TINSLAY 62 (bottom right)

COURTESY OF THE U.S. SENATE 18

SIMON UPTON 144

JONNY VALIANT 60 top left, 140, 282 (bottom left)

ALBERT VECERKA/ESTO 278 (top left)

SIMON WATSON 257

ANNA WILLIAMS 57

CHRISTIAN WITKIN 92

ROMULO YANES 55 (bottom left)

INDEX

A

Abdominal aortic aneurysm tests, 189
Abdominal bridges, 115
Abdominal curl-backs, 118
Aches and pains, 217
Acne, 244
Active adult housing, 356
Acupuncture, 214, 329
Affinity communities, 356
Affirmation file, 148
ALA fatty acids, 35
Alcohol, 230, 305, 312, 323
Alexander technique, 192
Allergies, 159
Almonds, 34
Alternative health remedies, 225
Alzheimer's, 124
Ankle alphabets, 99
Antidepressants, 334
Antioxidant-rich foods, 230
Antioxidant serum, 237, 243
Anxiety, 175
Apnea, sleep, 194
Appearance
  effect of aging on, 227
  hair, 254–57
  makeup, 246–53
  skin care, 229–43
  skin condition treatments, 244–45
Arm stretches, 95
Arthritis, 191, 329
Artistic pursuits, 156
Asbestos, 296
Aspirin, 318

Assisted Living Facilities (ALF), 357
Attention and focus, 170

B

Back
  best sleep positions for, 193
  pain, easing, 192–93
  strength exercises for, 112
  stretches for, 94, 95
Balance
  better-balance walk, 90
  daily exercises for, 183
  five moves for, 100–101
  improving, steps for, 98–99
  mix and match workouts, 121
Bathrooms, 261, 266, 274
Beans and legumes
  adding to diet, 33
  canned, buying, 44
  cooking from scratch, 33
  daily servings, 33
  health benefits, 33
  for healthy heart, 314
Bedrooms, 266, 294
Berries, 333
Biceps curls, 113
Bladder health, 214–15
Bloating, 211
Blood glucose, 315, 316
Blood pressure
  high, 312
  lowering, with yoga walk, 89

screening tests, 188, 189
  and vision, 334
Blood sugar levels, 334, 335
"Blue Zone" diets, 29
Body Mass Index (BMI), 43, 315
Bones
  bone density test, 189
  protecting, 322–26
  stronger-bones walk, 87
Botox, 251
Bowel movements, 183, 210
Brain. *See also* Memory
  -boosting foods, 128
  calisthenics, 135
  and creativity, 126–27
  exercising, benefits of, 124
  -health problems, preventing, 124
  lifetime learning for, 139
  mature, advantages of, 125
  and meaningful work, 154
  and meditation, 143
  mind-clearing walk, 90
  and physical exercise, 129
  and social games, 140, 165
  stimulating, strategies for, 133, 138–41
  and stress, 168–69
  thinking outside the comfort zone, 138
  vitamin B_{12} for, 132
Brazil nuts, 34

Breast cancer, 331, 332
Breast self-exams, 185, 188, 332
Broth, chicken, buying, 44
Bruises, 234
Bucket list, 157
Bunions, 222
Burnout, caregiver, 365–67
Buttocks stretches, 94, 95

C

Caffeine, 323
Calcium
    adding to diet, 37
    for bone support, 325
    daily servings, 37
    dietary sources of, 37, 40
    health benefits, 37
    non-dairy sources of, 37
    recommendations for, 40, 322
Calf raises, 114
Calluses, 222
Calories, empty, 46
Cancer, 219, 235, 330–32
Carbon monoxide, 295
Careers, 154
Caregivers
    balancing work and caregiving, 346
    building caregiving skills, 347
    choosing, 345
    conversations with elders, 339, 368–69
    nurturing spirits of elders, 362–64
    preparing for caregiving, 338
    preventing caregiver fatigue, 365–67
    and sibling conflicts, 348
    support groups for, 366

talking about death with elders, 368–69
Carpets, 292
Cataracts, 206
Catechins, 201
Cereal, buying, 44
Certified Aging-in-Place Specialist (CAPS), 261
Chair exercises, 118–21
Chemicals, household, 295–98
Chest stretches, 95
Chicken broth, buying, 44
Chili powder, 73
Chiropractic care, 192
Chocolate, 128
Cholesterol, 38, 188, 313
Chromium, 40
Cinnamon, 73
Cleansers, skin, 236, 242
Closets, decluttering, 278–79
Clothing storage, 278–79
Clutter, household, 268–69
Cognitive function. See Brain; Memory
Cohousing, 356
Colds, and sexual activity, 217
Collagen treatments, 252
Colonoscopy, 188
Colors, for homes, 288
Combustion gases, 295
Community activities, 164
Computer skills, 166
Conscientiousness, cultivating, 151–52
Constipation, 211
Continuing Care Retirement Communities (CCRC), 357
Convenience foods, 27, 28

Conversation skills, 141
Cooking
    essential equipment, 48
    in parchment, 69
    quick soups, 66
    roasting, 67
    stir-frying, 68
    vinaigrettes, 65
Core strength, 102–4, 121
Cosmetic enhancements, 250–53
Cosmetics, 240, 246–49
Crackers, buying, 44
C-reactive protein (CRP) test, 320
Creativity, 126–27

D

Dancing, 77
Death, talking about, 368–69
Death certificate, 371
Dentures, 209
Depression
    antidepressants for, 334
    and bone loss, 324
    identifying, 174
    preventing, with pets, 159
    reducing, with sex, 217
    from social isolation, 164
    and strokes, 317
Dermatologists, 233
DHA fatty acids, 35, 128
Diabetes, 315–16
Digestive health
    common gut woes, 212–13
    home remedies for, 211
    monitoring changes in, 71, 210
Diverticular disease, 212

Doctors
  choosing, 307
  communication with, 308
  keeping medical records
    with, 303, 310
  second opinions from,
    308
  specialists, seeking out,
    309
Do Not Resuscitate (DNR)
  Order, 344
Drugs. See Medications
Durable power of attorney
  (POA), 343
Dust, controlling, 294
Dysport, 251

E

Ears
  hearing acuity, 335
  hearing tests, 189
Eating
  adopting "Blue Zone"
    diets, 29
  for better vision, 205,
    334
  brain-boosting foods,
    128
  for cancer prevention,
    333
  for caregiver health, 367
  for changing nutritional
    needs, 70–73
  colorful fruits and
    vegetables, 50, 230
  eight major food groups,
    31–39
  for healing process, 73
  healthful cooking
    techniques, 48, 65–69
  healthful nutritional
    choices, 43–47, 305
  for healthy skin, 230

  impact on health, 28
  for joint health, 329
  mindful, practicing, 46
  planning better meals,
    28–30
  for preventing heart
    disease, 314
  real vs. processed food,
    27–28
  U.S. government
    guidelines, 30
  vitamin and mineral
    needs, 40–41
Eczema, 244
Education and learning,
  138, 139, 141
Elderly parents. See also
    Caregivers
  end-of-life paperwork for,
    341, 343–45
  financial issues, 340
  hiring help for, 349–51
  honoring passing of, 372
  hospice care for, 371
  housing options, 337,
    352–59
  insurance needs, 342,
    360–61
  moving in with adult
    children, 355
  nurturing spirits of,
    362–64
  palliative care for, 370
  talking about death with,
    368–69
Electrolytes, 201
Emotional balance, 149
Employment, 154
End-of-life wishes, 342
Endurance
  gradual progression,
    goals for, 91
  mix and match workouts,
    121
  walking for, 83–84

  a week's worth of walks,
    86–90
Entryways, 261, 270
EPA fatty acids, 35
Equipment, kitchen, 48
Estrogen, 317
Exercise. See also Walking
  "accidental," 78
  aerobic, effect on brain,
    129
  and arthritis, 329
  for better hearing, 335
  for bone health, 323, 326
  for caregivers, 367
  chair-based workouts,
    118–21
  combining travel with,
    17, 79, 109
  for core strength, 102–4
  and dog owners, 159
  for feet, 222
  finding something you
    love, 327
  and gardening, 80–82
  general health benefits,
    76, 305
  with a group, 165
  and head injuries, 129
  for healthy skin, 232
  for improving strength,
    106–20
  for increased energy, 198
  for increasing endurance,
    83–91
  indoor activities, 77
  interval training, 111
  for joints, 191, 328
  for maintaining flexibility,
    93–97
  mix and match workouts,
    121
  new sports, 105
  outdoor activities, 77, 324
  for preventing cancer,
    330

Exercise (continued)
  progressing gradually, 91
  target heart rate, 91
  varying routine, 84
  and workout intensity, 84
Exfoliants, 242
Experience Corps, 155
Eyes
  age-related problems,
    206–7
  dry, moisturizing, 205
  eye cream, 243
  eye exams, 188, 204
  eyeglass prescriptions,
    204
  goggles and glasses for,
    204, 334
  healthy diet for, 205
  makeup for, 249
  noting changes in vision,
    207
  protecting vision, 334

F

Facial lines, treating,
    251–53
Facial masks, 236
Facial massage, 241
Fall-proofing the home,
    262–65
Family
  moving elderly parents in
    with, 355
  sharing meals with,
    176
  staying connected to,
    162–63
Fatigue, 198, 365–67
Fats. See also Omega-3
    fatty acids
  healthy, 38, 39, 230
  unhealthy, 38, 39, 324
Fecal incontinence, 210

Fecal occult blood test,
    188
Feet
  buying right shoes for,
    220
  checking weekly, 184
  fitness exercises, 222
  improving circulation to,
    220
  keeping clean, 220
  massaging, 98
  preventative care for, 222
Fiber, 71, 201, 230
Finances, personal, 340
Fish
  canned, buying, 44
  for healthy brain, 128
  for healthy heart, 314
  for healthy vision, 334
  sardines, serving ideas,
    64
Fish oil capsules, 128, 331
Fitness. See also Exercise;
    Walking
  foot exercises, 222
  gardening, 80–82
  improving balance,
    98–101
  improving strength,
    106–20
  increasing endurance,
    83–91
  maintaining flexibility,
    93–97
  personal trainers, 326
  staying active every day,
    75–80
  strengthening your core,
    102–4
  trying new sports, 105
  yoga, 92, 109, 143
Flame retardants, 298
Flexibility
  assessing, 93
  daily exercises for, 183

massages for, 93
mix and match workouts,
    121
pre-exercise warmup, 93
relax and recharge
    stretches, 96–97
whole body stretches,
    94–95
Flexitarian diet, 315
Flooring, 290–93
Floss, 208
Fluoride, 209
Flu shots, 186, 203
Folate, 40
Folic acid, 335
Food additives, 230
Foot care. See Feet
Foreign languages, 138
Formaldehyde, 298
Fostering a child, 155
Fraternal organizations,
    164
Friends, 165, 366
Fruits
  adding to diet, 31
  berries, 333
  for better vision, 334
  colorful, 50, 230
  daily servings, 31
  dried, buying, 44
  frozen, buying, 31
  health benefits, 31, 50,
    230, 333, 334
  for healthy skin, 230
Funeral home, 371
Furniture, arranging,
    280–83

G

Games, social, 140, 165
Gardening, 80–82
Gardens, indoor, 284–87
Garlic, 333

Gastroesophageal reflux
   disease (GERD), 213
Geriatric care managers,
   349–50
Geriatricians, 307
Germs, 200
Ginger, 73
Glaucoma, 206
Glucose tests, 316
Gluten sensitivity, 211
"Golden Rules" for
   successful aging,
   22–23
Grains, whole, 32, 314
Grandmother Hypothesis,
   155
Gratitude, 177
Greenhouse projects, 356
Greens, leafy, 128, 333
Grief, 175, 369
Gum, sugarless, 208
Gum disease, 185, 317

H

Hair, 254–57
Hallways, 261
Hammertoes, 222
Hamstrings, 94, 115
Hands, washing, 200
Happiness, 149
Hardwood flooring, 293
HDL cholesterol, 38
Head injuries, 129
Health. See also
      Preventative care
   aches and pains, 190–93
   maintaining, blueprint
      for, 200–222
   practicing prevention,
      182–89
   and sleep, 194–99
Health-care proxy, 341,
   344

Health clubs, 93
Health insurance, 342,
   360–61
Hearing acuity, 335
Hearing tests, 189
Heart attacks, 317–18
Heartburn, 211
Heart disease
   and daily aspirin, 318
   and dental hygiene, 317
   foods to fight, 314
   gender differences, 318
   and pulse rate, 317
   risk factors, 317
   and sexual activity, 217
   signs of heart attack,
      318
   and speed walks, 86
Heart rate, target, 91
Heat-related illnesses, 82
Hepatitis vaccinations, 187
High blood pressure, 312
High-fructose corn syrup,
   312
Hiking, 17, 79
Hip stretches, 94, 95
Hobbies, 156, 165
Home
   chemical hazards, 295–98
   cleaning, pleasure in, 299
   closets, 278–79
   color palettes, 288
   controlling dust in, 294
   decluttering, 268–69
   elder-friendly, 352, 354
   entryways, 270
   flooring, 290–93
   furniture arrangement,
      280–83
   gifting, to adult children,
      355
   home offices, 276–77
   houseplants for, 284–87
   kitchens, 272–73
   lighting for, 289

safety-proofing, 262–67
   small living spaces, 282
   smart design features,
      260–61
Home health aides, 350–51
Hormone replacement
   therapy (HRT), 218,
   331
Horseback riding, 105
Hospice care, 371
Hospital stays, 321
Hot flashes, 324
Houseplants, 284–87
Humidifiers, 233
Hyaluronic acid, 251
Hydration
   for better digestion, 71
   with coconut water, 201
   for fighting fatigue, 198
   fluids intake for, 71
   for healthy brain, 128
   for healthy skin, 233
   indication of, 183
   for stronger immune
      system, 201
Hypertension, 312

I

Immune system, 200–201,
   203
Implants, dental, 209
Incontinence, 210, 214,
   215
Indigestion, 211
Inflammation, chronic,
   320
Insurance, 342, 360–61
Interval training, 111
Iron, 70
Irritable bowel syndrome
   (IBS), 211, 213
Isolation, 164
Itching, 234

J

Joints, 191, 328–29

K

Kegel exercises, 214
Kitchens
    cooking equipment, 48
    organizing, 272–73
    safety-proofing, 267
    universal design features,
        261
Kneeling leg extensions,
    115
Knowledge, and the
    elderly, 149, 155
Kostyra, Martha, 19, 20,
    153, 283, 353, 373

L

Lactose intolerance, 37,
    211
Languages, foreign, 138
Lasers, for skin, 253
Laughter, 170–71
Laundry areas, 275
LDL cholesterol, 38
Learning and education,
    138, 139, 141
Leg exercises, 95, 119, 120
Life insurance, 342, 361
Life stories, 178–79
Lighting, indoor, 205, 289
Living rooms, 267
Living will, 341, 344
Loneliness, 159
Long-term care insurance,
    342, 360
Looks. See Appearance
L-theanine, 199
Lunges, 114

M

Macular degeneration, 207
Magnesium, 323
Makeup. See Cosmetics
Mammograms, 188, 331
Martini stretch, 120
Massages, 93, 203, 241
Meals, rethinking, 47
Meals, sharing, 176
Medicaid, 342, 361
Medical records, 303, 310
Medical reminders, 184
Medicare, 342, 360, 361
Medications
    for anxiety, 175
    for arthritis, 329
    and dosages, 309
    effect on food intake, 71
    and gastrointestinal
        system, 210
    and hearing loss, 335
    and incontinence, 214
    for joint pain, 191
    managing prescriptions,
        223
    and memory, 136–37
    for osteoporosis, 324
    side effects, 71, 136–37,
        210, 214, 223, 309, 335
Medicine chest, 224–25
Meditation, 143, 168, 170,
    366
Mediterranean diet, 29
Melatonin, 199
Memory
    boosting, with sleep, 142
    challenging, tips for, 130
    consolidating learning
        into, 143
    loss of, preventing,
        130–32
    medications that impair,
        136–37
    myths about, 134

Memory care programs,
    357
Meningitis vaccination,
    187
Mental illness, 174
Mentoring a child, 155
Metabolic syndrome,
    317
Mindful eating, 46
Mindfulness, practicing,
    170
Minerals, dietary sources
    of, 40–41
MMR vaccination, 187
Moisturizers, 237
Mold, 297
Monitoring devices, at-
    home, 354
Morning rituals, 176
Mouth, dry, 209
Muscles, 190, 328
Music, 179
MyPlate, 30

N

Nails, 184
Naps, 142, 203
Natural health remedies,
    225
Negativity bias, 169
Neighborhood groups,
    164
Niche housing, 356
Night cream, 243
Nitrogen dioxide, 296
Noise pollution, 319
Nut butters, 44
Nutrients. See also
    Vitamins
    dietary sources of,
        40–41
Nuts and seeds, 34, 44,
    314

O

Office, at-home, 276–77
Oils, cooking, 39, 44, 314
Okinawans, 29, 47, 151
Omega-3 fatty acids
    for arthritis pain, 191, 329
    for fighting breast cancer, 331
    in fish, 128
    health benefits, 35, 128, 230
    for healthy skin, 230
    three types of, 35
Onions, 333
Oral health
    brushing teeth, 208
    and cardiovascular problems, 317
    cleaning tongue, 208
    dentist appointments, 208
    flossing, 208
    implants and dentures, 209
    and medications, 209
    signs of gum disease, 185
    treating dry mouth, 209
Oral history projects, 179
Osteoporosis, 324
Outdoors, safety-proofing, 267
Outlook
    adopting positive rituals, 176–77
    adopting positive view of aging, 146–50
    embracing "older and wiser," 149
    embracing technology, 166–67
    learning to move on, 173
    maintaining sense of purpose, 151–61
    taking long-view perspective, 178

P

Pains and aches, 190–93, 217
Palliative care, 370
Pantry items, 44
Paprika, 73
Pap smears, 188
Parchment-steaming foods, 69
Pasta, 32, 44
PBDES (polybrominated diphenyl ethers), 298
Peanuts, 34
Pecans, 34
Pedometer, 78
Pelvic exams, 188
Perceptions, negative, rephrasing, 150
Periodic limb movement disorder (PLMD), 194
Personal Health Record (PHR), 310
Personal histories, 178–79
Personal trainers, 326
Perspective
    fresh, finding, 170
    long-view, 178
    positive, benefits of, 147
Pesticides, 297
Pets, 159, 161
Physician Orders for Life-Sustaining Treatment (POLST), 344
Pilates ring, 109
Pistachios, 34
Pneumonia vaccine, 186
Poetry, 131
Posture, 85, 99
Posture-enhancing walk, 88
Power of attorney (POA), 340, 343

Prediabetes, 316
Prescriptions. See Medications
Preventative care
    avoiding "Big Three" health risks, 311
    bones, 322–26
    cancer, 330–33
    diabetes, 315–16
    goal of, 304, 306
    hearing, 335
    heart, 314, 317–18
    high cholesterol, 313
    hypertension, 312
    joints, 328–29
    nonnegotiable rules for, 305
    strokes, 319–20
    taking charge of, 306–10
    vision, 334
Probiotics, 201
Processed foods, 27, 28
Prostate, enlarged, 218–19
Prostate cancer, 219
Prostate Specific Antigen test, 189
Protein, 36, 73, 325
Psoriasis, 245
Pulse rate, 317
Purpose, maintaining sense of, 151–61
Push-ups, 113

Q

Quadriceps, 328

R

Radon, 298
Recipes (breakfast)
    Avocado-Pear Smoothie, 53

Recipes (breakfast)
(continued)
Blueberry–Green Tea
Smoothie, 53
Broiled Grapefruit, 54
Cantaloupe with
Ricotta and
Pistachios, 55
Carrot-Ginger
Smoothie, 53
Hard-Cooked Egg
Whites with
Avocado, 55
Hot Rice Cereal with
Almonds and Raisins, 55
Martha's favorite green
juice, 52
Oatmeal with
Blueberries, Walnuts,
and Bananas, 54
Peach-Raspberry
Smoothie, 53
Scrambled Eggs with
Spinach and
Tomatoes, 54
Whole-Grain Toast with
Goat Cheese and
Raspberries, 55
Yogurt Parfait, 54
Recipes (desserts and
snacks)
Chili-Lime Popcorn, 58
Cinnamon-Poached
Apples with Toasted
Walnuts, 63
Dark Chocolate and
Mixed Nuts, 59
Edamame with Chile
Salt, 58
Honey-Roasted
Plums, 63
Kale Dip with Blanched
Peas, 58
Pineapple with Ginger
Yogurt Sauce, 63

Watermelon and
Coconut Sorbet
Parfaits, 63
Whole-Grain Cracker
with Hummus and
Cheddar, 59
Recipes (dinner)
Almond-Crusted
Chicken Breast with
Spinach, 60
Broiled Tofu and Snow
Peas, 62
Brown Rice with
Black Beans and
Avocado, 61
Chicken, Snap Pea, and
Peanut Stir-Fry, 68
Herb-Filled Omelet, 60
Meatloaf with Green
Beans, 61
Mushroom and Fontina
Quesadilla, 61
Pasta with Green Beans
and Tuna, 60
Roasted Vegetable Salad
with Goat Cheese, 61
Salmon and Zucchini
Baked in Parchment, 69
Salmon Burger with
Spinach, 62
Seared Chicken with
Carrots, 62
Seared Salmon with
Bulgur, 60
Trout with Escarole and
Olives, 62
Recipes (lunch)
Baked Sweet
Potatoes with
Toasted Nuts and
Oranges, 56
Barley, Mushroom, and
Dill Salad, 56
Lentil and Bulgur Soup, 66
Martha's favorite salad, 57

Miso Soup, 59
Poached Chicken,
Escarole, and Pear
Salad, 56
Roasted Fall
Vegetables, 67
Tropical Salad, 59
Tuna and White Beans, 58
White Bean Salad
with Spicy Roasted
Tomatoes and
Broccoli, 56
Religious institutions, 164
Religious rituals, 369
Residential options for
seniors, 356–59
Resilience, cultivating,
168–75
Resistance bands, 109
Restless legs syndrome
(RLS), 194
Retirement, 154
Reunions, 165
Rice, buying, 44
Rituals, adopting, 176–77
Rituals, religious, 369
Rosacea, 245
Rugs, 292

S

Salads, preparing, 65
Salmon, canned, 44
Salt, buying, 44
Salt substitutes, 70–71
Sardines, serving, 64
School reunions, 165
Screening tests, 188–89
Seafood, 35, 128. See also
Fish
Sexual health, 216–19
Shoes, 220, 221, 291, 329
Shots and vaccinations,
186–87

Shoulder raises, 113
Shoulder stretches, 95
Sibling conflicts, 348
Side-stepping, 99
Sir-frying, 68
Skilled Nursing Facilities
    (SNF), 357
Skills, mastery of, 148
Skin
    buying cosmetics for,
        246–47
    cancer, signs of, 235
    -care routine, Martha's, 239
    checking for moles, 185,
        234
    conditions, treating,
        244–45
    cosmetic enhancements,
        250–53
    effects of aging on, 228,
        231
    exams, 189
    facial massages for, 241
    healthy diet for, 230
    makeup routine for, 248–49
    morning routine for,
        236–37, 239
    nighttime routine for,
        242–43
    peels and facials for, 233
    protecting, 232–33
    -related health problems,
        234
    sensitive, and cosmetics,
        240
    structural layers, 229, 231
    tags, 245
    tone, improving, 253
    wrinkled, repairing, 253
Sleep
    best positions for, 193
    and blood pressure, 319
    changing needs for, 194
    deprivation, effect of, 195
    getting enough, 142

health benefits, 142
for healthier brain, 142
healthy, guidelines for,
    196–97
insomnia, natural
    remedies for, 199
naps, 142, 203
patterns, shifts in, 194
rituals for, 177
and sexual activity, 217
and skin health, 229
Smart design, 260–61
Smoking, 232, 305, 317,
    323, 330, 334
Snacks, 42, 58–59, 72
Sneezing, 200
Social engagement
    benefits of, 141, 156
    for caregivers, 366
    expanding social circle, 165
    maintaining social
        connections, 152–53,
        162–65
    and virtual social
        networks, 166
Sodium, 36, 312, 335
Sores, on feet, 222
Soups, preparing, 66
Spices, 44, 73
Spiritual counselors, 369
Sports, companion, 165
Squats, 114
Stairways, 261
StoryCorps, 179
Strength training
    for bone health, 323
    chair exercises, 118–21
    changing routines, 110
    classic strength circuit,
        112–15
    interval training, 111
    Martha's favorite
        workout, 117
    mix and match workouts,
        121

planning workouts, 106
resistance training, 107
using good form, 110
weight machines, 106–7
Stress
    altering reaction to, 169
    effect on energy levels,
        198
    and heart disease, 317
    and immune system,
        203, 305
    managing, 143, 168, 305
    reducing, general tips
        for, 168
    reducing, with
        meditation, 366
    reducing, with sex, 217
Stretches, 94–97
Strokes, 319–20
Sunglasses, 204, 334
Sunscreen, 232, 237
Supplements
    for bone health, 325
    for fighting breast cancer,
        331
    for insomnia, 199
    for joint pain, 191
    for mental clarity, 132
    for skin health, 233
Swelling and discoloration,
    234

T

Tai Chi, 99
Target heart rate, 91
Taste, changes in, 70–71
TDAP vaccine, 186
Tea, 42, 199, 230, 324
Teaching, 155
Technology, 166–67, 354
TED (Technology,
    Entertainment, and
    Design), 139

Teeth, 185, 208. *See also* Oral health

Testicles, 185, 188

Tetanus shot, 82, 186

Thyroid, swelling of, 185

Thyroid test, 188

Tomatoes, 44, 333

Toners, 236

Tongue, brushing, 208

Tools, gardening, 82

Traditions, new, 165

Trans fats, 39

Travel
benefits of, 158
brain-boosting effects, 141
combining with exercise, 17, 79, 109
for physical health, 158

Triceps dips, 112

Triglycerides, 313

Tuna, canned, 44

Turmeric, 73

U

Ulcers, 212

Universal design, 260–61

Urine, 183

U.S. Senate Special Committee on Aging, 18–21

V

Vaccines, 186–87

Valerian, 199

Vegetables
adding to diet, 31
for better vision, 334
colorful, 50, 230
cruciferous, 333
daily servings, 31
Fall, Roasted, 67
frozen, buying, 31
health benefits, 31, 50, 230, 333, 334
for healthy skin, 230
leafy greens, 128, 333

Vigils, 369

Village model communities, 356

Vinaigrettes, preparing, 65

Vision. *See also* Eyes
changes in, 207
protecting, 334

Vitamin A, 40, 323

Vitamin B_6, 40

Vitamin B_{12}, 41, 132

Vitamin C, 41, 233, 331

Vitamin D, 41, 201, 233, 322, 325, 328, 331

Vitamin E, 41, 201, 331

Vitamin K, 41, 323

Vitamins
absorption of, 70
for bone health, 322, 325
for boosting immunity, 201
B vitamins, 70, 198
dietary sources of, 40–41
for fighting breast cancer, 331
for fighting fatigue, 198
for healthy skin, 233
for joint health, 328
for mental clarity, 132
multivitamins, 233

Vocabulary, 141

Volunteering, 154, 155, 164

Volunteers, for elders, 351

W

Waist/hip ratio (WHR), 43, 185

Walking
combining travel with, 17, 79
energy-boosting effects of, 198
for foot health, 221
health benefits, 75, 83
increasing intensity, 84
to let off steam, 173
pedometers for, 78
taking new routes, 75, 133, 141
target goals, 83–84
a week's worth of, 86–90

Walnuts, 34

Water, 71, 128, 198, 305

Weight
fluctuating, and skin health, 232
healthy, 43, 305, 328
and joint pain, 191, 305
tracking, 43, 184
and type 2 diabetes, 315
weight-loss walk, 86

Weight machines, 106–7

Whey protein, 73

Windshield wiper exercise, 118

Wisdom, 149, 155

Wood floors, 293

Work, and caregiving, 346

Work, meaningful, 154

Worry, 172

Wrist and ankle rotation, 119

Wrist fractures, 324

Y

Yoga, 89, 92, 109, 143

Z

Zinc, 40

Zoster (shingles) vaccine, 186